community nutrition and individual food behavior

mary ann bass

University of Tennessee
Knoxville, Tennessee

lucille wakefield

Florida State University
Tallahassee, Florida

kathryn kolasa

Michigan State University
East Lansing, Michigan

with contributions by

carolyn lackey

Michigan State University
East Lansing, Michigan

kitty r. coffey

Carson Newman College
Jefferson City, Tennessee

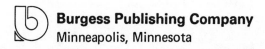

Burgess Publishing Company
Minneapolis, Minnesota

Editor: Kay Kushino
Production Editor: Elisabeth Sövik
Production Manager: Morris Lundin
Art Director: Joan Gordon
Designer: Paula Gibbons
Sales/Marketing Manager: Travis Williams

Copyright © 1979 by Burgess Publishing Company
Printed in the United States of America
Library of Congress Catalog Card Number 78-67116
ISBN 0-8087-0299-8

0 9 8 7 6 5 4 3 2 1

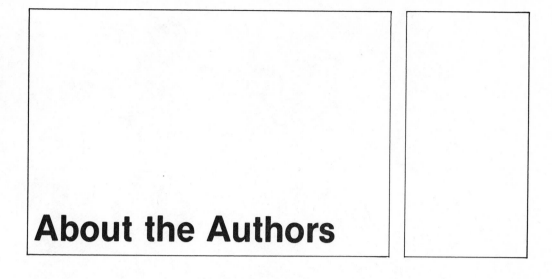

About the Authors

MARY ANN BASS, Ph.D., R.D., is director of Community Food and Nutrition Services in Knoxville, Tennessee, and a lecturer in the department of anthropology at the University of Tennessee. She has also taught at the University of Kansas and has taught short courses at the universities of Nebraska, Wyoming, Vermont, and Louisiana. She has been actively involved in the development of a meals-on-wheels feeding program, in community education programs with WIC, Headstart, and school lunch, and in a university-coordinated undergraduate program in dietetics and a graduate program in sociocultural aspects of food and nutrition. Current projects include research and educational programs concerned with the development of food behavior, obesity, and diabetes among American Indians and people in eastern Tennessee and in a small village in Mexico.

LUCILLE M. WAKEFIELD received her Ph.D. from Ohio State University. Since 1975, she has taught at Florida State University, where she is professor and head of the foods and nutrition department. She previously taught at Kansas State University and the University of Vermont. Dr. Wakefield is active in a variety of professional societies, and has written twenty journal articles on various aspects of nutrition.

KATHRYN M. KOLASA is assistant professor in the department of food science and human nutrition and community health science at Michigan State University. She received her Ph.D. in food science from the University of Tennessee in 1974. Dr. Kolasa was a General Foods Fellow from 1971 to 1973, and has conducted field research in Mexico, Nicaragua, Poland, eastern Tennessee, and Michigan. Her most recent study was conducted in Africa.

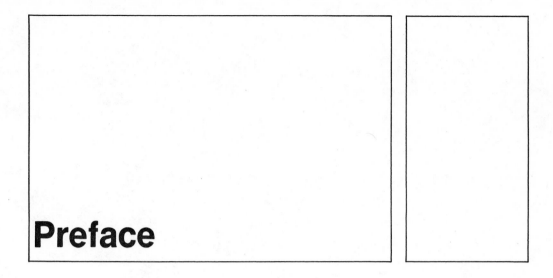

Preface

This book was written to fill a need for a textbook dealing with the complexity of people's behavior in relation to food. Interest in this topic and a growing recognition of its importance have led to the development of courses in the sociocultural aspects of food, cultural foods, community nutrition, and the development of foodways.

It is only recently that the study of people's food behavior has taken its place along with the physical and chemical aspects of nutrition as an important element in the education of food and nutrition professionals. Gilbert Levielle, Eva Wilson, Neige Todhunter, Marian Lowenberg, Grace Goertz, and others have recommended that food behavior be included in the study of food and nutrition. The American Dietetic Association, in the competencies it requires for dietetic students, includes the skill of assessing a person's food behavior and applying knowledge of the sociocultural aspects of food behavior to dietary counseling. And a committee of respected food and nutrition professionals has recommended concepts they think should be included in the study of human behavior in relation to food.

We have tried to approach the study from a broad perspective, so that students will see how the influence of research on the policies and actions of professionals is related to food behavior and hence to the nutritional status of the individual.

Mary Ann Bass
Lucille Wakefield
Kathryn Kolasa

Contents

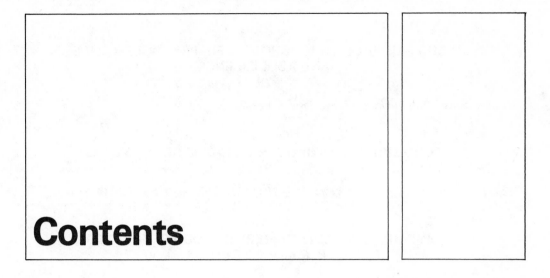

Chapter 13

PROGRAMS AND AGENCIES PROVIDING NUTRITIONAL SERVICES AND EDUCATION
182

STUDENT EXERCISES
203

INDEX
241

CHAPTER 1

Foodways, Food Behavior, and Culture

Food behavior is a fascinating and complex subject. Like all specialized areas of study, it has its own vocabulary, words and phrases that provide a brief way of referring to complex ideas and relationships. Such terminology is indispensable, but it can become a source of confusion when people attach different meanings to the same term or use different terms to express the same concept. It is therefore a good idea to begin any discussion by defining the terms on which it will be based.

Foodways refers to the human population's adaptation to the environment through uniform and diverse activities related to food selection, food procurement, food distribution, food manipulation, food storage, food consumption, and the disposal of uneaten food. Many of these activities are uniform across cultures, but others are specific to a particular culture. For example, all people must eat and, to do so, must put food into their mouths (uniformity); however, what people eat and how they eat it vary from one culture to another (diversity).

The parameters of a community's foodways are the same as those of the food behavior of individuals in the community. *Food behavior* is an individual's response to stimuli related to the selection, procurement, distribution, manipulation, storage, consumption, and disposal of food. (Some people use the term *food habits* rather than *food behavior*. Strictly speaking, however, habits are repetitive acts done without thinking, whereas behavior includes both habits and acts that require thought.) Food must be (1) available, (2) safe (at least for the short term), (3) sufficiently nourishing to sustain life and permit successful reproduction, and (4) acceptable as determined by the group and then by the individual. All food must meet the foregoing criteria, in sequence, in order for human beings to exist. (See figure 1.)

FOOD BEHAVIOR AND CULTURE

Food behavior in the United States is complex and diversified because people of many cultural origins are living in proximity and making rapid advances in technology. Yet diverse as ethnic backgrounds may be, most social scientists agree that there is in the United States a body of traditional knowledge and beliefs — a national lore — that

1

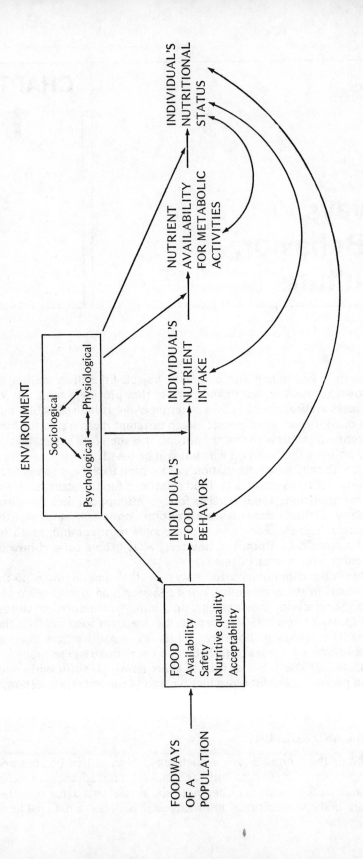

FIGURE 1. Factors that affect food behavior at any given time.

is transmitted informally and that has its origins in Western European culture. Arensberg and Niehoff (1975) described this lore in *The Nacirema* (p. 364).

> It is usually characterized as that of the middle class, having its origins in Western European culture. The language is English, the legal system derives from English common law, the political system of democratic elections comes from France and England, the technology is solidly from Europe, and even more subtle social values, such as egalitarianism (though modified) seem to be European derived. Thus, it seems justifiable to characterize the middle class value system of the United States, as derived originally from Europe but modified to suit local conditions, as the core of American culture.

People born in the United States have been conditioned by the national culture to some extent. The middle class has probably been influenced the most. This does not mean that there are no subcultural streams, but that, irrespective of region, national origin, race, class, or sex, certain points of likeness will occur more frequently among people within the United States than among groups of peoples in other countries.

It would be incorrect to assume that there are no differences in food behavior within the United States. There are ethnic, regional, urban-rural, and individual differences. Many people assume that all Americans eat the same way. People tend to understand and judge the actions, beliefs, and values of others according to the culture of their own group and to think of their own group as the norm and as superior to other groups. This attitude is called *ethnocentrism*. It leads to positive evaluation of one's own group and to less positive, or even negative, evaluation of other groups when their practices are different. For example, beef is an important food for people in the United States. It is difficult for United States citizens to understand or accept the starvation of children in India, where many beef cattle are present but are not used for food. This attitude of "my culture is better than yours" does not take into account whether the land and climate of India would support beef to be used as food. People notice only that cattle live while people starve because their religion prohibits eating beef.

Buchwald (1976), in an article on the Peace Corps, satirized the way we view other cultures. He described the reactions of a Peace Corps worker from Thailand to the United States. The Peace Corps worker said that, compared to the Thai standard, living standards were very primitive in Hoboken, New Jersey. When asked if he ate the food, he replied: "I tried but it wasn't easy. The Hoboken people refuse to raise any food themselves and they must buy it at supermarkets frozen and wrapped in cellophane." The Peace Corps worker then related how he had tried to teach the people to grow their own food so they wouldn't have to spend money, but "they were too set in their ways."

Miner (1956) described the daily activities of Americans as one would describe those of any culture. His discussion of the actions involved in the use of the bathroom shows how those actions could be considered ritualistic by someone of another culture. Overgeneralization from within our own frame of reference about what people of other cultures should do can lead to wrong conclusions.

Generally, people think that everyone eats as they do. Pangborn and Bruhn (1971) noted that California college students knew little about the foods of ethnic groups with whom they had daily contact. It doesn't seem to matter what ethnic background Americans have — they all believe they eat like everyone else.

A nutrition instructor related the following incident, which occurred when she asked women of different nationalities to talk about their food preferences to her class in food and culture. One student, particularly interested in Mexican cuisine, asked Ti, a Latino Enpaide, what she ate everyday. Ti seemed a bit taken aback and replied, "I eat what you do!" The instructor, more subtly, conducted a 24-hour recall with Ti and then with the student. Ti had eaten twelve tortillas, most as food pushers. The student (of Italian descent) had had no tortillas but had eaten several servings of pasta. Ti was correct because both ate carbohydrates, but the form was quite different.

The prerequisite for understanding how a person's response to the environment is related to food consumption is acceptance of the fact that culture influences food behavior and all that a person is or does. The question then arises, what is culture? Culture is a logical, integrated, holistic phenomenon in which the various subsystems fit together in meaningful patterns (Foster 1962). *Holism,* or *wholism,* refers to the theory that whole entities, as fundamental components of reality, have an existence other than as the mere sum of their parts. Culture has been described as an integrated sense-making system that (1) is continually changing, (2) has a value system, (3) is composed of learned behavior, (4) provides for reasonable, efficient interaction among people, (5) contains symbols that are understood by the group, and (6) emphasizes specific activities (Foster 1962; Haviland 1974; Hiebert 1976).

Food behavior can be defined within a culture. That is, if one element of the culture is modified, then the food behavior of individuals will probably change in some way. For example, suppose the local factory changes its shift so that instead of working from 10:00 a.m. to 7:00 p.m. employees work from 7:00 a.m. to 3:00 p.m. Female employees may now buy dinner food that requires more preparation time, because they have more time to prepare dinner. They may purchase fewer snack foods because their families must go to bed earlier in order to rise earlier. The food behavior of the families will alter accordingly.

Now let us look more closely at the six aspects of culture.

1. Culture Is Continually Changing

Culture is dynamic, continually changing because of the action and interaction of human beings with their environment. Although the elements of food behavior — selection, procurement, manipulation, storage, distribution, consumption, and disposal of food — remain the same, individuals will modify the manner in which they carry out these functions. Two examples of cultural change in food behavior can be seen in the history of coffee drinking and the attitude toward bran cereals.

The best cup of coffee, many believe, is the one that has been brewed from the finest freshly ground coffee beans. Instant coffee was introduced in 1909 to be used by the "less discriminating" coffee drinker. The culture also encouraged the attitude that no loving wife, no proper hostess, would serve her husband or guests instant coffee. Little change occurred in the coffee-processing industry until 1964, when freeze-dried coffee was introduced. Freeze-dried coffee was a technological innovation that combined the flavor of perked coffee, the convenience of instant, and the status of an expensive item. While homemakers still chose, prepared, and drank coffee, many changed their manner of doing so. A woman is no longer "second-rate" because she uses instant coffee. And, more recently, the use of instant freeze-dried coffee has been encouraged by cost-conscious homemakers because there is no wasted leftover coffee as there often is with perked.

Bran cereal, when first introduced, had a low status. It was used as a natural laxative. Low status, low-key marketing, and moderate pricing continued until the 1970s brought the return-to-nature movement. Bran cereal then acquired greater prestige. Industry gave the packaging of many bran cereals a face-lifting and increased both the price and the intensity of marketing. Recent research has indicated a need for more fiber in the Western diet and some physicians have recommended that people add half a cup of bran to their daily diet. The return-to-nature movement and the medical findings caused the change in marketing techniques. The sales, the prestige, and the price of bran cereals have all increased as a result.

2. Culture Has a Value System

Standards of "good" and "bad" behavior in certain situations are a part of one's culture and as such are transmitted to each succeeding generation, modified through cultural changes. Foods are labeled as being good for you or bad for you even though they all are accepted as food by the culture. "Junk food" is a term used widely in the United States to describe foods having high starch, sugar, or fat content — and therefore relatively high caloric content — but containing very few other nutrients. To be overweight is "bad" in the United States. Therefore, foods that provide calories but no redeeming nutrients are considered "bad" or "junk"; yet they are relished by many, as the large quantities sold indicate. Perhaps, then, they are considered treats, something beyond what one requires to survive. The general acceptance of "junk food" as a part of our culture was demonstrated in the nationally distributed cartoon "Peanuts." One of the characters is away at camp and is writing a letter home. Another character walks up and says, "What does PSJF mean?" and the first character replies, "Please send junk food." A song called "Junk Food Junkie" made the popular-record charts in 1975 while at the same time concerned parents of schoolchildren were waging limited campaigns to bar "junk food" from the school lunchroom. Texas banned "junk food" in the mid-1970s and Michigan, too, has attempted to limit the sale of "nonnutritious" foods in the schools — at least until half an hour after the lunch period ends.

In a recent class of graduate and senior students in food and nutrition and food and lodging, the students were asked to give an example of a "bad" food. In unison the class replied, "Junk foods." When they were asked to name such foods, Coke, candy, and potato chips were mentioned immediately. One student reported the results of interviews with college students about breakfast habits. It was noted that several students drank Coke at breakfast. The class responded negatively to this, but when asked what an appropriate drink would be, they replied, "Coffee." When asked why coffee instead of Coke, their reply was that Coke is a "junk food" and not something you have for breakfast, because breakfast is an important meal. Yet, coffee and Coke are both foods of low nutrient density. Values of "good" and "bad" had little to do with these students' scientific knowledge of the composition of the food items in question or with the fact that both drinks are used as stimulants.

Hsu (1975) considered self-reliance to be the American core value. He proposed that the values of achievement, success, activity, work, humanitarianism, efficiency, democracy, and individual personality are all expressions of, or spring from, this core value. He also pointed out that the psychological expression of valuing self-reliance is the fear of dependence. Perhaps some of the problems with our system for distributing food to people in the lower socioeconomic classes of our communities can be traced back to this value. Mead (1971) and Linton (1937) also discussed the American character and the value system of Americans. Understanding a community's value system and working within it are necessary conditions for the success of any community nutrition project.

3. Culture Is Composed of Learned Behavior

How is food behavior learned? Like any other aspect of culture, food behavior is learned through enculturation. *Enculturation* is the process by which culture is transmitted from one generation to another (Haviland 1974). It is generally divided into three categories: cultural cues or nonverbal behavior, informal education, and formal education.

Children receive cultural cues when their mothers frown at them for holding their forks with their fists instead of between the fingers or for slurping their soup or eating nonfinger foods with their fingers. The frown is a nonverbal cue to the children that their behavior is not appropriate. A smile, on the other hand, would be a reinforcing nonverbal cue.

Food behavior is learned informally. Women interviewed in numerous surveys have said that their mothers taught them "how to cook." They weren't taught from a systematic course outline; they learned by watching their mothers and listening to directions — all in an informal manner.

Some members of our culture do receive formal education in food behavior. Courses in home economics, environmental education, physical education, bachelor survival, and health provide information that encourages specific food behaviors.

The way an individual acts or reacts in situations involving food is learned in all of these ways. Culture influences food behavior because people who have been enculturated in the same society share beliefs and expectations about what will happen if they behave in certain ways. By the time children receive formal education, they already possess a set of food behaviors that will be expanded, reinforced, or modified throughout the rest of their lives.

In the United States, it is culturally desirable to be strong, healthy, young, and thin. It is also culturally desirable to be clean and long-lived. Products, such as health foods and vitamins, that are advertised as helping one to acquire the desired qualities are likely to be accepted by people. A nutritionally sound diet must be presented within the framework of culturally desirable qualities. Achieving and maintaining optimal nutritional status, however, requires more than swallowing a magic pill; it demands conscious thought, planning, and effort.

4. Culture Provides for Reasonable, Efficient Interaction among People

If a culture's methods of procuring and distributing food prove unreasonable or inefficient, the interactions among people will be affected and rioting may occur. This has happened in many of the developing countries.

In a diversified society some people produce food and other process and distribute it; some prepare food, and others dispose of the waste. Persons not directly involved in providing and managing the food supply perform paid services so that they can buy food. As a society increases in complexity and population, all of the activities related to food become more complex, and there arises a danger that the society will not meet the food-related needs of all segments of the population. Distribution of food is a problem in our own society today.

5. Culture Contains Symbols That Are Understood by the Group

Language is recognized as the most important symbolic aspect of culture, but food, too, can be symbolic. It can be a symbol of wealth or poverty, of ethnicity or "melting-pot" Americanism. A box of candy given on Valentine's Day is a symbol of affection. A pretzel fashioned in a special shape and eaten during Lent symbolizes repentance. An Easter egg symbolizes rebirth and hope. Until the late 1960s, the Roman Catholic church in North America forbade its members to eat meat on Friday. Many Catholics were amused by staunch Protestants who would not eat fish on Friday in a public place lest they be mistaken for Roman Catholics. Bread and wine, too, are religious symbols for many people.

Within a culture there are regional, ethnic, and subcultural differences in the terminology associated with food. For instance, in much of the southeastern United States, "creamed potatoes" means potatoes mashed with butter, with milk or cream added. In other parts of the nation, potatoes prepared in this manner would be known as "mashed potatoes," and "creamed potatoes" would refer to potatoes boiled, with a white sauce added. In the southeast, this dish would be called "boiled potatoes." As long as the term used conveys clearly to others what the speaker or writer means, there is no problem.

It is essential that food and nutrition professionals know and understand the food-related symbols (including language) used by the people they are working with. If the term "meat" means "fatback," "streak of lean," or mostly lean muscle tissue, the food and nutrition professional must know that. Other terminology may be equally important. If "evening" is used to denote the time after midday rather than the early part of night, food and nutrition workers may find themselves in the position of one of the authors of this book. An appointment for an interview had been made for Tuesday evening. The author appeared at the home about 7:00 p.m. and was met by an unhappy homemaker, who said, "I waited all evening for you and you didn't come." Evening was afternoon, 7:00 p.m. was night! Needless to say, the interview began in a negative atmosphere. The reverse situation could easily occur with a person from the southeastern region in a midwestern setting.

6. Culture Emphasizes Specific Activities

The emphasis in United States culture is on technology. Mechanization is increasing daily, and nowhere is this more evident than in food production. Because of our complex technology, in our culture only a few people are required to produce the food supply. Technological advances affect many aspects of each of the four parameters of foodways (i.e., availability, safety, nutritive quality, and acceptability).

THE FUNCTIONS OF CULTURE

If a culture is to survive, certain basic needs of its members must be met. The extent to which a culture meets those needs will determine its ultimate success. Success is defined according to the values of the majority of people in the culture. Outsiders may consider a culture unsuccessful at the same time that most of its members view it as successful. A culture must provide for the production and distribution of the goods and services necessary to maintain life; it must ensure biological continuity through the reproduction of its members; and it must socialize new members so that they can become functioning adults. The felt physical and psychological needs of the members have to be met. And, in addition, relationships between people within the culture and outsiders must be maintained (Haviland 1974).

One role of the community food and nutrition worker is to help fulfill the functions of culture. For example, if a community considers adequate food a "right" of all people, the worker may become involved in redistributing the food supply. In the course of a normal day a food and nutrition worker might receive a phone plea from the local soup kitchen or emergency food distribution center, "We're out of food — can you help?" The worker remembers that an ambitious student group planted a large garden in the spring. It is now harvest time. Perhaps the gardeners have a surplus they would contribute. Permission is obtained from the garden organizers to tack up a sign and leave a collection bin for surplus food at the garden entrance, and a soup kitchen volunteer is assigned to bring the produce from the garden to the soup kitchen. In this way a community food and nutrition worker may help provide the food necessary for life and at the same time aid people in helping each other to meet some of their psychological needs.

CULTURAL SYSTEMS

A *system* is a combination of parts forming a complex whole. In its dynamic aspect, the parts move in relation to each other and interact with the environment. The human body, for example, is a system made up of many subsystems (the lymph, the circulatory, etc.). Each of these subsystems is itself a system that performs a function as well as interacts with other systems to form the human body, a holistic entity. A culture, too, is a system composed of many subsystems. The individuals within a culture interact with each of the subsystems and with the culture as a whole. The philosophical, ideological, social (e.g., education and family), economic (e.g., mass media and industry), technological, and political subsystems interact with each other and influence the total cultural system as it in turn influences the parts (figure 2). As an individual progresses through life, the influence of each of these subsystems or forces varies.

The Family

The *family* is a system of the highest organization. Whatever happens to one member influences every other member to a greater degree than happens in other social systems. If one family member has diabetes, is obese, or has cancer, the way in which the others function and eat is affected.

Bubolz and Paolucci (1976) have noted that there is a relationship between the resources available to a family and the family's behavior. With regard to the family they state,

> We further assume that optimum development of humans is dependent upon the harmonious adaptation of humans to their total environment. We assume also that resources are finite and limited and that there must be greater equity in the distribution of resources. The family is assumed to be a major resource transformation system — a major consumer of resources and major creator and developer of human resources.

A family is defined as individuals with personal attributes organized as a corporate unit. Throughout this book references will be made to the family's influence upon the individual's food behavior.

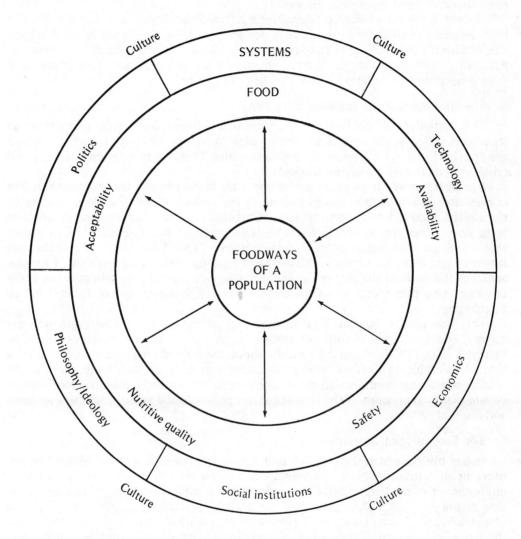

FIGURE 2. Factors that influence the foodways of a population.

The Educational System

Since the formation of the land-grant colleges, institutions of higher learning have given attention to the production, distribution, storage, and consumption of food products. As a result of activities in these areas, the United States has one of the safest, most abundant food supplies in the world.

Formal nutrition education from kindergarten through the twelfth grade has not been available to all children. Legislative action is evolving a program to provide food and nutrition education in the classroom for all children. Informal education, however, has always existed because what, how, when, and where to eat have been transmitted from generation to generation within families and groups.

The Philosophical and Ideological System

The United States, unlike most countries of the world, has a great many religious sects represented in its population. Many religions have some food restrictions, which are practiced in varying degrees by their adherents. Thus, for some people, dietary and religious practices are closely intertwined.

Manipulation of the physical environment by human beings for their comfort and convenience is a basic premise of culture in the United States. The major culture of the United States is based on the Judeo-Christian religious tradition and emphasizes technology. Thus, some people point to Bible passages like Genesis 1:26 to justify manipulation and exploitation of the environment: "Then God said, 'Let us make man in our image, after our likeness; and let them have dominion over the fish of the sea, and over the birds of the air, and over the cattle, and over all the earth and over every creeping thing that creeps upon the earth.' " Today, however, this attitude seems to be changing.

It is also part of our ideology to take care of the poor, to feed those who are hungry, and this conflicts with our knowledge that many of our resources are finite. Pimental et al. (1975) expressed concern about the limited energy and land resources that are available to increase food production, especially protein production, as the world's population continues to grow. The contradictions and conflicts in our welfare system are an expression of the conflict of our philosophical values with our economic and political systems.

The Technological System

It has been a widely held belief that technology can solve any problem and improve upon natural products. Technology can be an asset or a liability. For example, improvement of seed grain, fertilizer, production, storage, distribution, and manipulation techniques has vastly expanded the availability, safety, nutritive quality, and acceptability of foods. However, a substitute cheese product now on the market has the flavor and texture of cheese but is made from vegetable oils, thereby being acceptable as a substitute and cheaper (more available) but of different nutrient content. Unfortunately, it does not supply the high-quality protein or calcium of natural cheese and may increase the saturated fat in the diet. Thus, it may not be as safe a food for certain individuals as natural cheese would be.

Human beings procure food by four methods. Progress from one method to another means that less renewable energy and more finite, or nonrenewable, energy is used.

1. Hunting, fishing, and gathering were accomplished using renewable human energy.
2. Agriculture at first used renewable human and animal energy. Today mostly finite energy in the form of fossil fuel is used.
3. Engineered or fabricated foods (natural food products manipulated in some way to make them more acceptable or more available) require a still larger proportion of finite energy.
4. Synthesized foods (foods made up from the chemical components) require even more finite energy in their production.

The increased complexity of producing food requires a complex technology that depends on a constant source of finite energy.

The Economic System

Economics influences all aspects of food behavior from selection to consumption. In a complex culture such as that of the United States, the economic system controls both the food supply and food distribution to a great extent. The effect of marginal income on food intake is documented in many studies (U.S. Department of Health, Education and Welfare 1972; Burroughs and Huenemann 1970; Driskell and Price 1974; Hootman et al. 1967; Kelsay 1969; Larson et al. 1974; Simpson 1969).

The Mass Media

Probably no subsystem influences our food behavior more than the mass media, a product of our technology and a part of our economic system. Generally accepted functions of the mass media in the United States include (1) surveillance, (2) analysis of events from a broad and well-informed perspective (as in a commentary or news analysis), (3) transmission of the culture to new members (the mass media act as both agents and indices of cultural change), (4) entertainment, and (5) selling of products. In relation to food behavior, the third and fifth functions of the mass media — transmission of culture and selling of goods — are of the greatest interest.

The effect of the mass media on the public, in particular on children, is controversial. Roberts and Schramm (1971) remind us that the media are merely "message multipliers" whose effects depend on audience use. Messages relayed by newspapers, magazines, and other printed materials, and by radio, television, and telephone must gain attention before the receiver can interpret and act on them.

Each form of the mass media plays a unique role in American culture. Newspapers are vehicles for news, events, and advertising. The role of the newspaper may take on less or different significance for those who do not subscribe than for those who do. Magazines are intended for a more selective audience than are newspapers, radio, and television; their content and advertising are directed to specific interests. Radio, on the other hand, is an immediate medium. Commercials and instantaneous news broadcasts may interrupt a program at any time. Television, in particular commercial daytime television, may take on added significance for persons not employed outside the home. Some broadcasters say that television is a personal window on the world.

Commercial Television. The fast and widespread penetration of television throughout America has been a cause of great concern resulting in many studies. Entertainment, violence, instruction, news, values, and attitudes are all projected on its screen. Researchers have not been able to define the long-term impact of television on the behavior and attitudes of the American public. Many suggest, however, that incidental learning may take place during program watching. (Roberts and Schramm 1971).

Each season the broadcast literature devotes a great amount of print to the budgets, scripts, stars, and ratings for commercial prime-time television. Relatively little is written about daytime commercial television and its programs aimed at homemakers. It is hardly a debatable point that many women watch one or more "soaps" or stories each day. The popularity of the stories, first on radio (Herzog 1944) and now on television, bolstered by more than a million dollars in advertising yearly, documents the point (Forkan 1974). Steiner (1963) reported that 30 percent of the women he interviewed enjoyed the afternoon better than any other part of the day, primarily because of television viewing. Nixon (1972), one of the most prominent "soap opera" writers for television, defended the "soaps." " 'Soaps' receive ridicule and criticism," Nixon stated, "however, they disseminate vital messages to people in need of information — people not likely to read periodicals or newspapers and apt to turn off documentary programs."

Television Advertisements. Inseparable from commercial television is the television ad. Meyers (1963) defined advertising as a "mass paid communication whose ultimate purpose is to impart information, develop attitudes and induce action that is beneficial to the advertiser." On the average, 10 to 20 percent of television air time is filled with advertisements. Twenty-four percent of the women in Steiner's study (1963) reported obtaining information from television commercials. It is generally believed that television ads do work — they do sell products. And they have been effective in teaching nutrition, too (Brent 1974).

Dominick and Rauch (1972), interested in the cultural transmission of woman's role in society, studied network television ads. Seventy-five percent of all ads picturing females were for bathroom or kitchen products. Fourteen percent of the ads, viewed over a 2-week period in that study, positioned the female in the kitchen. Fifty-six percent of the women were portrayed as housewives and mothers.

The placement and timing of food commercials on television is very important to advertisers. Some firms specialize in advertising techniques that make food ads noticed (Ogilvy and Mather 1972). Meyers (1963) studied adjectives with special connotations for specific types of products. Those for food included *adolescent, adult, aromatic, basic, children, economical, necessary, satisfying, substantial,* and *tasty.* Again, the techniques effective in food advertising are known, but the why and how of producing results have not been illuminated. Broadcasters and advertisers recognize that the content of programs and ads are keys to success.

Food and Mass Media Studies. A few studies have defined the sources of food information used by homemakers.

Fliegel (1961), in a food consumption study of nationality groups in Pennsylvania, examined sources of information about food. While radio and television reached the largest number of people, few homemakers obtained new ideas about food from those sources. It is interesting that 74, 72, 81, 52, and 6 percent of the women reported being exposed to food information by radio, television, daily newspapers, "women's magazines," and organized groups, respectively. However, only a small percentage of those women reported using that information. In general, informal sources (e.g., friends and neighbors) were cited as the main sources of new ideas about food. (In response to these data one might ask, Where do the friends and neighbors obtain their information? and postulate transmission by some form of mass media.)

Homemakers participating in the North Central Regional Study of the nutritional status of preschool children reported obtaining nutrition information from magazines (63 percent), newspapers (48 percent), books (47 percent), television (34 percent), radio (21 percent), extension and government bulletins (17 percent), and other lay sources (3 percent) (Fox et al. 1970).

Sanjur and Scoma (1971) investigated the communication channels operative for low-income black homemakers in northern New York. Ninety-eight percent of these homemakers watched television and 97, 92, 91, 76, and 70 percent, respectively, obtained information from friends, church, radio, newspapers, and magazines or books. Thirty-five percent listed ads as a useful source of food information.

Emmons and Hayes (1973) studied the nutrition knowledge of mothers in upstate New York and found that most of them relied on newspapers, radio, magazines, and television for information.

While these studies report sources of food information for homemakers, they do not outline what kind of food and nutrition information, if any, is carried by those sources. It would be valuable for food and nutrition professionals to know what kind of information is learned from the mass media. Winick (1973) says we can assume that exposure to television advertising gives young children some ideas about the world and some impressions of family, work, and sex roles, as well as selling them products. Consumer groups, such as Children's Foundation and Action for Children's Television (ACT), are trying to influence aspects of the mass media that relate to children.

The Political System

People, although they may live alone, do not exist as isolates in our society. The political system regulates and controls many activities that affect their lives. Even the foodways of a population are directly related to its politics.

Decisions made by government officials have direct implications for the availability, safety, nutritive quality, and acceptability of the food supply (Pimental et al. 1975; Bass and Wakefield 1974). In our system of government, laws made by Congress that affect the four parameters of food behavior are made in the public arena and may be subject to pressures from special-interest groups. The regulation of production and marketing is an example of this. Prices paid to the farmer must be kept at a level that will encourage food production, but international trade in food commodities is another factor that must be reckoned with. The quality and wholesomeness of products is controlled by the federal government in interstate commerce, but it may not be controlled within a state. Transportation affects the availability, safety, nutritive quality, and acceptability of food; hence, anything affecting transportation can affect the market, which in turn affects the individual. Food is a political issue, from its production (or restriction of production) to its transport and storage and finally to its marketing distribution and price.

The politics of food distribution for schools, breakfast programs, food stamps, and food programs for the aged are of concern to many citizens. Social welfare programs, school health programs, and housing are also problem areas for political consideration. Where problems exist, political action can help bring about change. Before such action is undertaken, however, a nutritional assessment should be made to determine whether there is reason for the community to be concerned about the nutritional aspects of the problem. An educational program may be needed to sensitize the local citizens and government to specific nutritional problems in the community.

The forces of technology, economics, politics, and social institutions are all involved in the politics of food (figure 3). Special-interest groups from all of these areas are at work within the community, bringing pressure to bear to achieve results that are beneficial to them. Many times the results are also beneficial to society, but often they are not. Community food and nutrition professionals must be aware of the various special-interest groups within the community and learn to deal with them.

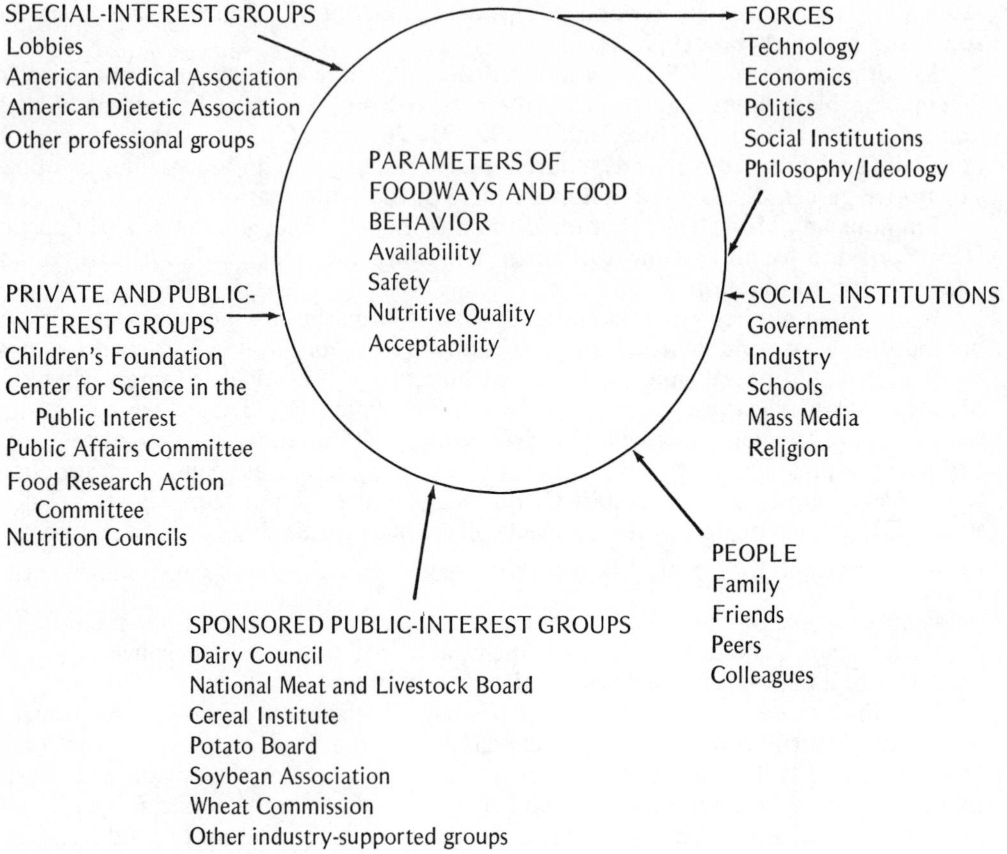

SPECIAL-INTEREST GROUPS
Lobbies
American Medical Association
American Dietetic Association
Other professional groups

PARAMETERS OF
FOODWAYS AND FOOD
BEHAVIOR
Availability
Safety
Nutritive Quality
Acceptability

FORCES
Technology
Economics
Politics
Social Institutions
Philosophy/Ideology

PRIVATE AND PUBLIC-
INTEREST GROUPS
Children's Foundation
Center for Science in the
    Public Interest
Public Affairs Committee
Food Research Action
    Committee
Nutrition Councils

SOCIAL INSTITUTIONS
Government
Industry
Schools
Mass Media
Religion

SPONSORED PUBLIC-INTEREST GROUPS
Dairy Council
National Meat and Livestock Board
Cereal Institute
Potato Board
Soybean Association
Wheat Commission
Other industry-supported groups

PEOPLE
Family
Friends
Peers
Colleagues

FIGURE 3. The politics of food.

ACCULTURATION AND TRANSMISSION OF FOOD BEHAVIOR

Acculturation

In light of the interest in the "new ethnicity" being demonstrated in the United States, it is important to explore the concept of acculturation. Descriptions of the American food pattern vary from observer to observer, just as the pattern varies from rural to urban areas, from deserts to mountain regions, and from house to house. Foods, food preferences, and general food behaviors have been brought to the United States from every part of the world. The last part of the "old life" that immigrants to a new land will give up is their food behavior, providing the old foods or their ingredients (or reasonable susbstitutes) are available. Immigrants may be pressured to conform to language, dress, and other customs, but in the privacy of their homes they can select, prepare, and enjoy foods that meet either old or new cultural expectations.

Adapting to the forces at work in an alien environment is a learning process termed *acculturation*. Before the Black Revolution of the 1960s, the acculturation process in the United States was governed by the melting-pot theory. Immigrants and other subgroups were encouraged by the dominant American culture to lose all their distinctive characteristics, to be in a sense "boiled down" to become "new Americans."

For some groups, the alteration of food behavior required to maintain health and well-being would be large. For example, if a Miskito Indian from the eastern coast of Nicaragua came to study at a midwestern American university, an almost complete change in food behavior would be necessary. The Miskito eat cassava and plantain daily, use coconut meat and coconut milk as common ingredients in prepared foods, and frequently consume saltwater fish — all rare items in the fast-food restaurants, vending machines, and cafeterias of a large university. If the Miskito student learns to choose fast-food hamburgers, french fries, and carbonated beverages for three meals a day, every day, the student's nutritional status and well-being are likely to deteriorate. Failure to adapt to a generalized Basic Four food pattern based on the local food supply may be extremely detrimental.

It is simple to identify people who must change their diets drastically in order to become acculturated to American life. More difficult to identify are people who arrive in this country with a core diet of foods readily available here but who are nevertheless required to change some aspect of their food behavior, or the people who move from ethnic centers like the Polish neighborhoods in Hamtramck, Michigan, or Buffalo, New York, or Chicago, Illinois, into the larger American culture and must modify their food behavior to fit the general patterns of food consumption in the United States. How does a change in environment affect the food attitudes, beliefs, and habits of people living in the United States? This question is one that community food and nutrition workers need to ask and research.

Transmission of Food Behavior

It is believed that all groups teach their offspring about food and that, at least in part, food behavior is culturally transmitted. Culture, including customs, attitudes, and values, is usually transmitted from one generation to the next. The community food and nutrition professional must discover what food practices are being passed along in this way.

Spindler (1959) discussed the transmission of the American culture and its two basic values, tradition and emergence. He noted that cultural transmission is difficult to perceive in our complex and changing society. Often the conflicts of a culture and its values are also transmitted to children, and then the cultural trait that the parents wanted preserved is lost. Jennings and Niemi (1968) noted that the transmission of certain values from parent to child, specifically political values, can be observed in late adolescence. In general, their hypothesis that the closer children feel to their parents the more susceptible they become to parental values was found to be untrue. Rather, the children used their parents as role models if they were neither too permissive nor too strict.

The transmission of food behavior from parent to child has often been alluded to in the literature on food behavior. Many researchers suggest that food behavior and food habits are stable and resistant to change, due in part to their establishment early in life. (However, observations indicate that this statement cannot be applied to children of immigrants to the United States.) "Socio-cultural experiences dominate the learning of food behavior because all societies attempt to pass on traditional foodways and all children tend to imitate or model their behavior on that of others" (U.S. Department of Health, Education and Welfare 1968). LeGros Clark (1968) stated that food behavior may be transmitted to each new generation and become entangled in the culture but is still susceptible to change. The transmission of food behavior and the factors effecting changes are of interest to educators trying to preserve good food behavior and modify poor food behavior (National Research Council 1943).

While the total family, the society, and the mass media play both formal and informal roles in the transmission of foodways, the mother has traditionally been seen as the primary transmitter. In many cultures, the mother has been the pivot of family life (Bloch 1976). Research in the United States during the 1940s (Lewin 1943; de Give 1943; and Cussler 1943) indicated that it is through the mother that cultural influences come to the child. It is the mother who teaches the child what foods are desirable, satisfying, delightful, good for one, not to be eaten with other foods, and so on. The mother has been viewed in this culture as the repository for food lore. Sims, Paolucci, and Morris (1972) viewed the mother as a central figure in the nuclear family, as the major link between the outside environment and other family members, being typically responsible for preparing and distributing food to the rest of the family.

How universal and enduring is this maternal effect on the food behavior of children as they mature? The literature is scarce. Hellersberg (1946) found that students' food patterns showed an astounding correspondence with those of their mothers. De Give (1943) viewed the role of the mother in relation to food behavior continuing throughout life and indicated that the mother transmits the cultural heritage in two principal ways — she is the source of nutrition information for the child and she is the daughter's cooking teacher. Later the mother gives advice to the grown daughter in matters of food, and as a grandmother she advises in the feeding of a newborn.

There are situations, such as immigration, that change the process of transmitting food behavior. The immigrating process breaks the continuity with the past. Perhaps the role of women changes in the upheaval of changing environments. For example, Bloch (1976) compared women living in a rural village of Poland with similar women who had moved to the United States. She found that the domestic roles of the women in the United States had changed immensely and affected the entire family life. The mother, once the pivot of family life, in America became just another member of the family intent on earning a living wage.

It has been suggested that several generations of immigrants to the United States, including the Polish Americans, did not transmit their cultural attitudes, beliefs, and food knowledge to their children. Chrobot (1976), for example, thinks that most American children and grandchildren of ethnic Americans have little or no knowledge of their heritage.

If one were to interview the children of an ethnic American of Polish descent and ask them to describe the Polish dietary, they might say that Polish foods include *kapusta* (sauerkraut), *golabki* (stuffed cabbage), *babka* (holiday bread or coffee cake), *czarnia* (duck blood soup, sometimes called chocolate soup by children), *paczki* (donuts), *chrusciki* (bow tie pastries, also known as angel wings) and *pierogi* (dumplings filled with ground meat or cheese or sauerkraut and potatoes or plums or berries). If asked why Polish people saute bread crumbs in butter and pour them over vegetables, they might reply, "I guess it tastes good," rather than recounting for you the belief that bread is the holiest of all edibles and that Polish people have never wasted bread — not even crumbs. Bread crumbs were collected and used to thicken gravy, line baking pans, or season foods.*

*Personal communication from Halina Ujda.

An attempt to document the food behavior of various ethnic groups in the United States was completed in the 1940s by the Committee on Food Habits (National Research Council 1943; Benet and Joffe 1943). These materials were developed to give insight and background material to aid nutritionists and social service and community workers who must work with the food problems of subcultures.

Accounts of Polish Americans depicted them as a fairly homogeneous group, generally of peasant background. Their core diet was composed of grains (rye, wheat, buckwheat, and barley), potatoes, cabbage, legumes, and green vegetables, and supplemented with milk, cheese, sour cream, eggs, home-raised pork, fruits, berries, wild mushrooms, and fish. Salt, sugar, tea, and coffee were not core food items for the Polish people, since in Poland they were all imported items. For the Polish immigrants who settled in urban areas, acculturation meant adopting white sugar and flour and abandoning rich vegetable soups, bean soups, and cottage cheese dishes. Disruption of a meal pattern that provided adequate nutrition as well as disruption of a society based on the family living on the land occurred.

The eating pattern of the Poles before coming to America has been described by Strybel (1975). They ate a hearty breakfast. At rising they might take milk soup or white coffee with sausage, ham cheese, cottage cheese and chives, eggs, and bread and butter. Later in the morning there would be a break for sandwiches, apples, cake, and hot tea. The main meal of the day, eaten between 2:00 and 4:00 p.m., consisted of soup, meat, potatoes, salad or hot vegetable, and dessert. The evening meal was usually served around 8:00 p.m. and included cold cuts, eggs, sour milk, and grain or blintzes. The American Dietetic Association has prepared a booklet entitled *Cultural Food Patterns in the U.S.* (1976), which describes the diet of Polish Americans. Though the diet is similar to that found in Poland, some changes have been noted in the way fruits and vegetables are prepared and used.

Arguments have been made for an integrated pluralist America. It has been suggested that Americans should take the most pleasurable components of their folk culture and of the urban culture and become integrated pluralists in an American mosaic, that is, preserve some of the history, culture, tradition, and differences while accepting modernism. People cry out in despair as they travel throughout the United States and other places of the world and find McDonald's hamburgers; yet they are thankful for the convenience, speed, safety, and cleanliness the chain represents. The community food and nutrition professional who assists the new American in changing food behavior while maintaining some continuity with the past will foster a successful acculturation.

REFERENCES

Arensberg, C. M., and Niehoff, A.1975. American cultural values. In *The Nacirema*, ed. J. P. Spradley and M. A. Rynkiewich. Boston: Little, Brown.

Bass, M. A., and Wakefield, L. M. 1974. Nutrient intake and food patterns of Indians on Standing Rock Reservation. *Journal of the American Dietetic Association* 64:29.

Brent, C. 1974. TV commercials can teach nutrition. *Journal of Home Economics* 66 (3):21.

Bubolz, M. J., and Paolucci, B. 1976. An ecological systems approach to the family: Preliminary conceptualization. Presented at the National Council on Family Relations, 19-20 October 1976, New York.

Buchwald, A. 1976. Peace Corp backlash. In *Cultural anthropology*, ed. P. Hiebert. Philadelphia: Lippincott.

Burroughs, A. L., and Huenemann, R. L. 1970. Iron deficiency in rural infants and children. *Journal of the American Dietetic Association* 57:122.

Dominick, J. R., and Rauch, G. E. 1972. The image of women in network TV commercials. *Journal of Broadcasting* 16:259.

Driskell, J. A., and Price, C. S. 1974. Nutritional status of preschoolers from low-income Alabama families. *Journal of the American Dietetic Association* 65:280.

Emmons, L., and Hayes, M. 1973. Nutrition knowledge of mothers and children. *Journal of Nutrition Education* 5:134.

Fliegel, F. C. 1961. *Food habits and national background.* Bulletin 684. University Park: Pennsylvania State University Agricultural Experiment Station.

Forkan, J. P. 1974. Soapers still pack 'em in despite game growth. *Advertising Age* 45 (6):10.

Foster, G. 1962. *Traditional cultures and the impact of technological change.* New York: Harper and Row.

Fox, H. M.; Fryer, B. A.; Lamkin, G. L.; Vivian, V. M.; and Eppright, E. S. 1970. Family environment. *Journal of Home Economics* 62:241.

Haviland, W. 1974. *Anthropology.* New York: Holt, Rinehart and Winston.

Herzog, H. 1944. What do we really know about daytime serial listeners? In *Radio research,* ed. P. F. Lazarsfeld and F. N. Stanton, pp. 3-33. New York: Duell, Sloan and Pearce.

Hiebert, P. 1976. *Cultural anthropology.* Philadelphia: Lippincott.

Hootman, R. H.; Haschke, M. B.; Roderuck, C.; and Eppright, E. S. 1967. Diet practices and physical development of Iowa children from low-income families. *Journal of Home Economics* 59:41.

Hsu, F. 1975. American core value and national character. In *The Nacirema,* ed. J. P. Spradley and M. A. Rynkiewich. Boston: Little, Brown.

Kelsay, J. L. 1969. A compendium of nutritional status studies and dietary evaluation studies conducted in the United States. *Journal of Nutrition* 99 (supplement 1, part 2):123.

Larson, L. B.; Dodds, J. M.; Massoth, D. M.; and Chase, H. P. 1974. Nutritional status of Mexican-American migrant families. *Journal of the American Dietetic Association* 64:29.

Linton, R. 1937. One hundred percent American. *American Mercury* 40:427.

Mead, M. 1971. *And keep your powder dry.* New York: William Morrow.

Meyers, L., Jr. 1963. Relation of personality to perception of television advertising messages. In *Television and human behavior,* ed. L. Arons and M. A. May, pp. 208-218. New York: Appleton-Century-Crofts.

Miner, H. 1956. Body ritual among the Nacirema. In *The Nacirema,* ed. J. P. Spradley and M. A. Rynkiewich. Boston: Little, Brown 1975.

Nixon, A. D. 1972. In daytime tv, the golden age is now. *Television Quarterly* 10 (1):49.

Ogilvy, and Mather. 1972. How to create food advertising that sells. *Advertising Age* 43 (28):9.

Pangborn, R., and Bruhn, C. 1971. Concepts of food habits of "other" ethnic groups. *Journal of Nutrition Education* 2:106.

Pimental, D.; Dritschilo, W.; Krummel, J.; and Kutzman, J. 1975. Energy and land constraints in food protein production. *Science* 190:754.

Roberts, D. F., and Schramm, W. 1971. Children's learning from the mass media. In *The process and effects of mass communications,* ed. W. Schramm and D. R. Roberts, pp. 596-611. Urbana: University of Illinois Press.

Sanjur, D., and Scoma, A. 1971. Food habits of low-income children in northern New York. *Journal of Nutrition Education* 3:85.

Simpson, O. 1969. *A nutritional survey to document the extent of malnutrition in a rural Georgia county.* Office of Economic Opportunity. Atlanta: Southern Rural Action.

Steiner, G. A. 1963. *The people look at television.* New York: Knopf.

U. S. Department of Health, Education and Welfare. 1972. *Ten-State Nutrition Survey 1968-70: Part IV. Biochemical.* DHEW publication no. (HSM) 72-8132.

Winick, C.; Williamson, L.; Chuzmic, S.; and Winick, M. 1973. *Children's television commercials: A content analysis.* New York: Praeger.

Acculturation and Transmission of Food Behavior

American Dietetic Association. 1976. *Cultural food patterns in the U.S.* Chicago: American Dietetic Association.

Anonymous. 1976. Poland — No sugar daddy. *Time,* 30 August 1976, p. 49.

Bakanowski, C. R. A. 1968. My memoirs — Texas sojourn. *Journal of Polish American Studies* 25 (2):106.

Benet, S. M., and Joffe, N. 1943. Polish food patterns. Washington, D.C.: National Research Council, Committee on Food Habits.

Block, H. 1976. Changing domestic roles among Polish immigrant women. *Anthropological Quarterly* 49 (1):3.

Brown, E. L. 1967. College students look at the basis for their food habits. *Journal of Home Economics* 59:784.

Carpenter, N., and Katz, D. 1929. *A study of acculturation in the Polish group of Buffalo.* University of Buffalo Studies 7, no. 4, pp. 103-133. Buffalo, N.Y.: University of Buffalo Press.

Chrobot, L. F. 1976. *Toward a definition of the integrated pluralist, or why we should not all be just "American."* Monograph 18. Orchard Lake, Mich.: St. Mary's College.

Cussler, M. R. 1943. Cultural sanctions and the food pattern in the rural Southeast. Ph.D. thesis, Radcliffe College (Cambridge, Mass.).

de Give, M. L. 1943. Social interrelations and food habits in the rural Southeast. Ph.D. thesis, Radcliffe College (Cambridge, Mass.).

Dembinska, M. 1971. Historical research on food consumption in Poland. *Ethnologia Europaea* 5:130.

Fliegel, F. C. 1961. *Food habits and national background.* Bulletin 684. University Park: Pennsylvania State University Agricultural Experiment Station.

Gowaskie, J. D. 1976. *Polish community in America: An annotated and classified bibliographic guide.* Franklin, N.Y.: Burt.

Hall, D. E. 1938. Discussion at section meeting on culture and personality. *American Journal of Orthopsychiatry* 8:618.

Hellersberg, E. F. 1946. Food habits of adolescents in relation to family training and present adjustment. *American Journal of Orthopsychiatry* 16:34.

Janasik, B. 1963. Polish American lenten customs. *Journal of Polish American Studies* 20 (2):97.

Jennings, M. K., and Niemi, R. G. 1968. The transmission of political values from parent to child. *American Political Science Review* 62:169.

Jerome, N. 1969. Northern urbanization and food consumption patterns of southern-born Negroes. *American Journal of Clinical Nutrition* 22:1667.

Joffe, N. F. 1943. Food habits of selected subcultures in the United States. In *The problem of changing food habits,* pp. 99-102. National Research Council, Bulletin no. 108. Washington, D.C.: National Academy of Sciences.

Keefe, E.; Bernier, D.; Brenneman, L.; Gilvone, W.; Moore, J.; and Walpole, N. 1973. *Area handbook for Poland.* Washington, D.C.: Government Printing Office.

Kolasa, K. M. 1974. Foodways of selected mothers and their adult daughters in upper east Tennessee. Ph.D. thesis, University of Tennessee (Knoxville).

Krolikowski, Z. 1976. More Indian corn. *Poland* 6 (262):11.

LeGros Clark, W. 1968. Food habits as a practical nutrition problem. *World Review of Nutrition and Dietetics* 9:56.

Lewin, K. 1943. Forces behind food habits and methods of change. In *The problem of changing food habits,* pp. 35-65. National Research Council, Bulletin no. 108. Washington, D.C.: National Academy of Sciences.

Litman, T. J.; Cooney, J. P.; and Stief, R. 1964. The views of Minnesota school children on food. *Journal of the American Dietetic Association* 45:433.

Ludanyi, A. 1976. Polish jokes and American destinies. *Phi Kappa Phi Journal* 56 (3):44.

Mackun, S. 1964. The changing patterns of Polish settlements in the greater Detroit area: Geographic study of the assimilation of an ethnic group. Ph.D. thesis, University of Michigan (Ann Arbor).

Marshall, K. K. 1976. A taste of Poland. *Sokol Polski* (Pittsburgh), 15 October 1976, p. 8.

Mead, M. 1964. *Food habit research: Problems of the 1960s.* National Research Council, publication 1225. Washington, D.C.: National Academy of Sciences.

Miller, F. H. 1896. *The Polanders in Wisconsin.* Parkman Club Papers, no. 10. Milwaukee: Parkman Club.

National Research Council. 1943. *The problem of changing food habits.* Bulletin no. 108. Washington, D.C.: National Academy of Sciences.

Roucek, J. S. 1937. *Poles in the United States of America.* Gydnia, Poland: Baltic Institute.

Sims, L. S.; Paolucci, B.; and Morris, P. M. 1972. A theoretical model for the study of nutritional status: An ecosystem approach. *Ecology of Food and Nutrition* 1:197.

Spindler, G. D. 1959. *The transmission of American culture.* Cambridge, Mass.: Harvard University Press.

Strybel, R. 1975. Nazdrowie — Or health of our heritage. *Dziennik Polski* (Detroit), 26 April 1975, p. 2.

Thomas, W. I., and Znaniecki, F. 1918. *The Polish peasant in Europe and America.* Chicago: University of Chicago Press.

U. S. Department of Health, Education and Welfare. 1968. *Determination of concepts basic to an improved foods and nutrition curriculum at the college level.* Washington, D.C.: U. S. Department of Health, Education and Welfare, Office of Education, Bureau of Research.

Williams, C. 1968. Life history of a Polish immigrant. *Journal of Polish American Studies* 25 (2):86.

Zand, H. S. 1960. Polish American folkways. *Journal of Polish American Studies* 18 (1):34.

Zand, H. S. 1961. Polish American profile. *Journal of Polish American Studies* 18 (2):94.

Zieleniewicz, A. 1971. *Poland.* Orchard Lake, Mich.: Center for Polish Studies and Culture, Orchard Lake Schools.

CHAPTER 2

Food Classifications and People

FOOD CLASSIFICATIONS

Food is, of course, the matter which nourishes the body. But it is much more than that. In every society, it has served various functions in addition to nourishing the body. People classify food according to (1) its actual use by the body, (2) its actual use in society, and (3) its perceived use by the body and in society. (For example, in our society potatoes are (1) a source of energy and minerals for the body, (2) a food for snacks or meals, and (3) perceived as fattening and as a "filler" food for meals.) Such classification is the result of interacting cultural, social, economic, technological, political, and historical factors. Anyone engaged in delivering food and nutrition services must understand how those who are being served classify specific foods.

Food classifications are transmitted through cultural cues and informal and formal education. The manner in which people regard foods has been classified formally by researchers in a variety of ways. A community food and nutrition worker might use a formal classification scheme to identify the roles of specific foods in a community. This information could then be used in planning ways to modify food behavior. Examples of formal classifications devised by professionals after observing food behavior or determining nutritional needs or surveying consumers' use of food will be discussed subsequently.

Linton (1936) classified as *core foods* those foods observed to be used most often and consistently. He classified as *secondary foods* the foods that were used less often and less consistently but that still were important in the diet. And foods used only to supplement the diet periodically he called *peripheral foods*. A person's intake of core foods is the most difficult to alter. For many people in the United States bacon and eggs for breakfast has been the pattern, and concern about cholesterol in eggs and nitrites in bacon has caused few to change that pattern beyond perhaps trying a low-cholesterol egg substitute.

A classification of food based on observations of food behavior and applicable worldwide was presented by Jelliffe (1967). According to this classification, foods are divided into five categories.

1. *Cultural superfood* is the dominant staple food item and often is the main source of calories. Its production and preparation take most of the time of the people. The religion, mythology, and history of the people reflect the importance of this food in their culture. It is often the food fed to young children. Wheat and corn might be considered cultural superfoods in the United States.

2. *Prestige foods* are served at important occasions or to important people. They are expensive foods or foods that are difficult to obtain. Usually they are of animal origin, such as steak and lobster, the prestige foods in the United States.

3. *Body-image foods* are associated with the workings of the body. Foods that provide a balance and that contribute to good health are included in this group. The yin-yang ideology of Zen macrobiotics and the balance of "hot" and "cold" foods* in the diets of people of Indian or Mexican ancestry, of slimming and fattening foods, and of diets based on the Basic Four food groups are examples.

4. *Sympathetic magic foods* are foods thought to have special properties that impart desired characteristics to the person who eats them. For instance, there are those who think that eating walnuts provides one with more brains, that ingesting rare steak makes one stronger, or that imbibing a solution of gelatin strengthens and beautifies the fingernails.

5. *Physiological group foods* are foods restricted by the culture to or for persons of a particular age or sex or condition (e.g., pregnancy). The culture may dictate that commercial baby food is for babies but not for toothless old people who find it tasty and convenient. Some pregnant women in the United States eat cornstarch and clay to meet a perceived physiological need. Milk is often perceived as a child's food.

Another way to classify foods is by determining the nutritional needs of people and grouping the foods they commonly eat into categories to meet those needs. The nutritional needs of the United States population were used to structure a food classification system, the Basic Four Food Guide. The meat, milk and dairy products, fruits and vegetables, and breads and cereals groups were defined in the 1950s as a teaching tool and this food classification system is now taught throughout the United States. However, the Basic Four only describes one aspect of food behavior in the United States, that related to the body image, or the balancing of foods to meet nutritional needs. And observation of American food behavior does not reveal the Basic Four to be a classification that people can use without express planning.

Food can also be classified according to actual consumer use. In recent years, Americans have been surveyed for their attitudes, beliefs, and feelings about food. Schutz et al. (1975), for example, asked American consumers to make judgments about food and then classified foods into five groups based on the consumers' judgments.

1. *High-calorie treats* included wine, pies, cakes, and dips. They were considered appropriate foods to serve to guests and on special holidays. They were not considered appropriate for persons wanting to lose weight or not feeling well. Schutz et al (1975) reported that wholesome snacks (carrots, celery, fruit) were regarded as suitable for everyday eating and for eating alone rather than with others. McConnell (1974) found applesauce, pudding, and carrot sticks to be foods that the high school students in her sample associated more with sick than with well people.

---

*"Hot" and "cold" do not refer to physical temperature but to certain qualities that a culture assigns to foods.

2. *Specialty meal items* included chitterlings, liver, chili, and kidneys. These foods were described as not appropriate for a variety of situations. Yet, they are known to be eaten regularly by certain ethnic groups.

3. *Common meal items* included chicken, roast beef, and steak, which were the foods ranked highest in this category. As a group, these foods were considered nutritious and appropriate for all age groups. They were thought suitable for guests and were used for the dinner meal, not for breakfast or dessert.

4. *Refreshing foods* included flavored gelatin desserts, cottage cheese, orange juice, and milk. These foods were described as appropriately served cold and served in the summer. They were thought to be nutritious and easy to digest but were not considered appropriate entrees. It is interesting to note that flavored gelatin desserts appear on this list, although in nutrient density they rank much below any of the other items unless they are prepared with fruit juice.

5. *Inexpensive filling foods* included peanut butter, bread, potato chips, and candy bars. These foods were not considered appropriate when one needs to lose weight or to "feel creative."

In a different way, Schutz et al. (1975) found that the uses of food could be grouped into the categories of utilitarian, casual, satiating, and social.

THE FUNCTIONS OF FOOD IN CULTURE

All people use food to facilitate certain activities within their society. Such uses of food can be described in a variety of ways. Van Schaik (1964) and Leininger (1969) have described some of the functions of food in a society. We shall discuss these functions and others here.

1. *Food satisfies hunger and nourishes the body.* People must have food enough to supply the nutrients necessary to maintain and reproduce life.

2. *Food is used to initiate and maintain personal relationships and business associations.* In a community people may be asked out to dinner or to another person's home for a meal to initiate a friendship or a business relationship. These relationships may be nurtured by a reciprocating invitation.

3. *Food is used to determine and demonstrate the nature and extent of relationships.* Casual relationships are maintained by infrequent and casual contact such as invited participation in a large social gathering once or twice a year. A much closer relationship may be created by intimate contact through more frequent small dinner parties.

4. *Food is used as a focus to bring people together for a specific purpose.* For example, dinners may be held at prices designed not only to cover the cost of the meal but also to obtain money for a charity or a political party or a new church or school building.

Sociability and friendship may be associated with certain foods (Moore 1957; Steelman 1974). Food can even define the occasion, as cake with candles means a birthday party (Gifft, Washbon, and Harrison 1972). Prestige foods may be served to impress guests, while more common foods will be served to close friends. Steelman (1974) found that in Louisiana chicken and barbecued pork, although rated low on the status scale, tended to be a popular dish to serve family and friends. The "steak cookout" seemed to be enjoyed most by those who could afford it. According to Gifft, Washbon, and Harrison (1972), "offering to share food with another connotes the offering of a bit of oneself."

5. *Food is used to express love or concern.* To show her concern, a mother may prepare the favorite food of a family member who is under stress. A neighbor may take a prepared meal to a family next door when there is illness or a death in the family.

6. *Food is used by individuals to set themselves apart from their peers.* A person may choose to eat food prepared in a manner different from that of the peer group in order to attract attention or to emphasize individuality. Some vegetarians and health food enthusiasts may do this.

7. *Food is used to set a group of people apart or to signify that a person belongs to a particular group of people.* Certain religious sects restrict specific foods. The Jewish religion prohibits the eating of pork; the Black Muslims are not allowed to eat pork or certain vegetables, such as collard greens. Catholics were not allowed to eat meat on Fridays until the 1960s. Seventh-Day Adventists may be vegetarians. Others may choose to be vegetarians to signify their commitment to solving the world food problem.

8. *Food is used to help people cope with psychological and emotional stresses.* The compulsive eater and the person who eats either excessively or not sufficiently when under stress are examples. Some people react to stress by over-eating, which may result in obesity. Others react by undereating, which may result in anorexia nervosa.

9. *Food is used to reward, punish, and otherwise influence the behavior of others.* The mother who hands a child a cookie to keep the child quiet or who takes away dessert because of undesirable behavior or who promises a candy bar if the child will help her in some way is using food to reward, to punish, and to influence behavior. Candy and other sweets may be given to children on special occasions when they are "good" or withheld when they are "bad" (Pumpian-Mindlin 1954; Moore 1957). Teenagers often use food as a self-reward for having come through a difficult and stressful situation (Axler and Schwarz 1972).

10. *Food is used as a status symbol.* (See Bleibtreu 1973.) Joining a gourmet dining club or going out to eat in an exclusive restaurant are ways of using food as a status symbol. One's choice of foods can be a way of enhancing one's self-image or of impressing others (Gifft, Washbon, and Harrison 1972). Cussler (1943) and de Give (1943) found that certain foods were highly esteemed by subjects in rural southeastern Georgia. In Steelman's 1974 study of black homemakers and white homemakers from northern and southern Louisiana, foods considered by southern Louisiana homemakers to have high status, such as steak and roast beef, were similar to foods listed as expensive by respondents from northern Louisiana. Homemakers in northern Louisiana were more concerned with status differences than were the homemakers in southern Louisiana. Whites in southern Louisiana frequently rated crayfish as a high-status food. Blacks, especially those in southern Louisiana, frequently rated rice as a high-status food, probably because it was often served with meat. Kolasa and Bass (1974) found that prestige levels of foods appeared to exist in Hancock County, Tennessee. Gifft, Washbon, and Harrison (1972) suggested that the recent American interest in foreign cookery might indicate that "novelty" can increase the prestige of foods. It was noted by Bleibtreu (1973) that food often indicated a person's social class position.

11. *Food is used to bolster self-esteem or to gain recognition.* Comparing the cakes or the baked dishes at a potluck supper or preparing "your" dish for a company meal are examples. Some people refuse to share recipes for this reason.

12. *Food is used by governments or groups of people as a political and/or economic weapon.* The trade embargo against Cuba in the late 1960s is an example. The embargo, in turn, affected the availability of sugar in the United States, with the result that the price of sugar went up and people began searching for less expensive sweeteners in order to keep certain foods acceptable to United States citizens. The distribution of surplus nonfat dry milk in Central America is another example of this use of food.

13. *Food is used to prevent, diagnose, and treat physical illness.* The glucose tolerance test (in which the body is overloaded with the sugar glucose) is used to detect and diagnose diabetes, a metabolic disorder. Certain foods are added to or dropped from the diet to prevent diabetes in those with a tendency toward it. As a treatment for diabetes, the amounts of carbohydrates, fats, and proteins in the diet are carefully monitored.

14. *Food is used to prevent, treat, and diagnose psychological illnesses and mental retardation.* Classes in food preparation are used as therapy in many psychiatric treatment centers. Metabolic deficiencies that result in mental retardation can be treated by eliminating from the diet foods containing the substance that the body is not able to metabolize.

15. *Food is used as a focus for heightened emotional experiences.* We all know of festivals that feature food — maple syrup, cherries, strawberries, asparagus, and so forth. Human beings do not thrive when their emotional level stays the same day after day; excitement is a necessary part of well-being. Food plays a central role in most of our holidays. Such use of food is important to each person, both as an individual and as a member of a community.

In attempting to modify the eating patterns of an individual or a group, the community food and nutrition worker must take into account all of these functions of food. Several studies have noted food being used in the United States in some of the ways we have listed.

According to Eppright (1947), memory and association increased the appeal of holiday food and of the pies which mother made. In the study by Steelman (1974) mentioned earlier, tradition was important to respondents in all four subcultural groups in Louisiana. Foods which could be identified as ones their mothers and mothers-in-law had prepared were the most traditional items in their diets — foods that were often thought of nostalgically and that were entrenched in the subculture. To many adults in the South, the words *fried chicken* bring to mind Sunday dinner with relatives and friends or the preacher, whereas children in the South today may associate *fried chicken* with a family outing to Colonel Sanders' Kentucky Fried Chicken or with the idea that mother is too busy to cook dinner. Not only do the meanings attached to food items vary by subculture, but so does the time of day thought appropriate for eating certain foods. For example, in the United States it is common for people in rural areas to eat their main meal at midday, while in urban areas people usually have their main meal in the evening.

Taylor (1975) found that middle-class black women did not think of the foods often associated with blacks in the South as foods having prestige. Foods associated with the South in general were considered to have greater prestige. McConnell (1974) also found that the rural students she studied did not prefer or give positive meanings to the foods associated with the South. Yet, both groups listed those foods in dietary recalls of food eaten the previous day. In both instances, the foods in question offered sources of needed nutrients and contributed to a well-balanced diet.

Sometimes the meanings attached to foods are detrimental to the well-being of a group of people rather than beneficial. Cabbage, greens of many varieties, and sweet potatoes have been important in the diet of southerners. Because these vegetables are good sources of vitamins and minerals, their nutritive value should be emphasized and their continued use encouraged. Too often food and nutrition professionals emphasize adding new vegetables to the diet and do not stress the importance and value of the vegetables that are already being eaten. Broccoli, asparagus, cauliflower, and spinach are fine vegetables, but they are no better, and should be given no more prestige, than cabbage, turnip greens, collard greens, and poke salat (a wild green eaten in the South). Moreover, as noted by McConnell (1974), the self-esteem both of individuals and of groups is linked to food. Aid in producing and preserving greater quantities of foods that are already a part of the foodways of a group of people will result in making available safe, nutritious foods that are acceptable to the people.

REFERENCES

Axler, B. H., and Schwarz, A. 1972. Selling students. *School Foodservice Journal* 26 (3):45.

Bleibtreu, H. K. 1973. An anthropologist views the nutrition profession. *Journal of Nutrition Education* 5:11.

Cussler, M. T. 1943. Cultural sanctions and the food pattern in the rural Southeast. Ph.D. thesis, Radcliffe College (Cambridge, Mass.).

Cussler, M. T., and de Give, M. L. 1952. *Twixt the cup and the lip.* New York: Twayne.

de Give, M. L. 1943. Social interrelations and food habits in the rural Southeast. Ph.D. thesis, Radcliffe College (Cambridge, Mass.).

Eppright, E. 1947. Factors influencing food acceptance. *Journal of the American Dietetic Association* 23:579.

Gifft, H. H.; Washbon, M. B.; and Harrison, G. G. 1972. *Nutrition, behavior, and change.* Englewood Cliffs, N.J.: Prentice-Hall.

Jelliffe, D. 1967. Parallel food classifications in developing and industrialized countries. *American Journal of Clinical Nutrition* 20:279.

Kolasa, K., and Bass, M. A. 1974. Participant-observation in nutrition education program development. *Journal of Nutrition Education* 6:89.

Leininger, M. 1969. Some cross-cultural universal and nonuniversal functions, beliefs and practices of food. In *Dimensions of nutrition: Proceedings of the Colorado Dietetic Association Conference,* ed. J. Dupont. Boulder: Colorado Associated University Press.

Linton, R. 1936. *The study of man: An introduction.* New York: Appleton-Century-Crofts.

McConnell, S. 1974. Selected food preferences and some connotative meanings of foods by high school students in Hancock County, Tennessee. M.S. thesis, University of Tennessee (Knoxville).

Moore, H. B. 1957. The meaning of food. *American Journal of Clinical Nutrition* 5:77.

Pumpian-Mindlin, E. 1954. The meaning of food. *Journal of the American Dietetic Association* 30:576.

Schutz, J. G.; Rucker, M. H.; and Russell, G. F. 1975. Food and food use classification systems. *Journal of Food Technology* 29:50.

Steelman, V. P. 1974. *The cultural context of food: A study of food habits and their social significance in selected areas of Louisiana.* Bulletin 681. Baton Rouge: Louisiana State University Agricultural Experiment Station.

Taylor, V. 1975. Food preferences, food intake and food prestige of some selected black women in Knoxville, Tennessee. M.S. thesis, University of Tennessee (Knoxville).

Van Schaik, T. 1964. Food and nutrition relative to family life. *Journal of Home Economics* 56:225.

	CHAPTER
	3

The Individual and Food Behavior

People view the world around them in different ways. We might say that they have a variety of *concepts* about their environment. (A *concept* is an idea of something formed by mentally combining all of its characteristics or particulars.) Concepts are creations of language and culture, and different cultures have their own conceptual sets. For example, there is only one word for snow in the Sun Belt, whereas the Eskimo have several. It is important to the Eskimo to know whether snow is dry or wet, but to persons in the Sun Belt it is only important to know whether or not there is snow.

A person's behavior can be thought of in terms of three zones of relative intimacy. Every culture allows an individual certain ideas and activities that fall within the most *intimate* zone. Most of a person's food habits are in this zone. The second, less intimate, zone is called the *personal* zone and includes primary grocery shopping. The third zone is the *social* zone (some types of grocery shopping may be in this zone). Figure 4 illustrates the three zones. Activities involving the selection, procurement, distribution, storage, consumption, and manipulation of food and the disposal of waste fit into all three zones. Identifying which zone a proposed modification of activity would affect is important in dietary counseling.

FOOD HABITS

Food habits are acquired through the processes of acculturation and enculturation, or socialization (learning to do what is expected of one within one's own culture under particular circumstances). They are in the intimate zone. The use of the fork and knife in transferring food to the mouth is a habit, a repetitive action that is largely automatic or done without thinking. Some people habitually reach for the salt before tasting their food. They do this without knowing whether the food needs salt or not and with no thought as to how salty it may already be. A mother may eat food left on her children's plates without even realizing she is doing it, because she has been taught not to waste food.

Responses to physiological individuality can become habits. One such response is the eating of food at specific times to alleviate hunger and low blood sugar. Conversely,

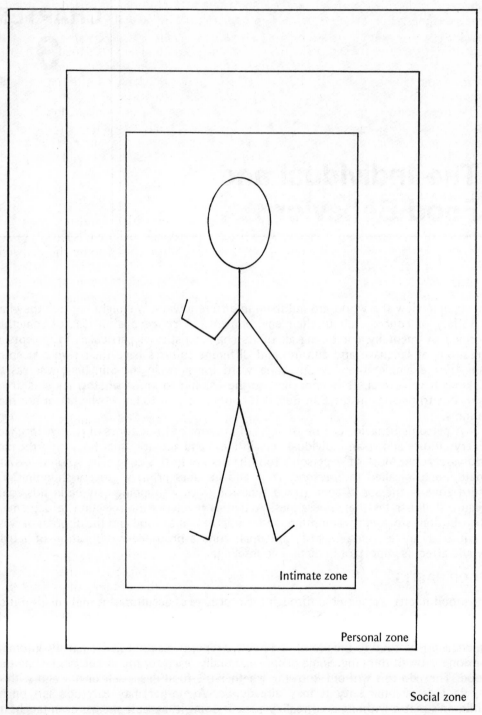

Intimate zone

Personal zone

Social zone

FIGURE 4. The three zones of behavior. Adapted from P. Hiebert, *Cultural anthropology* (Philadelphia: Lippincott, 1976).

long-term patterning of food intake may result in a physiological need for food at specific times. For example, coffee is addictive. Many people physiologically and psychologically require its stimulating effect to become alert. Persons eating at the same times every day for many years may become ill if they are prevented from eating at those times. Actions like these are very much a part of the individual, and modifying them means taking personality into account. Other aspects of food behavior are in the personal zone or the social zone and are less difficult to modify.

A food habit is food behavior, but not all food behavior is habit. For example, tasting food, deciding it needs a certain amount of salt to achieve the flavor one desires, and salting it accordingly is a behavior that is not a habit. *Food habits* are repetitive, characteristic acts, largely automatic, that an individual completes in order to satisfy a real or imagined need for food.

THE MEANINGS OF FOOD

People's beliefs and values concerning food and nutrition influence their food behavior in a given situation. Some Americans, for instance, believe it is harmful to eat fish with milk. Meanings are given to food by the culture and also by the individual because of past association with the food. One may have a negative or a positive attitude toward a food because of its association with a place, a person, or an event. A child entered in a blueberry-pie-eating contest who gets an upset stomach may never eat blueberries again.

According to Krech, Crutchfield, and Ballachey (1962), the connotative meaning of a word or concept includes all the ideas, attitudes, and feelings that a person associates with that word or concept. Fewster, Bostian, and Powers (1973) devised a method for measuring the connotative or implied meanings of foods. Their method included an instrument adapted from a behavioral science research technique, the semantic differential.

A study by McConnell (1974) measured some connotative meanings of food for sixty-one male and ninety-seven female high school students in Hancock County, Tennessee. The method used was of the type developed by Fewster, Bostian, and Powers (1973). It was found that spinach and most meats were associated with masculine images, while salads and nonmeat entrees were associated with feminine images. Foods associated with the words *teenager* and *young* were the preferred foods of the high school students, while less-preferred foods were associated with *baby*, *adult*, and *old*. Applesauce, pudding, and carrot strips were foods associated more with a sick person than with a well person. Taylor (1975) found that black women ranked high on their preference lists foods that had connotations of prestige for them.

Few studies have measured the connotative meanings of foods, but there have been numerous observations that foods do have implied meanings. Findings of psychological research indicate that every food is invested with meaning and that these meanings are a part of our cultural heritage (Moore 1957; Babcock 1961). Gifft, Washbon, and Harrison (1972) suggested that meanings attributed to food are learned and that they result from sociocultural, psychological, sensory, and intellectual experiences. According to Stare and Trulson (1966), feelings and attitudes about food are deeply rooted in a person's nature and culture.

At an early date, Mead (1943) recognized the need to study the meanings that different cultures attach to food. The two sociologists Cussler (1943) and de Give (1943) were among the first to investigate why people in the rural Southeast (Georgia, South Carolina, and North Carolina) choose the foods they eat. Cussler emphasized the cultural sanctions of the food pattern and de Give studied the social interrelations and food habits. Lewin (1943) studied groups in Iowa to find some answers to the question Why do people eat what they eat? Dickins (1945) and Dickins and Fergusen (1958), in their studies in Mississippi, have looked for the reasons underlying food use and consumption. When reviewing research projects having to do with consumer attitudes and beliefs about a particular food product, Bayton (1967) found that little effort had been made to investigate the relationship between attitudes and beliefs and consumption of the product. On the assumption that connotative meanings are associated with specific foods, Steelman (1974) questioned four subcultural groups in two Louisiana communities (black homemakers and white homemakers in northern and southern Louisiana communities) to determine what foods were associated with concepts related to tradition, convenience, frugality, health, social status, and sociability.

According to Eppright (1947), "Food with man is not just food; it is the crossroads of emotion, tradition and habit." Food feeds the ego, not merely the body (Cussler and de Give 1952; Pumpian-Mindlin 1954; Babcock 1961; Lowenberg et al. 1974). The symbolic meanings of food are often more important to people than the rational meanings (Pumpian-Mindlin 1954; Moore 1957; Gifft, Washbon, and Harrison 1972).

Since from the day of birth eating requires the cooperation of the child and another person, it becomes an interpersonal experience charged with emotional complexities (Bruch 1963; Menzies 1970). Invariably, a mother will convey to her child her own deep-seated attitudes toward food and its symbolic meaning for her (Babcock 1961; Bruch 1963). Milk, every person's first food, usually becomes psychologically connected with comfort and security, especially if early experiences with the mother or other person who fed the infant were satisfactory (Pumpian-Mindlin 1954). The early studies by Cussler and de Give (1943, 1952) indicated that people have strong emotional attitudes toward milk. De Give (1943) suggested that in many cases, in the Georgia community she studied, weaning would cut the child off entirely from milk, not just from the mother's milk. Moore (1957) suggested that the central role of the mother is teaching what foods, when, how much, why, and with what feelings one must eat.

Age and maturity are implied by certain foods. In America we associate olives with sophisticated or adult taste and peanut butter with childhood, especially the active and impulsive aspects of childhood (Moore 1957). Today the hamburger has an almost universal appeal for teenagers (Axler and Schwartz 1972).

Food also has sexual connotations. According to Bleibtreu (1973), there are masculine and feminine foods. For many individuals meat symbolizes masculinity (Moore 1957; Schafer and Yetley 1975). The housewife is so concerned with pleasing her husband that she makes meat the center of the meal. Even though vegetables are usually considered feminine food, the potato is an exception. It is thought of as hearty and suitable for the masculine taste. In contrast, a nonmeat salad is considered the epitome of femininity (Moore 1957). Perhaps this has changed in some areas as men have become more conscious of physical fitness. At a midwestern university cafeteria one man in three had salad for the entree at lunch.

Foods take on different meanings for a person during times of stress. Frustration or loneliness may be used as an excuse to indulge in a favorite high-calorie dessert, while anxiety may cause one to desire a food one has not eaten for a while but which is reminiscent of a time when life was more orderly. During examination week students usually eat more or less than usual, especially between meals. These snacks are often the high-calorie foods not included in their eating pattern. Boredom may send someone who is not even hungry to look for a particular food—or maybe just any food. Teenagers may show their resentment of advice by refusing to eat foods they accepted earlier and that they really like (Gifft, Washbon, and Harrison 1972). Illness may cause a person to desire some food that connotes security or love, or one that has not been thought about for a long time (Pumpian-Mindlin 1954). According to Babcock (1961) the ill individual, the emotionally immature adult, and the person tightly bound to culture through religious allegiances have an intense need to hold to earlier learned attitudes and facts about food. Gifft, Washbon, and Harrison (1972) stated that "the sum of the meanings attributed to any food by an individual at a given time will determine the food's relative acceptability to him."

SENSORY REACTIONS TO FOOD

Sensory reactions play a major role in food acceptance and preference (Todhunter 1973). Snyder (1931) studied taste deficiency in 440 subjects from 100 families. The bitter taste of *para*-ethoxy-phenylthiourea could not be detected by 31.5 percent of the subjects. When the parents could not distinguish this bitter taste, it was found that none of their children could distinguish it. This taste deficiency was not attributed to age, sex, or race, but to the inheritance of a single pair of recessive genes.

Sex and age alterations in taste preferences were studied by Laird and Breen (1939). These investigators used pineapple juice with five degrees of sweetness to study the preferences of males and females in the age groups of 12 to 18, 20 to 40, and 50 to 68 years old. They found that the preference curves for 12- to 18-year-olds paralleled the curves of the 20- to 40-year-olds, while the 50- to 68-year-old group preferred juice with a more tart, fruity taste. In all three age groups the women tended to prefer the tart taste and the men the sweet taste. It would be interesting to repeat this study today.

In a study by Korslund and Eppright (1967), children highly sensitive to one taste were also highly sensitive to three other primary taste sensations. Also, children with the lowest taste sensitivity tended to accept more foods and to approach eating with more enthusiasm than did those with the highest taste sensitivity. Jefferson and Erdman (1970) investigated the possible relationship of the food preferences and aversions of 13- and 14-year-olds to their taste sensitivity to sucrose, acetic acid, sodium chloride, quinine sulfate, and phenylthiocarbamide. There was no clear association between sensitivity to the five taste modalities and the number of food dislikes. There was, however, a significant correlation between a low threshold for phenylthiocarbamide and the percentage of foods disliked. Foods with a bitter quality, such as turnip greens and beets, were disliked significantly more often by subjects with a high sensitivity to the bitter taste of phenylthiocarbamide than by those with low sensitivity to it. Sex was not observed to affect food acceptance.

Schultz and Pilgrim (1953) reported an experiment with a large number of subjects in which the threshold for a sour taste was determined first in a relatively odor-free environment and then under the stimulation of a pleasant odor. Subjects with high thresholds in the odor-free environment had lower thresholds with odor stimulation, whereas subjects with low thresholds in the odor-free environment had higher thresholds with odor stimulation. It was suggested that this complex relationship might have gone undetected if it had not been for the large number of subjects.

An individual's perception of flavor depends upon past association with the food, upon the odor, texture or feel in the mouth, and taste (salty, bitter, sweet, sour) of the food, and upon perception of color and sound relative to flavor.

FOOD PREFERENCES

Food preferences are developed as a result of many factors in a person's environment. Pumpian-Mindlin (1954) described these factors as mainly cultural and familial. Strong likes and dislikes for certain foods have developed merely through association among members of a family and have little to do with the food itself. The many surveys done by Pilgrim and coworkers suggested that experiences in the early years of life, prior to age 16, are the major contributing factors in food preferences (Pilgrim 1961; Peryam 1963). According to Dickins (1965) the bases for food preferences are complex. She focused on the relationships of cultural, social, personal, and situational factors to food preferences and how these factors themselves are interrelated. Stare and McWilliams (1973) listed factors affecting a person's food preferences as (1) foods available in the locale, (2) foods preferred by other family members, especially by the parents, (3) foods purchased and prepared that reflect parental and cultural attitudes as well as family income, (4) foods permitted by religious or cultural dictate, and (5) foods whose taste, texture, or color appeal particularly to the individual. Brown (1967) suggested that food preferences would vary with experiences, much as attitudes vary and change.

The words *acceptance* and *preference* have been used interchangeably by many writers, but a distinction should be made. In studies of food likes and dislikes, it has been found that there is a difference between preference and acceptance. Before a food preference can evolve, an individual must find the food acceptable. *Acceptance* is the willingness to eat a food, while *preference* refers to an expressed choice (Hirsch 1974). Lantis (1962) mentioned that many Americans will accept foods that they may not prefer. Usually this would be because the food is convenient, inexpensive, and meets minimum standards of cleanliness and palatability. Eppright (1947) discussed food acceptance as a complex reaction influenced by several factors: (1) biochemical, such as hunger and appetite, (2) physiological, such as taste thresholds, ease with which sense organs are fatigued, and taste bud changes due to age, (3) psychological, such as memory and association, monotony, food aversions, and mental stability, (4) social, such as race, geographical conditions, economic conditions, technological advancements, and speed of transportation and communication, and (5) educational, such as group eating experiences.

Pilgrim (1961) described the components operative in food acceptance. Perception, the main component, was divided into the elements of physiology, sensation, and attitudes. Physiology referred to internal changes. Sensation was the influence of food (stimulus) on the organism (receptor). Attitudes meant attitudes toward food that were derived from aspects of the external situation, such as environment and learning. Both food and nonfood factors affecting perception could have been acquired recently or established for a long time. Even though each of the three elements was shown as contributing its own part to the perception and final acceptance of the food, there was much mutual interaction among them. Niehoff (1969) said that unfamiliarity was one of the most frequent problems affecting acceptance of new foods. Gifft, Washbon, and Harrison (1972) stated that acceptability would determine which of the available foods would be used by an individual and that acceptability was influenced by a network of elements. Kennedy (1952) suggested that acceptance or nonacceptance of a food was affected by an individual's food habits, which are determined by a variety of factors. He identified age and sex as two factors that had not been specified as important by other workers.

One early attempt to describe the vegetable preferences of junior high school children was a study by Dickins (1944) of 241 white and 392 black subjects in Mississippi. They were asked to choose three foods in each of six groups which contained mainly vegetables, breads, and milk. Butter beans were the most popular vegetable for both white and black children. String beans and field peas were next in popularity for the white children, collards and turnip greens for the black children.

Garton and Bass (1974) studied the food preferences and nutrition knowledge of ninety-eight deaf students and ninety-three hearing students, ages 12 to 20, in Tennessee. Foods preferred by the deaf students were similar to those chosen every time or often by 75 percent or more of the hearing students. Potatoes, green beans, peas, and corn were the vegetables given the highest preference ratings, while other green, red, and yellow vegetables received low preference ratings.

McConnell (1974) investigated the food preferences of high school students in Hancock County, Tennessee, and also studied the connotative meanings the students attached to certain foods. Rolls, french fried potatoes, chicken, soda pop, apples, oranges, mashed potatoes, strawberries, biscuits, milk, bananas, and pork chops were chosen every time or often by at least 75 percent of the students. Game meats and leafy green vegetables had the lowest preference ratings. She suggested that some foods associated with the South, such as turnip greens, black-eyed peas, okra, hominy, and butter beans, were low on the preference list. Einstein and Hornstein (1970) found that grits, black-eyed peas, lima beans, and iced tea were among the foods preferred by college students in the South.

Kolasa (1974), when studying the foodways of mothers and their adult daughters in eastern Tennessee, found that milk, fruits, greens, soup beans, and soda pop were liked by 75 percent of the women. The food preferences of mothers and their adult daughters were similar. The foods most disliked by the mothers were pizza, groundhog, and possum, while sardines, groundhog, souse meat, liver mush, beef liver, brussels sprouts, spinach, and parsnips were disliked by over 50 percent of their adult daughters.

Lackey (1974) instructed three groups of interested participants in food-purchasing practices. One group was from a rural area and two groups, one of which was a low-income group, came from urban areas. By the completion of the program, the participants had adopted some of the new food-purchasing practices but indicated that the food preferences of their families would determine their final food selections.

Pilgrim (1961), a long-time investigator with the Quartermaster Food and Container Institute for the Armed Forces, has conducted numerous surveys of men in the United States armed forces to determine if food preferences could be used to predict food consumption. Einhoven and Pilgrim (1960) found a significant correlation between food preferences and food consumption when foods were rated on a nine-point hedonic scale. Milk, grilled steak, ice cream, french fried potatoes, hot biscuits, and hot rolls were some of the best-liked foods. Mashed turnips, broccoli, asparagus, iced coffee, and cauliflower were some of the least-liked foods. The food preferences and the food preference frequencies of 573 servicemen from Fort Lewis, Washington, were reported by Meiselman (1972). The twenty-five foods most highly rated on the preference scale were the traditionally popular ones reported in earlier surveys of servicemen. It was found that the correlation between hedonic preference and desired frequency of serving was not a perfect one. Certain rich or "heavy" foods (e.g., grilled steak, fried chicken, and french fried potatoes) were highly preferred but infrequently selected, while other food items which were moderately preferred were frequently selected. Thirteen of the least frequently selected foods were also the least-preferred foods. Many vegetables, soups, combination and bean salads, stuffings, and certain "ethnic" foods were desired no more than three times per month.

The food acceptance of 100 young soldiers under an *ad libitum* regimen was studied by Vawter and Konishi (1958) for a period of 28 days. The subjects demonstrated a high preference for meat dishes, milk, hamburger and frankfurter buns, orange cake, and french fried potatoes. The least-acceptable foods were vegetables and cereals. According to Pilgrim (1961), there is evidence that the food preferences of people in the army correspond generally with those of the entire American population.

Kennedy (1952) investigated the food preferences of 144 pre-army-age California bosy for 258 food items. The 17- to 19-year-old subjects rated each item as "very good," "good," "moderate," "tolerated," "disliked," or "not tried." Foods receiving the highest ratings, in order of preference, were bananas, ice cream, strawberries, pies, peaches, beefsteak, turkey, pineapple, milk products, butter, and sweet corn. Some of the foods disliked by 20 percent or more of the subjects, in order of dislike, were buttermilk, kidney, turnip roots, eggplant, turnip greens, parsnips, brussels sprouts, and liver. Several green leafy vegetables headed the list for foods "not tried."

In cooperation with the Quartermaster Food and Container Institute, Eppright (1950) compared the food preferences of two groups of Iowa people, 17- to 18-year-olds and 46- to 50-year-olds. Milk was preferred and used more frequently by the younger group, and eggs were more highly favored by the older group. The older people had a higher preference for nearly all the vegetables, while the younger people had a higher preference for fruits. Cereals and desserts were highly preferred by the younger group, while puddings were the only dessert preferred by the older people. Women preferred vegetables and fruits and used them much more frequently than men, yet mild-flavored vegetables were more preferred by both groups than were strong-flavored ones. Food dislikes were more numerous among older men and younger women.

Lindgren (1962), also, was interested in age as a variable in aversions to food. Lindgren's food questionnaire included the twenty-eight foods used by Wallen (1948) in his studies of food aversions and an additional eleven foods, selected because of their relatively rare appearance in the middle-class American diet. The questionnaire was administered to 392 college students, who were to indicate foods that they disliked so much that they would not eat them. Scores were computed by counting the number of aversions, and it was found that the college students under 21 years of age tended to indicate dislike for more foods than did the students over 21. A similar trend was found by Smith, Powell, and Ross (1955) when studying the food aversions of college students at Bucknell University and of high school students in central Pennsylvania. Lindgren (1962) suggested that the inclination to make negative choices was characteristic of individuals in their late teens and that this tendency would lessen for adults in their twenties and older.

Leverton and Coggs (1951) surveyed the likes and dislikes of 1,882 boys and girls living on farms and in town in Nebraska. The young teenagers responded to forty-five different foods with "willing to eat often," "willing to eat once a week," "unwilling to eat," or "have never tasted to my knowledge." Except for commonly known fruits and vegetables, the foods were selected because of their low cost and good nutritional value or because they were associated with definite prejudices. White potatoes, apples, oranges, and whole wheat bread were the most popular foods. White potatoes, whole milk, and eggs were chosen more often by boys, while apples, oranges, raw tomatoes, lettuce, and green peas were chosen more often by girls. The foods that many of the children marked "unwilling to eat" were buttermilk, green peppers, greens, brains, parsnips, and turnips. A large number of children indicated they had never tasted rutabagas, brains, soybeans, dried peas, or oleomargarine. There were a few noticeable differences between the responses of children living on farms and those living in towns.

Schorr, Sanjur, and Erickson (1972) reported the food preferences of 118 students in grades seven through twelve in a small village in western New York. The foods liked most by at least 30 percent of the students were soda pop, milk, steak, hamburgers, pizza, chicken, french fries, ice cream, and spaghetti. Liver was liked least by over 40 percent of the students. Other foods that were disliked by more than 10 percent of the students were fish, squash, clams, coffee, spinach, cabbage, and beets. Ten percent or more of the students indicated they had never tasted nine of the foods, but all nine are considered to be delicacy items not common in the American diet.

Some studies have attempted to determine the factors influencing food acceptance and food preference.

Litman, Cooney, and Stief (1964) studied 558 girls and 481 boys in Minnesota public schools, between 10 and 22 years of age, to determine the factors that might be associated with their attitudes toward food. There was a high preference for milk, potatoes, bread, meat, butter, and eggs as foods for an ideal meal. Liver and several green and yellow vegetables were considered the least-desirable foods. The children commented that they would receive praise for eating vegetables and dairy products but would be scolded for eating candy, pastry, and too much ice cream and for drinking carbonated beverages and "adult" beverages like alcoholic drinks and coffee.

When interviewing 9- to 17-year-olds and their parents in Philadelphia, Peoria, and Atlanta, Walker, Hill, and Millman (1973) found that children seemed to prefer fruits over vegetables, the texture of raw fruits and vegetables over that of cooked ones, and sweet-tasting over tart or bland vegetables. The children's rejection of certain fruits and vegetables appeared to be based on prejudice relating to (1) early negative conditioning, (2) rejection of "baby foods," or (3) faulty generalization from an unfavorable attribute such as texture, odor, color, shape, or accidental associations.

Brown (1967), using a different approach, asked 101 nutrition students at the University of Illinois to describe their food preferences and to trace the history of those preferences. The foods listed under "like" were apples, beef, carrots, chocolate, french toast, hamburgers, ice cream, lobster, noodles, olives, potato chips, sour cream, and steak. Some of the foods that were liked by some students and disliked by others were broccoli, cauliflower, cottage cheese, eggs, hot dogs, spinach, squash, and tomatoes. The study revealed certain influences affecting the students' likes and dislikes: (1) the variety of foods served in the home, (2) the likes and dislikes of family members, (3) the appearance of foods, and (4) parental policies concerning foods.

Some years ago Hall and Hall (1939) studied foods that were disliked or unfamiliar to college students in the western part of the United States. Some of the ten foods disliked the most were buttermilk, glandular meats, several alcoholic beverages, oleomargarine, and parsnips. Women had more food aversions than did men, but women were also familiar with a wider assortment of foods than men were. Wallen (1943) studied the relationship of sex to food aversions in 545 college students in several sections of the United States and found that women were more likely than men to have food aversions. This could be because women are more sensitive to intense stimulation or because they may be subjected to fewer social pressures. Men are more reluctant to admit their food prejudices because of social pressures, and they eat disliked foods more than women do. Smith, Powell, and Ross (1955) found that female subjects in both senior high school and college had significantly higher anxiety scores and significantly more food aversions than male students had. The three most-disliked foods were brains, buttermilk, and kidneys. Students with high anxiety had more food aversions than students with low anxiety.

Einstein and Hornstein (1970) studied the food preferences of approximately 50,000 college students in the United States. Ice cream, soft rolls, beefsteak, hot biscuits, milk, and orange juice were liked by 92 percent or more of the students. The other most-preferred foods were certain meats, desserts, french fried potatoes, and tossed salad. On the list of extremely disliked foods were liver and a large number of vegetables. Some of the foods rated as "do not know" are known only in certain areas of the country (e.g., grits and kale) and some names (e.g., chicken cacciatore and veal scallopini) may not have been associated with the food. Regional differences were more pronounced in the South.

The food preferences and eating habits of 170 Texas Technological College women 17 to 25 years of age were studied by Lamb, Adams, and Godfrey (1954). Fried steak was the only food marked "well liked and enjoyed" by 100 percent of the dormitory residents. Whole milk, apples, oranges, and cookies shared the second position of preference for 97 percent of the residents. The foods "well liked and enjoyed" by 97 percent of the students not living in residence halls were roast beef, lettuce salad, cookies, and cherry pie. The strong-flavored vegetable group was disliked by a large number of the dormitory residents. Foods disliked by at least 30 percent of all the students were a variety of vegetables, soft-cooked eggs, buttermilk, and canned figs.

Young and La Fortune (1957) investigated the food preferences of 81 Cornell University freshmen women. The students responded to the 185 food items with "will not choose but will eat when served," "will eat frequently," "will eat occasionally," "will not eat," and "other—explain." Pot roast, hamburgers, beef stew, lamb, veal, chicken, oranges, peaches, pears, pineapple, apples, bananas, potatoes, corn, peas, lettuce, raw carrots, and ice cream were liked by all students. Foods receiving the most "will not choose but will eat when served" responses were liver, cottage cheese, oatmeal, spinach, and cabbage. The food dislikes did not seem to influence the adequacy of the diet. Buttermilk, oysters, heart, olives, and mushrooms received the most "will not eat" responses.

Schuck (1961) studied the food preferences of forty-two men and seventy-nine women (mainly freshmen) at South Dakota State College. Choices for responding to the list of sixty-one foods were "willing to eat often," "willing to eat once a week," "unwilling to eat," and "have never tasted." It was found that 90 percent or more of the students were "willing to eat often" milk, butter, strawberries, apples, peaches, pears, grapes, corn, beef, and fowl. There were nineteen vegetables considered to be acceptable as often as once a week by 10 to 30 percent of the students. Parsnips, turnips, green peppers, buttermilk, and spinach were the foods least acceptable to 30 percent or more of the students. It was found that women were willing to eat fruits more often than men but men were willing to eat more vegetables and meat frequently.

The acceptability of 126 menu items by University of Nebraska students was studied by Knickrehm, Cotner, and Kendrick (1969). Of the 1,479 students who returned usable responses, 932 were women and 547 were men. Fifty percent of the students said they would select some form of potatoes, fruits and vegetables, salad, and dessert at least twice a week. At least 25 percent of the students would not eat many of the vegetables, variety meats, meat-extended items, veal, and lamb.

Food preferences, then, are the result of the complex interaction of many factors, including past experiences, sensory response, attitudes, beliefs, values, and meanings associated with food. Figure 5 illustrates these interactions.

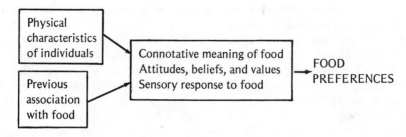

FIGURE 5. Interaction of factors that influence food preferences.

FOOD INTAKE PATTERNS

Preference for a food does not necessarily mean that the food will be eaten. Food intake patterns (a combination of food intake activities forming a consistent or characteristic arrangement) are formed by one's interaction with the environment throughout one's lifetime. Preference for a food is one of the factors involved in choosing food. Needham (1974) presented 3 days' worth of menus to high school students and asked them to select from the five meals available for each day the one they would choose if the meals were served. When the meals were served 2 weeks later, only 64 percent of the students chose the meals they had picked from the menus. Factors other than preference affected their actual selection.

Cultural heritage, food preferences, and the availability of the food are fundamental in establishing and molding the food patterns of individuals. When attempting to answer the question of what sociocultural factors affect food consumption, de Garine (1972) divided sociocultural factors into material influences and intangible influences. Various investigators have attempted to delineate some of the material and intangible influences on people's food intake patterns.

Dickins and Gillaspie (1953) analyzed the menu patterns of black and white families in the tenure groups of owners, renters, and sharecroppers in the Delta cotton areas of Arkansas and Mississippi. They found many combinations of menu items within the same meal, but when classifying these into several broad subgroups they found some typical patterns. For the morning meal, the typical pattern for the families of white owners and renters was meat, eggs, biscuits, coffee, and three extra items (such as butter, syrup, and jelly or preserves). For the families of black renters and sharecroppers, the typical morning pattern was meat, biscuits, coffee, and one or two extra items (such as syrup or boiled rice). There was no typical morning pattern for the white sharecroppers. The most common noon meal pattern for blacks in all three tenure groups and for white sharecroppers was vegetable and no meat, with two or three added items. For white owners and renters the noon meal of vegetable with meat, with five extra items, was the most usual. For the evening meal pattern, the vegetable and no meat, was typical for all race-tenure groups except the white owners, where the highest percentage contained meat and vegetable. For the black renters and share- croppers, the meat and no vegetable meal was about as common as the vegetable and no meat pattern. Corn bread and biscuits were the only menu items served at both noon and evening meals by the majority of the families in all groups. Between-meal snacks and packed lunches usually included foods from the bread, sweets, and fruit groups. Jerome (1967, 1969) found that when black families moved north they retained as many of their old food practices as possible until they became acculturated or the foods became unavailable.

The Household Food Consumption surveys of 1955-56 and 1965-66 gave extensive quantitative data about the food consumption of households (U.S. Department of Agriculture 1956, 1968). Data in these surveys are in terms of quantities of foods reported by families as used within a week. No information was obtained on how food was distributed among family members; therefore, some members of the family might not have had diets that met allowances even though the household diet met the 1963 Recommended Dietary Allowances for seven nutrients (U.S. Department of Agriculture 1970).

When the data for 1955 and 1965 were compared, it was found that little if any improvement had occurred in the 10-year period. In 1965, 48 percent of the households in the South had diets that met the Recommended Dietary Allowances as compared with 55 percent in 1955. The proportion with poor diets (24 percent) remained the same over the 10-year period (Adelson 1968). The nutrients most often below allowances were calcium, vitamin A, and ascorbic acid. These nutrient shortages were associated with the use of less than the recommended amounts of milk and milk products, vegetables, and fruits (U.S. Department of Agriculture 1970).

Clark (1970) discussed the many changes that have caused this deterioration in food consumption patterns in the South. Many of these changes seem to be virtually irreversible—the migration from farm to city, the decline in home production of food, the increase in the use of convenience and snack foods, the increase in meals eaten away from home and in irregular meals at home. The greater popularity of snack foods and beverages has been attributed in part to the increased proportion of children and youth in the population. In the South, it was found that children and youth used much less milk and fewer milk products, juices, and punches than the same groups in the North. The consumption of soft drinks was especially high in the South.

Van de Mark and Underwood (1971) studied the food consumption patterns of 100 teenage families (families in which both husband and wife were under 20). The results indicated that the race, annual income, and age of the homemaker had little effect on the diet of these young families. In all cases the dietary intakes of the husband and wife were low for milk, vegetables, and fruits. In the white families each member of the family consumed more milk than the corresponding member of the black families. Children of both white and black families received more-than-adequate quantities of milk but less-than-adequate amounts of meat, vegetables, and fruits.

Schuck and Tartt (1973) studied the food consumption patterns of low-income rural black households. They found that meats and grains were the principal sources of calories, with the contribution from meats sometimes exceeding that from grains, especially at the higher income levels. Seiders (1972) studied the adequacy of the diets provided by homemakers participating in the Expanded Food and Nutrition Education Program in selected counties in Tennessee and found that families who had vegetable gardens tended to have more adequate diets than families who did not have gardens.

Edwards et al. (1964) studied food consumed, meals missed, and snacks eaten as reported for a 24-hour period by 6,200 teenagers in North Carolina. Only 16 percent of the subjects ate a serving of green or yellow vegetables and only 35 percent had a serving of food rich in ascorbic acid. Although a majority of the students ate breakfast, 15 percent missed at least one meal during the 24-hour survey period. The teenagers in the seventh and ninth grades tended to select milk and nutritious snacks much more often than did those in the tenth and twelfth grades.

The traditional eating pattern of three meals a day seems to be disappearing rapidly (Bauman 1971; Fine 1971; Lachance 1973). For instance, Bauman reported that 30 to 50 percent of families in the United States have one or more members who periodically skip breakfast. About 75 percent of families do not eat breakfast as a family unit. As a result of this pattern, at least 50 percent of school-age children have either no breakfast or a nutritionally inadequate breakfast. Fine described eating today as a nonstop activity with a pattern of many minimeals. Ullensvang (1969) noted that our culture underwent rapid changes in the last decade and that all had a significant impact on food consumption patterns. Considerable evidence indicated that breakfast was still an important meal and that the big change had been in the pattern of eating and the foods consumed. Over 25 percent of all households in the United States were not serving a noon meal, and even the number of evening meals in the home was declining.

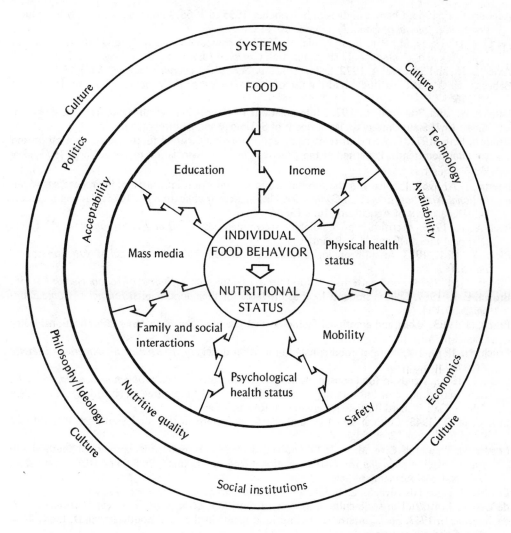

FIGURE 6. Interactions of personal characteristics and cultural subsystems that influence food behavior.

With the increase in mobility and the development of new food technology, regional differences in food consumption patterns will gradually disappear. New food products and new methods of food manipulation are appearing every day. Food products that have existed exclusively as elements of ethnic customs are either disappearing or being assimilated into our general culture. Because the population of the United States is diverse and mobile, people of different ethnic backgrounds, from different parts of the country, are continually intermingling and influencing each other's foodways. Figure 6 schematically depicts the interactions of some personal characteristics and cultural subsystems which affect an individual's food behavior. The holistic approach to food behavior takes into account these diverse phenomena.

REFERENCES

Adelson, S. F. 1968. Changes in diets of households, 1955 to 1965: Implications for nutrition education today. *Journal of Home Economics* 60:448.

Au Coin, D.; Haley, M.; Rae, J.; and Cole, M. 1972. A comparative study of food habits: Influences of age, sex and selected family characteristics. *Canadian Journal of Public Health* 63:143.

Axler, B. H., and Schwarz, A. 1972. Selling students. *School Foodservice Journal* 26 (3):45.

Babcock, C. G. 1961. Attitudes and the use of food. *Journal of the American Dietetic Association* 38:546.

Bauder, W., and Bruchinal, L. 1972. Interpolations of the original North-Hyatt scales. Lithograph. Ames: Iowa State University, Department of Sociology and Anthropology.

Bauman, H. E. 1971. Problems of researching and marketing fortified foods and its implication and consumption trends. Presented at the American Medical Association meeting, March 1971, New Orleans.

Bayton, J. A. 1967. Problems in the communication of nutrition information. In *Proceedings of the National Nutrition Education Conference.* Miscellaneous publication no. 1075. Washington, D.C.: U.S. Department of Agriculture, June 1968.

Beal, V. A. 1968. A critical view of dietary study methods. *Food and Nutrition News* 40 (3):1. (National Livestock and Meat Board)

Bleibtreu, H. K. 1973. An anthropologist views the nutrition profession. *Journal of Nutrition Education* 5:11.

Bowden, J. J. 1973. Food patterns and food needs of adolescents. *Journal of School Health* 43:165.

Brown, E. L. 1967. College students look at the basis for their food habits. *Journal of Home Economics* 59:784.

Bruch, H. 1963. Social and emotional factors in diet changes. *Nutrition News* 26:4. (National Dairy Council)

Bruch, H. 1970. The allure of food cults and nutrition quackery. *Journal of the American Dietetic Association* 57:316.

Clark, F. 1970. Trends in food consumption in the South. In *The food problem in Georgia,* ed. G. G. Dull. Report no. 2 of the Interdepartmental Institutional Committee on Nutrition, USDA-ARS. Athens, Ga.: Richard B. Russell Agricultural Research Center.

Cussler, M. T. 1943. Cultural sanctions and the food pattern in the rural Southeast. Ph.D. thesis, Radcliffe College (Cambridge, Mass.).

Cussler, M. T., and de Give, M. L. 1943. Outline of studies on food habits in the rural Southeast. In *The problem of changing food habits.* National Research Council, Bulletin no. 108. Washington, D.C.: National Academy of Sciences.

Cussler, M. T., and de Give, M. L. 1952. *Twixt the cup and the lip.* New York: Twayne.

de Garine, I. 1972. The socio-cultural aspects of nutrition. *Ecology of Food and Nutrition* 1:143.

de Give, M. L. 1943. Social interrelations and food habits in the rural Southeast. Ph.D. thesis, Radcliffe College (Cambridge, Mass.).

Dickins, D. 1944. Vegetable preferences of children show need for planning, even with abundance. *Mississippi Farm Research* 7 (9):7.

Dickins, D. 1945. Changing pattern of food preparation of small town families in Mississippi. Bulletin 415. State College: Mississippi State College Agricultural Experiment Station.

Dickins, D. 1965. Factors related to food preferences. *Journal of Home Economics* 57:427.

Dickins, D., and Fergusen, V. 1958. Knowledge of nutrition as related to the use of dairy products. *Journal of Home Economics* 50:25.

Dickins, D., and Gillaspie, B. V. 1953. Menu patterns in the delta cotton area. *Journal of Home Economics* 45:169.

Edwards, C. H.; Hogan, G.; Spahr, S.; and the Guilford County Nutrition Committee. 1964. Nutrition survey of 6200 teen-age youth. *Journal of the American Dietetic Association* 45:543.

Einhoven, J., and Pilgrim, J. F. 1960. *Food preferences of men in the U.S. armed forces.* Chicago: Quartermaster Food and Container Institute for the Armed Forces.

Einstein, M. A., and Hornstein, I. 1970. Food preferences of college students and nutritional implications. *Journal of Food Science* 35:429.

Eppright, E. S. 1947. Factors influencing food acceptance. *Journal of the American Dietetic Association* 23:579.

Eppright, E. S. 1950. Food habits and preferences: A study of Iowa people of two age groups. Research Bulletin 376. Ames: Iowa State College Agricultural Experiment Station.

Fewster, W. F.; Bostian, L. R.; and Powers, R. D. 1973. Measuring the connotative meanings of foods. *Home Economics Research Journal* 2:44.

Fine, P. A. 1971. Modern eating patterns—The structure of reality. Presented at the American Medical Association symposium (Eating patterns and their influence on purchasing behavior and nutrition), November 1971.

Garton, N. B., and Bass, M. A. 1974. Food preferences and nutrition knowledge of deaf children. *Journal of Nutrition Education* 6:60.

Gifft, H. H.; Washbon, M. B.; and Harrison, G. G. 1972. *Nutrition, behavior, and change.* Englewood Cliffs, N.J.: Prentice-Hall.

Gladney, V. M. 1972. *Food practices of some black Americans in Los Angeles County.* Los Angeles: County Department of Health Services, Community Health Services.

Hall, I. S., and Hall, C. S. 1939. A study of disliked and unfamiliar foods. *Journal of the American Dietetic Association* 15:540.

Hiebert, P. 1976. *Cultural anthropology.* Philadelphia: Lippincott.

Hirsch, N. L. 1974. Getting fullest value from sensory testing: Part 1. Use and misuse of testing methods. *Food Product Development* 8 (10):33.

Jefferson, S. C., and Erdman, A. M. 1970. Taste sensitivity and food aversions of teenagers. *Journal of Home Economics* 62:605.

Jerome, N. W. 1967. Food habits and acculturation: Dietary practices and nutrition of families headed by southern-born Negroes residing in the northern metropolis. Ph.D. thesis, University of Wisconsin (Madison).

Jerome, N. W. 1969. Northern urbanization of food consumption patterns of southern-born Negroes. *American Journal of Clinical Nutrition* 22:1667.

Kennedy, B. M. 1952. Food preferences of pre-army-age California boys. *Food Technology* 6:93.

Knickrehm, M. E.; Cotner, C. G.; and Kendrick, J. G. 1969. Acceptance of menu items by college students. *Journal of the American Dietetic Association* 55:117.

Kolasa, K. M. 1974. Foodways of selected mothers and their adult daughters in upper east Tennessee. Ph.D. thesis, University of Tennessee (Knoxville).

Korslund, M. K., and Eppright, E. S. 1967. Taste sensitivity and eating behavior of preschool children. *Journal of Home Economics* 59:169.

Krech, D.; Crutchfield, R.; and Ballachey, E. 1962. *Individual in society,* pp. 279-291. New York: McGraw-Hill.

Lachance, P. A. 1973. The vanishing American meal. *Food Product Development* 7 (9):36.

Lackey, C. J. 1974. Family food purchasing: A consumer education program. Ph.D. thesis, University of Tennessee (Knoxville).

Laird, D. A., and Breen, W. J. 1939. Sex and age alterations in taste preferences. *Journal of the American Dietetic Association* 15:549.

Lamb, M. W.; Adams, V. J.; and Godfrey, J. 1954. Food preferences of college women. *Journal of the American Dietetic Association* 30:1120.

Lantis, M. 1962. The child consumer. *Journal of Home Economics* 54:370.

Leverton, R. M., and Coggs, M. C. 1951. Food choices of Nebraska children. *Journal of Home Economics* 43:176.

Lewin, K. 1943. Forces behind food habits and methods of change. In *The problem of changing food habits.* National Research Council, Bulletin no. 108. Washington, D.C.: National Academy of Sciences.

Lindgren, H. C. 1962. Age as a variable in aversion toward food and occupations. *Journal of Consulting Psychology* 26:101.

Litman, T. J.; Cooney, J. P.; and Stief, R. 1964. The views of Minnesota school children on foods. *Journal of the American Dietetic Association* 45:433.

Lowenberg, M. E.; Todhunter, E. N.; Wilson, E. D.; Savage, J. R.; and Lubawski, J. L. 1974. *Food and man.* 2nd ed. New York: Wiley.

McConnell, S. 1974. Selected food preferences and some connotative meanings of foods by high school students in Hancock County, Tennessee. M.S. thesis, University of Tennessee (Knoxville).

Mead, M. 1943. The factor of food habits. *Annals of the American Academy of Political and Social Sciences* 225:136.

Meiselman, H. L. 1972. *Modern military man's food preference.* Natick, Mass.: Pioneering Research Laboratory, U.S. Army Natick Laboratories. Reprinted from *Activities Report,* vol. 24, no. 1, 1972.

Menzies, I. E. P. 1970. Psychosocial aspects of eating. *Journal of Psychosomatic Research* 14:223.

Miller, D. C. 1964. *Handbook of research design and social measurement.* New York: McKay.

Moore, H. B. 1957. The meaning of food. *American Journal of Clinical Nutrition* 5:77.

Needham, R. 1974. Food preference influences on meal selections of high school students at Central High School, Knoxville, Tennessee. M.S. thesis, University of Tennessee (Knoxville).

Niehoff, A. H. 1969. Changing food habits. *Journal of Nutrition Education* 1:10.

Peryam, D. R. 1963. The acceptance of novel foods. *Food Technology* 17 (6):33.

Phillips, D. E. 1975. Presweetened cereal patterns of older sib families and no older sib families: Child's preference, mother's perception of child's preference, and family purchase. Ph.D. thesis, University of Tennessee (Knoxville).

Pilgrim, F. J. 1961. What foods do people accept or reject? *Journal of the American Dietetic Association* 38:439.

Pumpian-Mindlin, E. 1954. The meanings of food. *Journal of the American Dietetic Association* 30:576.

Schafer, R., and Yetley, E. A. 1975. Social psychology of food faddism. *Journal of the American Dietetic Association* 66:129.

Schorr, B. C.; Sanjur, D.; and Erickson, E. C. 1972. Teenage food habits. *Journal of the American Dietetic Association* 61:415.

Schuck, C. 1961. Food preferences of South Dakota college students. *Journal of the American Dietetic Association* 39:595.

Schuck, C., and Tartt, J. B. 1973. Food consumption of low-income rural Negro households in Mississippi. *Journal of the American Dietetic Association* 62:151.

Schultz, H. G., and Pilgrim, F. J. 1953. Psychophysiology in food acceptance research. *Journal of the American Dietetic Association* 29:1126.

Seiders, R. 1972. Dietary adequacy of homemakers participating in Extension's Expanded Food and Nutrition Education Program in selected Tennessee counties. M.S. thesis, University of Tennessee (Knoxville).

Smith, W. I.; Powell, E. K.; and Ross, S. 1955. Food aversion: Some additional personality correlations. *Journal of Consulting Psychology* 19:145.

Snyder, L. H. 1931. Inherited taste deficiency. *Science* 74:151.

Stare, F. J., and McWilliams, N. 1973. *Living nutrition.* New York: Wiley.

Stare, F. J., and Trulson, M. F. 1966. The implantation of preference. In *Food and civilization,* ed. S. M. Farber, N. L. Wilson, and R. H. L. Wilson. Springfield, Ill.: Charles C. Thomas.

Steelman, V. P. 1974. *The cultural context of food: A study of food habits and their social significance in selected areas of Louisiana.* Bulletin 681. Baton Rouge: Louisiana State University Agricultural Experiment Station.

Taylor, V. 1975. Food preferences, food intake and food prestige of some selected black women in Knoxville, Tennessee. M.S. thesis, University of Tennessee (Knoxville).

Todhunter, E. N. 1973. Food habits, food faddism and nutrition. *World Review of Nutrition and Dietetics* 16:286.

Ullensvang, L. P. 1969. Food consumption patterns in the seventies. *Vital Speeches of the Day* 36:240.

U.S. Department of Agriculture. 1956. *Food consumption of households in the South.* Household Food Consumption Survey, 1955. Washington, D.C.: Agricultural Research Service and Agricultural Marketing Service.

U.S. Department of Agriculture. 1968. *Food consumption of households in the United States, spring 1965.* Household Food Consumption Survey, 1965-66. Washington, D.C.: Agricultural Research Service, Consumer and Food Economics Research Division.

U.S. Department of Agriculture. 1970. *Dietary levels of households in the South, spring 1965.* Household Food Consumption Survey, 1965-66. Washington, D.C.: Agricultural Research Service, Consumer and Food Economics Research Division.

Van de Mark, M. S., and Underwood, V. R. S. 1971. Dietary habits and food consumption patterns of teenage families. *Journal of Home Economics* 63:540.

Vawter, H. J., and Konishi, F. 1958. Food acceptance by soldiers under an ad libitum regimen. *Journal of the American Dietetic Association* 34:35.

Walker, M. A.; Hill, M. M.; and Millman, F. D. 1973. Fruit and vegetable acceptance by students. *Journal of the American Dietetic Association* 62:268.

Wallen, R. 1943. Sex differences in food aversions. *Journal of Applied Psychology* 27:288.

Wallen, R. 1948. Food aversions in behavior disorders. *Journal of Consulting Psychology* 12:310.

Young, C. N., and La Fortune, T. D. 1957. Effect of food preferences on nutrient intake. *Journal of the American Dietetic Association* 33:98.

CHAPTER 4

Food Behavior throughout Life — Pregnancy and Infancy

PREGNANCY

Growth of the Fetus

Pregnancy is neither an abnormality nor a natural state that will take care of itself as far as food and nutrition are concerned. The pregnant woman has increased nutritional needs and is responsible for providing the nutrients for the developing fetus. The nutritional state of the mother during pregnancy influences the health of the unborn child. Regions of the world with marked malnutrition have high rates of infants with low birth weight (Gordon 1975; Rush 1975; Leichtig et al. 1975).

In recent years, the prenatal growth of the child in relation to its environment has received much attention. Growth taking place at the cellular level may be classified into three types: (1) *accretionary,* an increase in intercellular substance, (2) *multiplicative,* an increase in the number of cells, and (3) *dimensional,* an increase in the size of the cells. These three types of growth go on more or less simultaneously. The rate of growth during the prenatal period is tremendous, though it slows down as term is approached. During the entire period of gestation, the environment of the fetus is that provided by the mother (Krogman 1972). Growth of the fetus is determined by its genetic code and the environment provided by the mother. This environment may be modified by physiological stress (other than pregnancy) and by psychological and sociological stress.

Stress

The diabetic mother-to-be, the grossly obese mother-to-be, and the pregnant woman with other physical problems will need to have that stress minimized as much as possible to avoid influencing both the prenatal and postnatal growth of the infant. Medication involved in the treatment of physical and psychological stresses on the mother can influence the growth of the fetus. Environmental pollution, such as fumes of paint, can be detrimental to the unborn child. The provision of needed nutrients during the first 3 months of prenatal life, when cell differentiation and growth are taking place at the most rapid rate, is a problem for many women because they may not yet know that they are pregnant.

44

Weight Gain

Weight gain during pregnancy has been a source of controversy among health care personnel (Pomerance 1972). Because of the tendency to place a high value on being thin, it also is of much concern to the pregnant woman. Most of the mother's weight gain during pregnancy can be attributed to increases in maternal and fetal tissues. Maternal tissue gains approximate 5 to 7 kilograms by the end of the third trimester (Lambert 1970). Maternal gains result from:

1. An increase in uterine tissue of approximately 1.0 kilogram.
2. An increase in breast tissue of approximately 1.5 kilograms.
3. An increase in circulating blood volume of approximately 1.5 kilograms.
4. An increase in maternal extracellular fluid of approximately 1.5 kilograms (Pitkin et al. 1972).
5. Storage of fat tissue in the mother of approximately 3.5 kilograms.

The rate of storage of fat is highest during the second trimester and is thought by some to be a cushion against possible malnutrition in the third trimester (Pitkin 1972; Thomson and Hytten 1973). Generally, this fat is lost between pregnancies.

Fetal tissues account for approximately 5 kilograms of weight increase. These tissues include the placenta (0.6 kilogram), the amniotic fluid (1.0 kilogram), and the fetus itself (3.4 kilograms).

The additional caloric needs of the pregnant woman were estimated by Thomson and Hytten (1973) as being 200 kilocalories per day for the entire period, or 350 kilocalories for the last two-thirds of the pregnancy.

Felig (1973) pointed out that low caloric intakes, that is, those designed for the patient to lose weight, are likely to be detrimental to the fetus. During 4-day fasts, blood glucose levels in pregnant women showed a greater drop than those of non-pregnant women. Since the fetus uses glucose, plasma alanine shifts to the fetus for conversion of exogenous substrate to glucose. Fetal tissues show increased ketones (forty times normal levels) during maternal fasts. Therefore, the evidence suggests that the pregnant woman should receive the caloric intake needed to maintain her weight during pregnancy with an expected increase of approximately 10.9 kilograms.

Thomson and Hytten (1973) believe that, with the exception of iron and folic acid, a pregnant woman can get all the nutrients she requires if her caloric needs are met with a well-balanced diet.

Klerman and Jekel (1973) stated that a greater-than-average gain in weight during pregnancy has not been shown definitely to have a negative influence on the health of the mother or the child. It may be associated with poor obstetric outcome, however, if it is due to the accumulation of fluids caused by toxemia or to poor nutrition (e.g., a high-starch, low-protein diet). Conversely, very small gains in weight were associated with poor obstetric outcome and might indicate poor nutrition, which would have a negative effect on pregnancy.

Nausea

Nausea occurs in approximately half of all pregnancies and usually lasts 6 to 8 weeks. The consumption of food in general or of foods containing specific nutrients may be affected during this time. The lowest energy intake is usually in the second month, when nausea is most frequent; however, since the greatest need for more calories is in the last two-thirds of pregnancy, there would be no problem if a well-balanced diet containing the necessary amounts of all nutrients were ingested. (The National Research Council's report on maternal nutrition [1970] stated that a majority of women reported a marked increase in appetite during the first trimester, which is not necessarily inconsistent with the common symptom of nausea in early pregnancy — many women feel ravenous once the wave of early-morning nausea has passed.) But hormonal and metabolically induced nausea can be so severe that the mother's food intake is drastically affected — to the point where the fetus may be harmed. Pregnancy does increase the nutrient needs of the mother, and care should be taken to see that those needs are met.

Psychological Aspects

Roberts (1977) has discussed the psychological tasks of the pregnant woman. The first task is fusion with her fetus, that is, accepting the pregnancy and relating to the embryo as a part of herself. The bond of mother-child relationship begins here. If the pregnancy is rejected, the woman may become depressed and fail to eat. Nausea at this time may further complicate matters.

The second psychological task is to relate to the fetus as a separate entity while maintaining the bond of fusion. Quickening or movement of the fetus is usually noted in the second trimester, and the greatest gain in weight usually occurs during this time. As the fetus develops into the third trimester, physical discomforts cause the mother to expend less energy and may also cause her to eat less.

The third psychological task, according to Roberts (1977), is for the woman to assume the mothering role, modeling herself on others. Rubin (1967) said that at the beginning she imitates without evaluating but, as she begins to evaluate, makes comparisons before adopting behavior as her own. It is at this period that she may be more amenable to changing her own food behavior and that of her infant, based on her knowledge of food and nutrition.

The psychological stability of the pregnant woman and also her personality type will be of vital importance in how she relates to food during her pregnancy.

Sociocultural Factors

Sociocultural influences on food behavior during pregnancy include religious observances. Matter and Wakefield (1971) found that while Hindus did not eat meat in any form and had lower intakes of protein, calcium, fat, and calories than Christians and Muslims in India, their hemoglobin levels were not significantly different. Other cultures encourage the pregnant woman to eat more meat and milk. Beliefs that the mother's eating certain food will harm the baby in some way abound in many cultures. For example, there are people in West Virginia who believe that eating tomatoes will cause the child to be deformed or that eating fish will give the child fish-shaped birthmarks (Shifflett 1976). Food and nutrition professionals need to know about such beliefs if they are to help pregnant women obtain the nutrients they need.

The Practice of Pica

The eating of substances not usually considered to be food is practiced by some women while they are pregnant (Anonymous 1960; Cooper 1957). Much of the literature on the subject has associated pica with low-income blacks in the South. However, in a study by Lackey, Bass, and Kolasa (1973) in east Tennessee, many of the white women of lower socioeconomic status practiced pica. Nationwide studies of the incidence of this practice among pregnant women of higher socioeconomic groups have not been conducted.

Pica has been mentioned in the literature since the sixteenth century (Cooper 1957). Whether it is a deviation from the more culturally acceptable practice among middle- and upper-class pregnant women of craving a specific food has not been investigated. Pliny, in the first century, remarked, *"Praecipiunt in malacia praegnantum,"* meaning roughly, "We knew she was pregnant since she was nauseated and begging for pickles" (Hochstein 1968).

Reasons given by women for eating clay and cornstarch are relief of nausea, relief of nervousness, tradition, fear that the baby will be marked otherwise, pleasure, "liked the crunchiness," "stimulated the appetite," "helped the baby to slide out easier," "made the baby a lighter color," "quieted hunger pains," "just craved it," desire for approval of peers, and "just wanted it so bad I couldn't stand it," (Cooper 1957; Edwards et al. 1964; Lackey, Bass, and Kolasa 1973).

Hochstein (1968) listed six hypotheses to account for the practice of pica by pregnant women.

1. *Psychological hypothesis.* (The pregnant woman uses pica to obtain attention. Kolasa observed pica being practiced openly by some women in Detroit; however, Lackey, Bass, and Kolasa (1973) found women in Tennessee who practiced pica in secret and did not want their husbands to know about it.)
2. *Anthropological hypothesis.* (Since the women were responsible for the gardening in most primitive societies, pica was the result of behavior taught by mothers to their daughters. If this is true, then all cultures would have this in their background, and people of greater sophistication would simply substitute other items, such as pickles, for clay and dirt.)
3. *Sensory hypothesis.* The eating of clay or dirt is done to decrease movements in the uterus, decrease intestinal mobility and thus stop nausea, get rid of worms, and decrease hunger. (Also, the women may like the flavor.)
4. *Microbiological hypothesis.* The acidity of the intestinal tract is influenced, providing for the growth of normal organisms and preventing the growth of pathogenic organisms.
5. *Physiological hypothesis.* The clay or cornstarch helps to correct disorders of the gastrointestinal tract and reduces the amount of saliva in the mouth. (Many women tend to salivate more during the first 2 months of pregnancy. For some this becomes a real problem and they have trouble with drooling or "spitting" when they are talking.)
6. *Nutritional need hypothesis.* Pica is practiced in order to provide some nutrient thought to be missing from the diet. (This has probably been the most popularly believed theory.)

The evidence to support any of these theories is lacking. Some research shows that certain types of clay impair iron absorption while other types do not (Talkington et al. 1970). Roselle (1970) and Edwards et al. (1964) found anemia to be associated with the practice of pica. O'Rourke et al. (1967) found no significant differences in hemoglobin levels, but they did find a statistically significant association of pica and the development of toxemia. Edwards et al. (1964), however, found no significant differences in the incidence of toxemia among women who practiced pica and those who did not. They did find that babies born to women engaging in pica had lower ratings of general condition at birth than babies whose mothers did not practice pica.

Socioeconomic Factors

Socioeconomic factors influencing the availability of food have been noted by Ellis (1973). In many slums, rural areas, and Indian reservations there are no large supermarkets. Prices are higher for the smaller variety of foods available. While it is debatable that knowledge of food and nutrition influences food behavior, access to such knowledge has been less for the poor. Inadequate income also decreases the ability to buy whatever food is available.

The size of her family influences the amount of work a pregnant woman must do and the emotional strain that she is under and may even limit the food available to her. A pregnant woman with two pre-school-age children would be likely to have a different food intake pattern than a primipara, whether she was of a low-income or a middle-income level.

The presence of extended-family members in the home, neighborhood, or city would mean that traditional food customs, beliefs, and attitudes toward pregnancy would have a greater hold on the pregnant woman. The educational level of the family, the ages of the various family members, and whether or not the woman is working outside the home are other factors that will affect her food behavior.

Affect on Women with Careers

Pregnant career women have role conflicts between the traditional expectations of how pregnant women should behave and their career demands. The expectations of family and friends also contribute to the pressures upon them. Many companies allow for maternity leave. Some force maternity leave without pay from the sixth month of pregnancy until 6 weeks after the infant is born, but others have liberal paid maternity leaves.

The pregnant career woman must make sure her diet provides the necessary nutrients, and she must plan her work in order to avoid becoming overtired. (The pregnant woman with several small children and a home to take care of has many of the same problems without some of the benefits many career women receive. In fact, the demands made on her by home and children may be even greater than those of a job outside the home would be.)

Affect on Teenagers

The physiological need for food is particularly acute for the pregnant teenager. Not only must she maintain her normal growth, she must also supply nutrients for the developing fetus. Her need for psychological ego bolstering also may be more acute during pregnancy, but her social situation may make it difficult for her to get positive support. The family ties are loosening as she begins to assert her independence. Indeed, even if she does eat at home, frequently the meals will be only hurried snacks on the way out the door. If she is married, of course, a large portion of her meals will be eaten in her own home or at least with her husband. Typically, she will prepare the meals herself, although she may know little about purchasing and preparing food or about nutritional needs. Yet, the young couple may be searching for information to aid them in providing an adequate environment for their baby.

The food behavior of young adolescents is sometimes considered bizarre. Kestenberg, Ehrenwalk, and Luce (1972) studied the eating practices of 996 pregnant girls, age 15 or younger, served by the Maternity and Infant Care Project in Chicago. Most of the girls were black. The diets of almost 45 percent were rated poor, 26 percent fair, and 30 percent good (based on the number of nutrients meeting the National Research Council's Recommended Dietary Allowances). One-fifth of the girls ate no more than two meals a day, with only 12 percent of these meal missers having a "good" diet. As expected, the intake of snack items and soft drinks was high, with a large proportion of the total calories being derived from these "junk" items. Forty percent of the diets were low in all food groups except the meat and bread groups; half or more were rated low in vegetables, milk, and milk products. They also found that the tendency to form poor food patterns was more pronounced among girls coming from poorer homes.

Frequently, pregnant adolescents are included in the widespread practice among physicians of placing prenatal patients on restricted diets to control weight gain. Several studies indicate the effect of this. A study in Iowa (Klerman and Jekel 1973) rated a majority of the pregnant girls' diets as poor in vitamin A and ascorbic acid and borderline in calories, protein, iron, and calcium. Caloric restriction significantly decreased the amounts of protein and iron, as well as the number of calories, which the girls consumed. Additional caloric restriction could have had pronounced ill effects.

Weight gain in pregnancy is conspicuously variable. Young women tend to gain slightly more weight than older women, primigravidas (women pregnant for the first time) slightly more than multigravidas (women who have been pregnant more than once), and thin women slightly more than fat women. In Western societies, housewives tend to be relatively sedentary. For them, the total "energy cost" of pregnancy for a healthy woman is approximately 40,000 kilocalories, representing an additional *daily* requirement of about 200 kilocalories. This is commensurate with a weight gain of 11.4 kilograms (25 pounds) for the 9-month period (National Research Council 1970).

Evidence indicates that the 11.4-kilogram weight gain "limit" set by many physicians may not be sufficient for the pregnant adolescent. Almost half of the subjects in the study groups of Klerman and Jekel (1973) gained more than that during pregnancy, based on the girls' own estimate of their weight before becoming pregnant. To adjust for normal adolescent growth during the 9 months of pregnancy, the following amounts were *subtracted* from the uncorrected weight gain to obtain a corrected weight gain due to the pregnancy: ages 11 to 13, 8 pounds; age 14, 7 pounds; ages 15 and 16, 5 pounds; and age 17, 3 pounds. After this correction, a smaller proportion of the girls in each age group gained more than 25 pounds. For example, in the youngest group, where the most active growth would normally have occurred, the number of girls gaining more than 25 pounds dropped from 46 to 32 percent. A few girls actually *lost* weight on that basis, and more than 10 percent of each group showed either a loss in weight or a gain of less than 9 pounds. Those who gained less weight seemed to be suffering from both physical and emotional malnutrition.

Others have suggested that, to allow for the mother's growth as well as that of the fetus, a weight gain of 13.6 to 15 kilograms (30 to 33 pounds) might not be too high for the pregnant adolescent (Seiler and Fox 1973).

Changes in Eating Practices

Changes in eating practices during pregnancy have been studied by Nobmann and Adams (1970). Of the 370 participants in their study, 217 ate more during pregnancy. Reasons given were appetite (54 percent), changes in living pattern (15.6 percent), pressure from family members (13.8 percent), physician's advice (8.3 percent), and health reasons (6.4 percent). Advice from professionals other than doctors accounted for the remaining less than 2 percent.

The 104 women who ate less while pregnant gave these reasons: reduced appetite (47 percent), nausea, vomiting, and gas (24 percent), changes in living pattern (21 percent), weight control (17 percent), mood and a liking for blander food (13 percent), physician's advice (9.6 percent), health (9.6 percent), pressure from family (2.8 percent), and cost of food (1.9 percent).

Appetite or lack of appetite was the major reason given for both increasing and decreasing the amount of food eaten. Changes in the living pattern played an important role in both cases, while the advice of the physician accounted for less than 10 percent of the changed eating habits in both cases. Family members were more apt to influence an increase than a decrease in the quantity of food eaten. It was interesting that the cost of food did not have much influence.

Influence of Sociological and Psychological Variables

In a study by Mason and Rivers (1970), the most significant variable in predicting ascorbic acid levels in the plasma of pregnant women was found to be the level of performance on the nutrition knowledge test. If a woman's score on the test was high, then it could be predicted that she would have a higher plasma ascorbic acid level. In this instance, knowledge does seem to influence food behavior. However, the subjects who scored higher on eight socioeconomic factors, four personality dimensions, three food and nutrition variables, and the initial hematocrit levels were apt to have the highest ascorbic acid plasma levels. Mason and Rivers were able to make the following predictions about subjects with high mean ascorbic acid levels during the latter half of pregnancy.

1. They were older.
2. They had high scores on fruit preferences and on the Gordon profile responsibility and ascendancy dimensions.
3. They had high scores on the nutrition knowledge test.
4. They had received dietary instruction.
5. They had incomes of more than $4,000.
6. They had low scores on the emotional dimensions of the Gordon profile and on the vegetable preferences survey.

The food behavior of the pregnant women with regard to foods high in vitamin C was influenced by nutritional knowledge and socioeconomic status. The first five points describe what could be expected of middle-class women. On most preference studies vegetables have ranked low. Luidahl (1976), in a similar study designed to identify variables that could be used to predict the intake of iron by pregnant women, found that only the high score on scoresheets showing the frequency of intake of an iron-rich food could be used.

Hansen, Brown, and Trontell (1976) found that pregnant adolescents who attended a special school were more likely to have infants whose weight at birth was normal than were girls who attended regular schools. The special school situation was relatively free of stress and the girls received considerable emotional support from the staff and from their peers and were motivated to eat properly.

In the 1950s, Jeans, Smith, and Stearns (1952) studied low-income pregnant women in Iowa and found bread and potatoes to be the common caloric mainstays in the women's diets. Many of the women reported eating six slices of bread and two servings of potatoes a day. Some of the women had received nutrition instruction but others had not. The food choices of the women who had been instructed in nutrition reflected their greater knowledge. Changes have taken place since this study two decades ago.

Darby et al. (1959), in an extensive study at Vanderbilt University, found that the kinds of foods eaten by pregnant women varied with the season of the year. The mean daily dietary intake of protein, calcium, phosphorous, iron, B vitamins, and calories was higher during the fall and winter.

The Women, Infants and Children Program of the federal government is making food available for low-income pregnant women and providing them with nutrition information. (See chapter 13.)

Additional research is needed to further examine environmental factors that influence the food behavior of pregnant women at all economic levels. The conceptual model in figure 7 shows some of the factors that have been noted in the literature.

INFANCY TO TWO YEARS OLD

Infants at birth have certain capacities that allow them to relate to food. Most newborn infants are able to suck and swallow and may respond to tastes and odors. Most of us have held a small baby in our arms and experienced its turning toward our chest with rooting motions. Dubignon and Campbell (1969) found that infants 48 to 90 hours old could distinguish milk from dextrose and that taste was the most likely basis for the discrimination. Another developmental component that influences an infant's food behavior is the ability of the tongue to move soft solids to the pharnyx for swallowing. When an infant pushes food forward with its tongue, it is sometimes interpreted to mean that the infant does not like the food; however, it may mean that the infant has not as yet developed the ability to move food to where it can be swallowed (Aldrich 1942; Gryboski 1965; Lewis and Couniham 1965).

The period of mouthing and licking objects is often referred to as "the stage when the baby puts everything in its mouth." Rhythmic biting movements and chewing are developmental and appear in different children at different ages. That these behaviors do not develop at precisely the same age in all children may be owing to differences in genotype, in environment, and in the developmental state at birth. The ranges in normal age for the occurrence of these behaviors are great.

Pediatricians' recommendations of the type and amount of solid food and the time at which it should be added to the infant's diet vary, depending on the child. The developmental stage of the child is an important consideration (Illingsworth and Lister 1964). Most of the digestive enzymes are present in both premature and mature infants. Lactase, the enzyme required for digesting lactose, the sugar in milk, is found in greater abundance in infants than in adults. However, the infant's level of development and its need for solid food are considered when deciding on the time to add solid food to the diet (Fomon 1974). Illingsworth and Lister pointed out that a baby should be given solid food as soon as it has learned to chew; otherwise, introducing solid foods later may be difficult. Deisher and Goers (1954), however, investigated the early and late introduction of solids into the diet of eighty-five infants and found that the time when solids were added to the diet did not seem to affect the child's acceptance of them.

The introduction of solids continues to be discussed today in reference to overfeeding the infant and to the quality of food being fed. Purvis (1973) noted that juice is usually offered at 1 month and cereals sometime during the first 3 months. By the seventh month, most infants are eating table foods.

Beal (1957, 1961), in a longitudinal study of infants in Colorado, found that the average child in the study did not willingly accept any solid food before 2½ months of age. Marked preferences for specific foods were observed. Fruits were especially liked by 70 percent of the infants throughout the first year. Bananas and applesauce were the favorites. Vegetables were less popular. Beets and spinach were disliked.

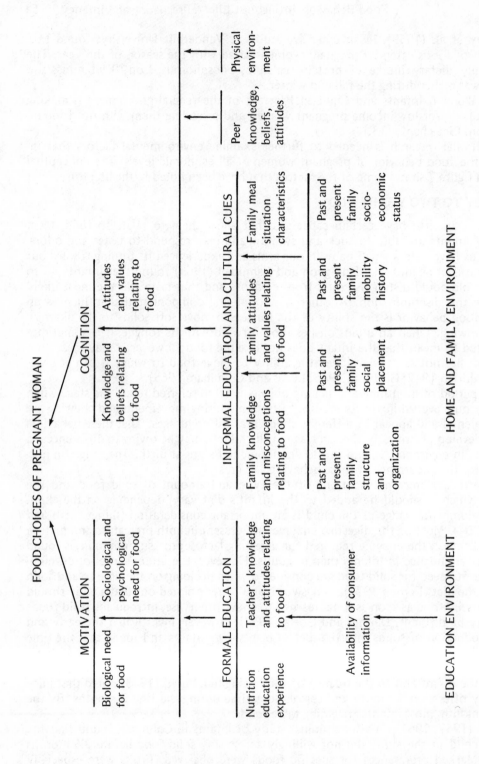

FIGURE 7. A conceptual model of the factors influencing the pregnant woman's choice of food.

Liver was disliked more than any other meat. Beal (1961) found that the intake of calories was higher for boys than girls after the second month but became markedly so only after 18 months of age. Boys consumed more milk than girls until the age of 18 months. After 1 year boys ate more meat, and between 1 and 3 years of age girls ate more eggs.

Breast-feeding or Bottle-feeding

The incidence of breast-feeding in the United States has been variously estimated as anywhere from 11 to 30 percent (Weichert 1975). Weichert believes that there will be fewer women breast-feeding babies in the future as the pool of possible role models diminishes even further. Jelliffe and Jelliffe (1971) have pointed out the uniqueness of human milk. The problems of bottle-feeding in less developed countries where women are following the role model in the United States are well known (Behar 1976). Breast-fed infants are less likely to develop respiratory and gastrointestinal infections and allergic reactions. Gerrard (1974) said that the best protection is achieved when the infant receives only breast milk for the first 6 months of life. He pointed out that this is particularly important in areas where contamination of cow's milk and other foods is likely and where medical facilities are inadequate.

Food and nutrition professionals have been appalled when they have encountered infants with gastrointestinal upsets probably due to poorly prepared formulas. However, since many drugs and other harmful substances may be passed through the mother's milk to the infant, a blanket policy of breast-feeding for everyone might be even more harmful to the infant. Each situation must be analyzed and all its elements considered, including the mother's health, the needs of the infant, and the environment.

Davis (1928) conducted a study to determine whether infants would, on their own, choose the foods that they needed to maintain good health. The infants chose from a wide variety of foods, both animal and vegetable in origin, that would adequately provide all the food elements known to be necessary for human nutrition. The foods were all simple "natural" ones. This study was the basis for much of the permissive or lax attitude shown during the past four decades toward the feeding of children. However, the provision of only simple "natural" foods was not taken into account. Davis (p. 679) found that the three infants studied for 6 months after weaning and one for 1 year after weaning were

> able from the first to select their own foods from a list of simple natural ones and in quantities to maintain themselves with apparently optimal digestive and good (as far as immediate results could be judged) nutritional results. They were omnivorous and in eating were governed not only by their caloric needs, but showed definite preferences, which, however, changed from time to time and were unpredictable.

Many have interpreted this to mean that one does not need to bother about a child's food behavior, that children will eat what they need when they need it. (See Murno 1966 for a discussion of the influence of Davis's research on children's feeding practices.)

Physical and Behavioral Changes

Infants increase tremendously in size, and behavior changes take place as more and more control is gained over activities. They become more independent and better able to initiate and sustain interaction with others (Smith and Bierman 1973). By the age of 2 years a child has grown from a weight of 2.7 to 3.8 kilograms (6 to 8.5 pounds) at birth to approximately 12.2 kilograms (27 pounds), and from a length of 48.5 to 53.3 centimeters (19 to 21 inches) to 81.2 to 88.9 centimeters (32 to 35 inches). Newborn infants usually have no teeth; by age 2 children are using sixteen to twenty deciduous teeth to eat. Children progress from being able to suck, breathe, and swallow in a coordinated way to being able to direct their vision, reach for objects, sit alone, crawl, walk, and talk. Since children are totally dependent on others during this time, how others react to them in feeding situations is very important. Krogman (1972) believes that the first postnatal year sets both the pace and the directions for the child's future growth and development. Table 1 lists nutrients needed for the first years of life.

TABLE 1. NUTRIENT NEEDS OF INFANTS

Age (years)	0.0-0.5	0.5-1.0	1-3
Weight (kg, lb)	6, 1	9, 20	13, 28
Height (cm, in)	60, 24	71, 28	86, 34
Energy (kcal)[a]	kg x 117	kg x 108	1,300
Protein (g)	kg x 2.2	kg x 2.0	23
Fat-soluble vitamins			
Vitamin A activity			
RE[b]	420[c]	400	400
I.U.	1,400	2,000	2,000
Vitamin D (I.U.)	400	400	400
Vitamin E activity[d] (I.U.)	4	5	7
Water-soluble vitamins			
Ascorbic acid (mg)	35	35	40
Folacin[e] (mcg)	50	50	100
Niacin[f] (mg)	5	8	9
Riboflavin (mg)	0.4	0.6	0.8
Thiamin (mg)	0.3	0.5	0.7
Vitamin B_6 (mg)	0.3	0.4	0.6
Vitamin B_{12} (mg)	0.3	0.3	1.0
Minerals			
Calcium (mg)	360	540	800
Phosphorus (mg)	240	400	800
Iodine (mcg)	35	45	60
Iron (mg)	10	15	15
Magnesium (mg)	60	70	150
Zinc (mg)	3	5	10

Source: Data from the National Research Council, *Recommended Dietary Allowances*, 8th ed. (Washington, D.C.: National Academy of Sciences, 1974).

[a]Kilojoules (kj) = 4.2 x kilocalories (kcal).

[b]Retinol equivalents.

[c]Assumed to be all as retinol in milk during the first 6 months of life.

[d]Total vitamin E activity estimated to be 80 percent as D-tocopherol and 20 percent other tocopherols.

[e]The folacin allowances refer to dietary sources as determined by *Lactobacillus casei* assay. Pure forms of folacin may be effective in doses less than one-fourth of the Recommended Dietary Allowance.

[f]Although allowances are expressed as niacin, it is recognized that, on the average, 1 mg of niacin is derived from each 60 mg of dietary tryptophan.

Food is the fuel for growth, and growth influences development. Both are involved in a person's food behavior throughout life. Figure 8 depicts the four postnatal growth curves as described by Scammon (Krogman 1972).

Neural growth includes the brain, the spinal cord, and the related bony parts of the skull. The complete optic system and the related bony parts of the skull, the upper face, and the vertebral column are included. Since 95 percent of neural growth is completed before a child enters elementary school at age 6 or 7, adequate nutrients in the diet are of utmost importance. *Genital* growth includes the primary sex apparatus and all secondary sex traits. Most growth in this area occurs between 10 and 18 years of age. The *lymphoid*, including the thymus, the lymph nodes, and the intestinal lymphotic masses, grows between the ages of 10 and 15 to twice what it will be at adulthood. The *general* growth curve includes the external dimensions of the body as a whole and the respiratory, vascular, digestive, and skeletal systems as well as the musculature, kidneys, and bladder. Growth is very rapid until about age 5, when it levels off until the age of 10 or 12 and then speeds up again (Krogman 1972).

As one looks at the nutrient needs and the food behavior of the individual, growth must be taken into account. As Krogman pointed out (1972, p. 8),

> there is a periodicity in growth which is a matter of relative speed (fast period, slow period) and area or region, leading to a differential growth (a time, for example, of height gain, or of weight gain; or of head-face growth and arm-leg growth). The basic idea is, simply, that the child does not grow "all of a piece," expanding as it were, radially from some central point.

The developmental and emotional changes taking place in a child are related to physical growth. Because food is a necessity of life, it is involved in each of these changes, and the child's food behavior is modified by each of these.

Cheek (1968) reminded us that the study of growth is the study of life itself, and Lafrancois (1973) remarked on the difficulty of trying to describe an infant as a more or less integrated whole whose intellect, emotions, and physical being interact. Krogman (1972) said that growth refers to proportionate changes in size, while development refers to increasing complexity and progress toward maturity. "Both processes are integrative, with growth perhaps somewhat more structural, development more functional, with the structure providing function" (p. 3). Table 2 shows some of the interactions of growth, development, and food behavior.

Approximately 30 percent of a person's life is spent in growth. In the biocultural growth complex there are four major aspects to be considered.

1. *Motor growth.* This includes both gross and fine motor coordination. Since food has to be obtained and put into the mouth and chewed, one can readily visualize how motor growth is related to eating.
2. *Growth of adaptative responses.* This requires directing the body's motor equipment toward the performance of a specific task and involves the neuromuscular coordination of the entire body. For example, one sees food, judges its distance, and picks it up.
3. *Language and physical forms of communication.* A child learns the name of a food and how to ask for it or reject it.
4. *Personal social development and adjustment.* The sum of a child's reactions to the environment is reflected in this aspect of biocultural growth. The child must learn how, when, and what foods are acceptable at what times in the environment.

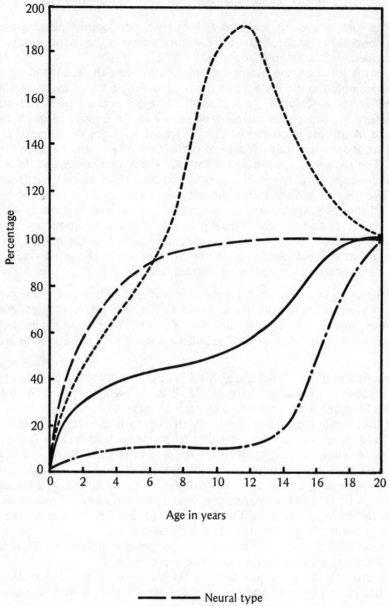

FIGURE 8. Scammon's postnatal growth curves. Adapted from W. M. Krogman, *Child growth*, Ann Arbor Science Library Series (Ann Arbor: University of Michigan Press, 1972).

TABLE 2. GROWTH, DEVELOPMENT, AND FOOD BEHAVIOR

Approximate Age	Source of Food	Oral Activities Related to Ingestion of Food	Neuromuscular Development	Variances
Conception to birth	Maternal blood stream			Nutritional status of the mother before conception; prenatal diet
Birth to 2 weeks	Colostrum or substitute	Sucking, swallowing, and rooting	Putting the hand or thumb in the mouth	
2 weeks to 3 weeks	Milk plus vitamins	Sucking, swallowing, and rooting	Putting the hand or thumb in the mouth	Breast- or bottle-feeding, thumbsucking, or pacifier; solid foods added for some infants
3 months to 5 to 8 months	Semisolid pureed food	Transfering of food voluntarily from front to back of mouth; biting	Helping to hold the bottle	Holding the baby while feeding it; letting the baby hold the bottle and feed itself in bed; variety of solid food; commercial or home-prepared baby foods
5 to 8 months to 2 years	Well-chopped food	Distinctive biting and ability to swallow small things	Ability to sit, reach for food, and convey it to the mouth; ability to drink from a cup and to use a spoon.	Weaning from the breast or bottle to a cup; some babies may have bottle or breast only at night until 3 years of age
2 years	Solids, non-simplified food	Chewing with the molars	Use of all utensils in eating	Appetite and growth slow

Source: Adapted from M. Breckinridge and M. Murphy, *Growth and development of the young child* (Philadelphia: W. B. Saunders, 1969).

The growth and developmental process begun in the infant continues throughout life, with physical growth being completed in the first 20 years. The foods available to a child and the interactions of the child with those who are responsible for feeding it are of utmost importance during these first 2 years of life. The problems and frustrations of feeding an infant are many. What to do when and how to do it are questions that must be answered for each infant (Anonymous 1973). The many cultural and ethnic beliefs about the feeding of infants must be known and taken into account by food and nutrition workers when feeding practices are discussed.

REFERENCES

Pregnancy

Anonymous. 1960. Clay- and cornstarch-eating women. *Nutrition Reviews* 18:35.

Anonymous. 1972. Longitudinal studies of diet in pregnancy. *Nutrition Reviews* 30:38.

Chang, B. 1974. Some dietary beliefs in Chinese folk culture. *Journal of the American Dietetic Association* 65:436.

Cooper, M. 1957. *Pica: A survey of the historical literature as well as reports from the fields of veterinary medicine and anthropology, the present study of pica in young children and a discussion of its pediatric and psychological implications.* Springfield, Ill.: Charles C. Thomas.

Darby, W. J.; McGainity, W. J.; Martin, M. P.; Birgforth, E.; Denson, P. M.; Kaser, M. M.; Ogle, P. J.; Newhill, J. A.; Stockholl, A.; Ferguson, M. E.; Touster, O.; McClellan, G. S.; Williams, C.; and Carmon, R. A. 1959. The Vanderbilt Cooperative Study of Maternal and Infant Nutrition: IV. Dietary, laboratory and physical findings in 2,219 delivered pregnancies. *Journal of Nutrition* 51:565.

Edwards, C. H.; McDonald, S.; Mitchell, J. R.; Jones, L.; Mason, L.; and Trigg, L. 1964. Effect of clay and cornstarch intake on women and their infants. *Journal of the American Dietetic Association* 44:109.

Ellis, E. O. 1973. Family: Nutrition and consumer problems. In *U.S. nutrition policies in the seventies,* ed. J. Mayer. San Francisco: W. H. Freeman.

Felig, P. 1973. Maternal and fetal fuel homeostasis in human pregnancy. *American Journal of Clinical Nutrition* 26:998.

Ferro-Luzzi, G. E. 1973. Food avoidances of pregnant women in Jamiland. *Ecology of Food and Nutrition* 2:259.

Gordon, J. E. 1975. Nutritional individuality. *American Journal of Diseases of Children* 129:422.

Hansen, M.; Brown, M. L.; and Trontell, M. 1976. Effects on pregnant adolescents of attending a special school: Nutritional status and outcome of pregnancy. *Journal of the American Dietetic Association* 68:538.

Hochstein, G. 1968. Pica: A study in medical and anthropological explanation. In *Essays on medical anthropology,* ed. T. Weaver, pp. 88-97. Southern Anthropological Society Proceedings, no. 1.

Jeans, P. C.; Smith, M. B.; and Stearns, G. 1952. Dietary habits of pregnant women of low-income in a rural state. *Journal of the American Dietetic Association* 28:27.

Kestenberg, J.; Ehrenwald, J.; and Luce, R. 1972. *The adolescent: Physical development, sexuality and pregnancy* New York: Mss Information Corporation.

King, C.; Cohenour, S. H.; Doris, M. S.; Calloway, D. H.; and Jacobson, N. 1972. Assessment of nutritional status of teenage pregnant girls: 1. Nutrient intake and pregnancy. *American Journal of Clinical Nutrition* 25:916.

Klerman, L. U., and Jekel, J. F. 1973. *School-age mothers: Problems, programs and policy.* Hamden, Conn.: Shoe String Press.

Krogman, W. M. 1972. *Child growth.* Ann Arbor Science Library Series. Ann Arbor: University of Michigan Press.

Lackey, C.; Bass, M. A.; and Kolasa, K. 1973. Study of pica among pregnant women in east Tennessee. Presented to the American Dietetic Association, Denver.

Lambert, R. A. 1970. Physiological changes during pregnancy. In *Maternity nursing today,* ed. J. Clavsen et al. New York: McGraw-Hill.

Leichtig, A.; Delgado, H.; Lasky, R. E.; Klein, R. E.; Engle, P. F.; Yorhorough, C.; and Habicht, J. 1975. Maternal nutrition and fetal growth in developing societies. *American Journal of Diseases of Children* 129:434.

Luidahl, W. A. 1976. Development of a mathematical model that will predict the mean daily dietary iron intake of pregnant women based upon sociological, psychological and physiological factors assessed to be related to the mean daily dietary iron intake. Ph. D. thesis, University of Tennessee (Knoxville).

Mason, M., and Rivers, J. 1970a. Factors influencing plasma ascorbic acid levels of pregnant women: I. Predicting second and third trimester levels. *Journal of the American Dietetic Association* 56:313.

Mason, M., and Rivers, J. 1970b. Factors influencing plasma ascorbic acid levels of pregnant women: II. Predicting changes in levels following dietary instruction. *Journal of the American Dietetic Association* 56:321.

Matter, S. L., and Wakefield, L. M. 1971. Religious influence on dietary intake and physical condition of indigent, pregnant Indian women. *American Journal of Clinical Nutrition* 24:1097.

Murphy, T. H., and Wertz, A. W. 1954. Diets of pregnant women: Influence of socioeconomic factors. *Journal of the American Dietetic Association* 30:34.

National Research Council. 1974. *Recommended Dietary Allowances.* 8th ed. Washington, D. C.: National Academy of Sciences.

National Research Council, Committee on Maternal Nutrition, Food and Nutrition Board. 1970. *Maternal Nutrition and the course of pregnancy.* Washington, D.C.: National Academy of Sciences.

Nobmann, D., and Adams, S. 1970. Survey of changes in food habits during pregnancy. *Public Health Reports* 85:1121.

O'Rourke, D. E.; Quinn, J. G.; Nicholson, J. O.; and Gibson, H. H. 1967. Geophagia during pregnancy. *Obstetrics and Gynecology* 29:581.

Pitkin, R. M.; Kaminetzky, H. A.; Newton, M.; and Pritchard, J. A. 1972. Maternal nutrition: A selective review of clinical topics. *Obstetrics and Gynecology* 40:773.

Pomerance, J. 1972. Weight gain in pregnancy: How much is enough? *Clinical Pediatrics* 11:554.

Roberts, F. B. 1977. *Prenatal nursing: The care of newborns and their families.* New York: McGraw-Hill.

Roselle, H. A. 1970. Association of laundry starch and clay ingestion with anemia in New York City. *Archives of Internal Medicine.* 125:57.

Rubin, R. 1967. Attainment of the maternal role: Part 1. Process. *Nursing Research* 16:237.

Rush, D. 1975. Maternal nutrition during pregnancy in industrialized societies. *American Journal of Diseases of Children* 129:430.

Schorr, A. L. 1973. Income maintenance. In *U.S. nutrition policies in the seventies,* ed. J. Mayer. San Francisco: W. H. Freeman.

Seiler, J. A., and Fox, H. M. 1973. Adolescent pregnancy: Association of dietary and obstetric factors. *Home Economics Research Journal* 1:188.

Shifflett, P. 1976. Folklore and food habits. *Journal of the American Dietetic Association* 68:347.

Talkington, K. M.; Gant, N. F.; Scott, E. D.; and Pritchard, J. A. 1970. Effect of ingestion of starch and some clays on iron absorption. *American Journal of Obstetrics and Gynecology* 105:262.

Thompson, M. F.; Morse, E.; and Morrow, S. 1974. Nutrient intake of pregnant women receiving vitamin and mineral supplements. *Journal of the American Dietetic Association* 64:382.

Thomson, A. M., and Hytten, F. E. 1973. Nutrition during pregnancy. *World Review of Nutrition and Dietetics* 16:22.

Thonangdul, I., and Anathayahul, K. 1975. Nutrition of pregnant women in a developing country — Thailand. *American Journal of Diseases of Children* 129:426.

Infancy to Two Years Old

Aldrich, C. A. 1942. Ancient processes in a scientific age. *American Journal of Diseases of Children* 64:714.

Anonymous. 1973. Dilemmas in infant feeding. *Lancet* 11:366.

Beal, V. A. 1957. On the acceptance of solid foods and other food patterns of infants and children. *Pediatrics* 20:448.

Beal, V. A. 1961. Dietary intake of individuals followed through infancy and childhood. *American Journal of Public Health* 51:1107.

Behar, M. 1976. A potent medicine. *Pan American Health* 7 (3-4):17.

Breckinridge, M., and Murphy, M. 1969. *Growth and development of the young child.* Philadelphia: W. B. Saunders.

Cheek, D. 1968. *Human growth.* Philadelphia: Lea and Febiger.

Davis, D. 1928. Self-selection of diets by newly weaned infants. *American Journal of Disturbed Children* 36:651.

Deisher, R. W., and Goers, S. S. 1954. A study of early and later introduction of solids into the infants diet. *Journal of Pediatrics* 45:191.

Dubignon, J., and Campbell, D. 1969. Discrimination between nutrients by the human neonate. *Psychonomic Science* 16:186.

Foman, S. 1974. *Infant nutrition.* Philadelphia: W. B. Saunders.

Gerrard, J. 1974. Breast-feeding: Second thoughts. *Pediatrics* 54:757.

Gryboski, J. D. 1965. The swallowing mechanism of the neonate. *Pediatrics* 35:445.

Illingsworth, R. S., and Lister, J. 1964. The critical or sensitive period with special reference to certain feeding problems in infants and children. *Journal of Pediatrics* 65:339.

Jelliffe, D., and Jelliffe, E. 1971. The uniqueness of human milk: An overview. *American Journal of Clinical Nutrition* 24:1015.

Krogman, W. 1972. *Child growth.* Ann Arbor Science Library Series. Ann Arbor: University of Michigan Press.

Lafrancois, G. R. 1973. *Of children: An introduction to child development.* Belmont, Calif.: Wadsworth.

Lewis, J. A., and Couniham, R. F. 1965. Tongue-thrust in infancy. *Journal of Speech and Hearing Disorders* 30:280.

Murno, J. 1966. A review of the 1928 research by Clara Davis. *Journal of Home Economics* 58:655.

Purvis, G. A. 1973. What nutrients do our infants really get? *Nutrition Today* 8 (5):28.

Smith, D., and Bierman, E. 1973. The biologic ages of man. Philadelphia: W. B. Saunders.

Weichert, C. 1975. Breast feeding: First thoughts. *Pediatrics* 56:987.

Food Behavior throughout Life — The Young Child

THE PRESCHOOL CHILD

Growth and Development

Various stimuli affect the growth and behavior of children between the ages of 3 and 6 years. Past experiences, physical needs, and environmental conditions combine during development to regulate patterns of individual behavior (Sherif and Sherif 1969). Piaget (1972) explained child development in terms of four factors — maturation, experience, social transmission, and equilibration. Development occurs in stages of physiological and psychological maturation, and as children mature, they become able to handle increasingly complex situations. Experience is a basic factor in the development of cognitive structures; from past experience, children begin to make associations with new experiences. Social transmission (enculturation) of such tools as language and education provides a structure that allows children to assimilate information. Equilibration is the process of self-regulation. Lowenberg (1965) believes that, throughout a child's development, food intake patterns can and do change as the child's psychological, mental, and physical development progresses.

Cognitive development influences the formation of food habits. Piaget (1972) described children of 4 to 7 or 8 years old as being in the period of intuitive thought. Mussen, Conger, and Kagan (1974) said that children's perceptions of what they hear, see, touch, smell, or feel may change as a function of their learning, labeling, and experience. Gibson and Gibson (1955) found that children were able to conceptualize more, verbalize their conceptions, and construct more complex representations, thoughts, and images as their cognitive development increased. Children become able to group objects together into classes according to their own perceptions of similarity. These advances may be related to improvements in language ability. Language development is important in verbal mediation, concept formulation, and problem solving. Thus, with increased abilities in understanding and communication, children possibly are better able to formulate and to express their food preferences.

Motor development plays an important role in the development of food patterns. According to Gessel et al. (1940), children of 4 to 5 years old are still developing fine motor skills. They are acquiring good eye-hand coordination and appropriate functioning of the fingers. Gutteridge (1939) stated that a child does not usually master these abilities until the age of 6 years. These studies are the basis for the feeding practices of the past three decades. Today writers like Spock and Lowenberg (1966) recommend giving finger foods to perschool children.

What children eat may influence their emotional responses to their social environment (Kerrey et al. 1968). Wakefield and Merrow (1967) studied 150 children from low-income families in Vermont, using nutritional status measurements, food recall records, personality tests, and interviews with each child's mother and teacher. The children in the average weight groups were better adjusted socially than the overweight or underweight children.

The physical needs of the body affect the development of the child (Kerrey et al. 1968). Children 4 to 5 years old have a slower rate of growth and weight gain than they had previously (Wilson, Fisher, and Fuqua 1975). Recommended nutrient intakes for children of this age are given in table 3.

By the age of 3, the average boy is a little over 91 centimeters (36 inches) tall and weighs over 13.5 kilograms (30 pounds); by age 5, he has grown to about 111 centimeters (44 inches) and 19.5 kilograms (43 pounds). Girls are slightly shorter and lighter (Ambron 1975; Watson 1973). Boys and girls develop at about the same pace during the preschool years and through childhood until puberty. Boys do have more muscle and girls more fatty tissue. (In both sexes the infant fatty tissue is replaced, but girls tend to retain it longer than boys.) After the second year appetite tapers off until about 5 years of age (Robinson 1973). Respiratory diseases and other childhood diseases reach a peak during this time (Watson 1973).

These aspects of child development indicate that the growth and maturation process influences the food a child eats and the food patterns which are forming. The stage of development determines the type of food that a child can handle. On the other hand, the foods themselves may serve to promote development. For example, finger foods may help in fine motor development of the fingers, mealtime manners may teach consideration of others, and new foods may be used to build vocabulary.

Development of food behavior is a part of the enculturation of children. Lowenberg (1965) stated that adults transmit cultural food patterns which inform children what foods are desirable, how to eat them, and what rules govern conduct while eating. Cultural cues, or nonverbal behavior, and informal education are the means through which this is accomplished.

Food Preferences and Flavor Perception

Several researchers have identified foods liked and disliked by preschool children (Ireton and Guthrie 1972; Sanjur and Scoma 1971; Eppright et al. 1969; Dierks and Morse 1965; Leverton and Coggs 1951; Vance and Temple 1933). Some types of food especially favored by 4- to 5-year-old children included mild-flavored foods, foods with a soft, jellylike texture, finger foods, and colorful foods. The food practices and attitudes established during the early years are believed to affect children's food choices and, consequently, their nutritional status throughout life (Kerry et al. 1968; Wagner 1954).

TABLE 3. NUTRIENT NEEDS OF CHILDREN

Age (years)	4-6
Weight (kg, lb)	20, 44
Height (cm, in)	110, 44
Energy (kcal)[a]	1,800
Protein (g)	30
Fat-soluble vitamins	
Vitamin A activity	
RE[b]	500
I.U.	2,500
Vitamin D (I.U.)	400
Vitamin E activity[c] (I.U.)	9
Water-soluble vitamins	
Ascorbic acid (mg)	40
Folacin[d] (mcg)	200
Niacin[e] (mg)	12
Riboflavin (mg)	1.1
Thiamin (mg)	0.9
Vitamin B_6 (mg)	0.9
Vitamin B_{12} (mcg)	1.5
Minerals	
Calcium (mg)	800
Phosphorus (mg)	800
Iodine (mcg)	80
Iron (mg)	10
Magnesium (mg)	200
Zinc (mg)	10

Source: Data from the National Research Council, *Recommended Dietary Allowances*, 8th ed. (Washington, D.C.: National Academy of Sciences, 1974).

[a]Kilojoules (kj) = 4.2 x kilocalories (kcal).

[b]Retinol equivalents.

[c]Total vitamin E activity estimated to be 80 percent as D-tocopherol and 20 percent other tocopherols.

[d]The folacin allowances refer to dietary sources as determined by *Lactobacillus casei* assay. Pure forms of folacin may be effective in doses less than one-fourth of the Recommended Dietary Allowance.

[e]Although allowances are expressed as niacin, it is recognized that, on the average, 1 mg of niacin is derived from each 60 mg of dietary tryptophan.

Food acceptance and preference depend partially on sensory evaluation of the food (Weisberg 1974; Sharon 1965). Although foods are evaluated in terms of all of the senses — taste, smell, touch, sound, and sight — flavor has the prominent role (Stone and Pangborn 1968). Flavor is generally regarded as consisting of taste, odor, and feel in the mouth (Caul 1951).

Feeney, Dodds, and Lowenberg (1966) administered threshold tests to fifty-three preschool children and their parents. No differences were found in the abilities of the parents (scores of the mother and father combined) and their child to detect low concentrations of sucrose. However, when the mothers and fathers were considered as subgroups, the mothers detected differences in the concentration of sucrose solutions at a significantly lower level than their children but the fathers' sensitivities were similar to their childrens'. Therefore, differences in threshold perhaps cannot be attributed solely to age.

The Influence of Television on Children

In addition to the physiological influences on food acceptance that have been discussed, advertising, especially television advertising, affects the food practices of Americans. Holden (1971) noted that advertising (1) brings new foods to the notice of trend seekers, (2) reinforces justification for new food behaviors, (3) serves to identify brands, (4) reminds people of the value of present food practices, and (5) establishes quality criteria for manufacturers to follow. Commercial advertising may have a great impact on the food practices of children because of the influence children have on their parents or whoever else provides food for them.

Advertising becomes effective when it relates to the needs and concerns of the audience by working within society's values, wants, and goals (Jelley and Hermann 1973). Advertising that appeals to both the "rational" and "emotional" levels of the audience may create some strong consumer desires.

Promoters of specific products use advertising to induce behavior change, which is closely connected with attitude change. Those who buy the family's food exhibit attitudes that correspond to their purchasing behavior, unless they are buying items they disapprove of. Pinson and Roberto (1973) stated that in some circumstances attitude change can precede behavior change. For example, a parent's perception of the validity of the advertising and of its effect on the parent's own attitude and behavior will help determine what food is bought for a child. Phillips (1975) found that a mother's perception of television's influence on her child's preferences for presweetened cereal was greater than the child's.

Because many food items are cheap and quickly consumed, individual items may not be considered to have a long-lasting effect. The household food purchaser may agree to buy a specific food without agreeing with its use in the family diet. Before buying food, a parent must consider several factors, including price, nutritive value, family preference, and the quality of the food (Opinion Research Corporation 1972). The availability of specific foods also has an influence on purchases.

In its early years, television penetrated most swiftly into homes where there were young children (Schramm, Lyle, and Parker 1961). Because of television's quick adoption into the American home, watching television has become a major factor in socializing the child. Over 95 percent of the homes in the United States have television, and in the average home it is on 5 hours and 45 minutes a day (Manoff 1973). Appell (1963) contended that television is a part of the environment of children and represents one aspect of their culture. According to Schramm, Lyle, and Parker (1961), the primary function of television in children's lives is to give them the passive pleasures of being entertained or of living in a fantasy. Other functions include the semination of information and, as already mentioned, socialization of the child.

Ward (1972) found that kindergarten children could not distinguish between the television commercial and the program, nor could they define the purpose of the commercials. Children may use the fantasy function of television to relieve stress and to try out ideas in a make-believe setting (Schramm, Lyle, and Parker 1961). Once absorbed in a program, younger children may be more influenced by television commercials than if they were not interested in the program.

The Family's Influence on the Child

In studying children's food consumption patterns, researchers have observed that various factors having to do with the family and mothers are related to food practices. A positive relationship between per capita income and nutritional status was found by Futrell, Kilgore, and Windham (1971). Kerrey et al. (1968) studied the nutritional status of 40 children 3-1/2 to 5-1/2 years old and concluded that the generally better nutritional status of the higher socioeconomic group was attributable to a higher nutrient intake, provided partly by vitamin supplements. Zee, Walters, and Mitchell (1970) found anemia and retarded growth to be common among the low-income black children they studied. Lack of food was listed as the main cause.

The education of the mother has been related to the food intake of the children. In the North Central Regional Study of the diets of preschool children, a positive correlation was found between the educational level of the mother and the calcium, iron, thiamine, riboflavin, and ascorbic acid intake of the children (Eppright et al. 1969). The mother's educational level was a more influential factor than the family's income. A positive correlation between nutrition knowledge and nutrition attitudes was also found in the North Central Regional Study.

Parents have both a direct and an indirect influence on the developing food preferences of their children. James (1961) found that foods liked by the parents were also liked by their children. The parents' food preferences influenced the children's knowledge of food and their dietary habits and, consequently, what they actually ate. Grissom (1957), too, found that parents influenced their children's food preferences. Feelings about food may contribute to the quality of children's relationships with their parents and other adults in an eating situation.

Various methods of preparing vegetables, and children's preferences for them, were compared by Dudley, Moore, and Sunderlin (1960). Preference influenced the children's intake of vegetables to a large extent. Ireton and Guthrie (1972) found that varying the method of preparation had no significant effect on a child's consumption of vegetables but that if children were rewarded for eating vegetables they would eat more of them.

Ilg (1948) stated that 4-1/2- to 5-year olds were less demanding and more receptive to foods that were available than were younger children. Children's food habits were influenced by the habits of other people and by other factors in their environment. Children imitated the family's food practices, which then became a part of their own (Beyer and Morris 1974). Glaser (1964) found that, according to parents, food acceptance at nursery school does carry over into the home.

Children's food behavior and attitudes are influenced by their families. Older siblings are in close contact with the child whose food preferences are developing. Cicirelli (1972) studied the effect of the male sibling versus the female sibling versus the nonsibling child-teacher on the child's food behavior. Female siblings were more influential than female nonsiblings or male siblings. Theoretically, the female sibling took the role of the mother: she was accustomed to telling the younger child what to do and the child responded more readily than older children. If the older brother was closer in age to the younger child, the younger child displayed hostility, competitiveness and jealousy and became defensive and resisted learning.

Within the family structure siblings have an effect on one another's behavior. It seems that even the presence of an older or younger male or female sibling may influence the 5-year-old child's personality and approach to personal interactions. Koch (1956) studied 384 children 5 to 6 years old from white families having 2 children in the family. She found that both the relative age and the sex of the sibling influenced the behavior of the children in her study. Children with a brother 4 to 6 years older were more aggressive than other pairs of siblings, except when the age difference was less than 2 years. The older children of the sibling pairs were more curious than their younger brothers or sisters. Children having siblings of the opposite sex, either 3 to 4 years older or younger, had more curiosity than children having a sibling of the same sex. This greater or lesser curiosity, related to the position and sex of the sibship, may influence the 5-year-old's desire to try new foods.

As the difference in age between the children in Koch's study increased, they played together less. Therefore, both children had more association with their peers and the mother became somewhat protective of the younger child. Depending on the manifestation of her protection, this relationship might have given the child either more or less influence on her food purchases.

Mothers of 5- to 6-year-old girls gave them a higher responsibility rating than mothers gave their 5- to 6-year-old boys (Koch 1956). Perhaps this is related to girls being given the consumer role earlier than boys because women are generally responsible for shopping. However, firstborn girls do not necessarily have a greater tendency toward the housewife role than other girls in the family (Edwards and Klemmock 1973). In fact, firstborn children are more likely to attain a position of eminence (Altus 1966). Perhaps the higher responsibility ratings given to the girls indicated overall achievement rather than specific role playing. The influence of ordinal position in the family with regard to food behavior and the development of food behavior needs to be investigated.

The Child's Influence on the Family

In a study of the food choices of women in Kansas, Cosper and Wakefield (1975) found that 64 percent of the motivation for food selection was due to family (36 percent) and personal (28 percent) preference. Within the family, the husband had the strongest influence on the food purchases of the wife, but children's food preferences were considered. Children about 5 years of age frequently attempted to influence food purchases, with cereal being requested often and parents yielding most of the time (Ward and Wackerman, 1972; Lamkin, Hielscher, and James 1970; Metheny et al. 1962).

Hammonds and Wunderle (1972) believe it is important to know the child's influence on family food purchases because foods intended for children must conform to parental attitudes of what is appropriate for a child. The food purchaser for the family controls what food is available in the home (Lewin 1943). Lackey (1974) found that the homemakers' food purchases were determined mostly by family preference and by convenience.

Wells and LoScuito (1966) used direct observation in a grocery store to investigate the specific conditions under which point-of-purchase decisions were made. They found that 35 percent of the shoppers were women alone, 16 percent were women with their children, 16 percent were women with their husbands, and 6 percent were women with other adults. Twenty-two percent of the shoppers were men and 4 percent were children. Mothers with young children apparently predominate in the 16 percent of the women shopping with children. Metheny et al. (1962) interviewed 94 mothers with 2-1/2- to 5-1/2-year-old children. Of these mothers, 54 percent were always accompanied to the grocery store by their children and another 34 percent sometimes took their children.

In their study, Wells and LoScuito found the influence of children to be strongest at the cereal counter. When children of all ages were considered, 59 percent made some attempt to influence the cereal purchase and 36 percent were actually successful. Of the younger children, it was reported that 91 percent requested specific foods — especially cereals (Metheny et al. 1962).

Perhaps one reason mothers take their young children to the grocery store is to begin the enculturation of consumerism. "The consumer role behavior does not blossom suddenly with the advent of adulthood — it is a product of learning that begins with childhood and develops throughout the life cycle" (McNeal 1965, p. 190).

McNeal (1965) interviewed 60 nonminority children in the age groups of 5, 7, and 9 years old from a middle socioeconomic class. The 5-year-old children had some money but generally sought satisfaction from their parents rather than directly from the marketplace. Their purchase suggestions were usually of a personal nature rather than family oriented like the suggestions of older children. Five-year-olds usually preferred grocery stores to other retail outlets, perhaps because children this age have begun to realize that grocery stores are another source (other than parents) of products giving immediate satisfaction.

When a 5-year-old's attempt to influence a purchase was unsuccessful, only one-half of the mothers offered explanations for their refusal. Older children received a reason, which increased in detail as the child increased in age. This acquainted them with factors that their parents considered when purchasing various products.

The combination of parental permissiveness and independence-seeking by the child fostered a rapid growth in independent consumer behavior between the ages of 5 and 9. Five-year-old boys were allowed to go to the store alone more often than 5-year-old girls and therefore had more freedom than the girls in making consumer decisions. By age 7, however, boys and girls were equal in this regard, and by age 9 girls did more shopping than boys. Boys' purchase suggestions remained of a personal nature, whereas girls were more apt to suggest purchases for the family. Because shopping was considered a feminine activity, the girls' opinions were more frequently asked and they enjoyed shopping more than the boys did.

The environment of preschool children is limited to the family, with the possible exception of nursery school. The food behavior of children this age will reflect the interactions within the family, certain influences from the outside (such as television), and also the personality and physiology of the children themselves.

SIX- TO TEN-YEAR-OLDS

The world of a child 6 to 10 years old is continually expanding. Before this time, children are essentially homebodies and their food behavior is therefore controlled to a great extent by the family atmosphere. It has been said that during middle childhood even the nicest children begin to behave in a most awful way. In reality, it is a period of broadening interests, of learning to make social contact, and of establishing intense friendships with other children (Hawkes and Pease 1962). It is the period when a child learns to read and becomes rather proficient at reading. In formal education the child progresses from the first through the fourth grade. For some children, school is the first experience of an environment that mother does not control. Some have not been exposed to food other than that prepared by their families or by family friends. School lunch with its unfamiliar foods — foods prepared differently and eaten with peers in a limited time and often in a crowded, noisy room — is a new experience.

School Lunch

School feeding programs appeared in New York City as early as 1853; however, today's school lunch program was begun in Boston in 1894 by the home economist Ellen H. Richards. By 1913, many city school boards were operating food-service programs in some of their schools.

The Seventy-fourth Congress enacted Public Law 320 in 1935, permitting the secretary of agriculture to purchase price-depressing surplus food from the market. Needy families and school lunch programs became excellent outlets for commodities purchased by the United States Department of Agriculture. Then, in 1944, Congress authorized specific funds for the operation of the school food-service and milk program, without regard to the surplus of agricultural commodities, and in 1966 the Child Nutrition Act provided for the National School Breakfast Program. A bill passed in 1971 made it mandatory for schools to use the income poverty guidelines of the Department of Health, Education and Welfare to determine which children are entitled to free or reduced-price breakfast and lunch.

In addition to using up surplus commodities, the National School Lunch Program has created opportunities for children to develop good nutrition habits. Indeed, school lunch has had an influence on the food behavior of Americans over the past 30 or 40 years (Anonymous 1971). Todhunter (1970) believes that children have a right to learn at school how to achieve and maintain good health. This includes learning the basis of desirable food behavior, which will serve them throughout life.

Many factors influence what children eat at school. Children come to school as individuals. They may come from homes of strong cultural background and many traditions, perhaps from a specific ethnic group. They may have definite taste preferences and may have been indulged by their parents so that they eat only what they like. They may watch television and be susceptible to advertising. There are social and economic factors, in addition to the immediate state of family finances, that influence behavior. Some children may have had a poor breakfast or none at all; others may have no money to buy lunch or may have spent their lunch money on snacks of low nutritive value. Children may have ideas about weight and body image. Or their nutritive needs may be quite different from the Recommended Dietary Allowances. All of these factors influence children's acceptance of the food provided by school feeding programs. Some factors will encourage sound food choices, while others will contribute to markedly undesirable ones. In other words, culture, ethnicity, socioeconomic factors, and psychological reactions may help or hinder a child in making nutritionally sound food choices.

One school food-service manager worked with the teachers at all grade levels to help plan learning experiences that would be reinforced when the children went into the cafeteria for lunch (Anonymous 1967). "Tasting parties" were held at which new foods made their debuts. Later, when small portions of those foods were served at lunch, they were no longer unfamiliar. Games and poster contests related to food heightened the children's curiosity and enthusiasm for learning. With a nutritionally balanced school lunch menu, the teacher stressed the importance of a good diet for a strong body and clear complexion. Students watching their weight were encouraged to choose fruit for dessert instead of cake and not to cut calories by skipping lunch. For some children the school lunch was their best and often only complete meal of the day. In schools where there were food programs for needy children, there were frequent reports of much-improved attendance records, greater participation in sports and other class activities, and less frequent occurrences of student dizziness and weakness formerly attributed to hunger. For these youngsters, a good lunch made education possible!

Elementary school children are usually better fed than preschool children or adolescents. Peer acceptance is extremely important at this time, and children need to be able to keep up with their classmates and to have a sense of accomplishment. They learn that certain foods are acceptable to the peer group, whereas other foods from a different cultural pattern, may be looked upon unfavorably; as a result, they may be unwilling to accept those foods at home. On the other hand, within a group, children are willing to try foods they are unacquainted with and which they would not try alone (Robinson 1972).

Group feeding along with an education program is a valuable method of improving food behavior. Alford and Tibbets (1971) conducted a nutrition education program at a camp for diabetic children. The education program in the dining hall included colorful cartoon posters emphasizing vegetables. A tasting demonstration introduced the children to many vegetables low in carbohydrates. Charts were used to illustrate the number of calories in relation to the nutrient content for various methods of preparation, such as potatoes cut and fried for chips, french fried potatoes, and baked potatoes.

In a study of the influence of nutrition education on fourth and fifth graders, 200 children participated in a study to determine the influence of a specially prepared and taught program on nutrition, diet, and related factors. Scores on a nutrition test were significantly higher for the experimental classes than for the control groups when retesting was done within a week after the instruction had been completed. However, no significant changes in diet due to the program were observed (Baker 1972).

A study made in the late 1950s of the food attitudes of fifty-one children, ages 5-1/2 to 11-1/2, obtained responses of "like," "dislike," and "indifferent" for twenty-five items. Many children said they liked a majority of the foods. Meat, ice cream potatoes, bread, crackers, milk, raw fruits, and cereals scored high in popularity. Fat meat, fish, cooked vegetables, cheese, meat mixtures, eggs, and cooked or canned fruit were the least popular (Breckinridge 1959).

Mass Media

Another very important factor in food choices is the mass media — television, radio, movies, books, magazines, comic books, and newspapers. Some of them (television, radio, magazines, and newspapers, for example) contain advertising material.

Food industry critic Robert Choate critized food advertisers. He said food advertisements had taught a generation how *not* to eat. In 1972, he was looking forward to the day when foods would be more accurately labeled so that advertisements would have to become more accurate. He believed that children watching advertisements for such products would inevitably gain an unbalanced perspective on their food supply (Cohen 1973).

Unpublished market surveys suggest that children's favorite flavors are probably chocolate, vanilla, and strawberry. Grape is the most popular fruit flavor. Flavor ranking, however, depends on the form of the product, so that chocolate may be very popular in candy or ice cream but not so popular in drinks (Winick, Williamson, and Chuzmir 1973).

If we judge the importance of the mass media in terms of the time children spend with them, we must admit that they loom large in children's lives. Probably the greatest influences upon children and young people are messages brought by radio and television, which together account for 80 to 90 percent of the time children spend with mass media. Two direct effects upon children's food habits are attributed to broadcasting. The first is the direct response to advertising and the second relates to food behavior developed as an "accommodation to radio and TV" (Tyler 1962). The influence of advertising on those who buy food for young children cannot be discounted either.

Clancey-Hepburn, Kickey, and Neville (1974) found that television was the young child's main source of advertising. Children 8 to 13 years old, who typically watch approximately 25 hours of television per week, are exposed to a great number of food advertisements. Gussow (1972), reporting to the Subcommittee on the Consumer of the Senate Commerce Committee, said that 82 percent of the commercials on children's television were for ingestible items. Of these commercials, 38.5 percent were for breakfast cereals. The Code Board of the National Association of Broadcasting, with whose rulings 60 percent of the nation's broadcasters comply, stated that, beginning 1 January 1975, advertising on children's programs on Saturday and Sunday should not exceed 10 minutes an hour and that advertising during the rest of the week should not exceed 14 minutes per hour (Anonymous 1975).

Television viewing and food requests were studied by Clancey-Hepburn, Kickey, and Neville (1974) in two groups of children. One group consisted of fifty children in the third to sixth grades and their parents, and the other of fifty-five third to sixth graders and their parents. The children were watching between 3.2 and 4 hours of television per day. The younger children (8- to 9-year-olds) viewed more than the older children. A positive correlation was found between the number of requests made by the child for specific items and the number of hours of Saturday morning television the child watched.

Exposure to television commercials affects attitude and behavior (Goldberg and Goan 1974). One hundred thirty-eight 8- to 10-year-old boys in the upper middle class watched a television program interspersed with commercials including 0, 1, or 3 commercials showing a specific toy. Following the program, each child was asked to solve a puzzle to win the toy. Increased exposure to the commercial showing the toy affected the boys' attitudes and behavior, causing them to work longer to try to solve the puzzle.

Robertson and Rossiter (1974) interviewed 289 primary school boys in the first, third, and fifth grades. They found that the persuasive intent of a commercial was the main determinant of the boys' response to television advertising. The older boys were better able than the younger ones to perceive the persuasive intent of the messages of television commercials. The age factor had two components, greater maturity and greater exposure to television commercials. Recognition of persuasive intent served as a cognitive defense to persuasion. Therefore, the older boys were less influenced by advertising, were less trusting of television commercials, and tended to make a decreasing number of consumption requests. The younger boys, who did not recognize the persuasive intent, were more persuadable. Two-thirds of the first graders indicated that they trusted all commercials, and one-half wanted all of the products they saw advertised.

McNeal (1965) studied 60 middle-class, nonminority children of both sexes, ages 5, 7, and 9. Beginning at age 5, there was increasing dislike and mistrust of television advertising, and by age 9 only 35 percent of the children asked their parents to buy products advertised on television. Girls developed skepticism toward advertising earlier than boys, but even for girls there was little mistrust at 5 years of age.

Ward (1972) interviewed sixty-seven children ages 5 to 12, and their mothers, in their homes. The children were asked to recall television advertisements of food products. The ability to recall complexities in the advertising increased with age. It was estimated that 37 percent of the commercials seen by 5- to 7-year-old children were for food. The younger children enjoyed commercials because they liked the product.

In 1970, Robert Choate aroused controversy about the ready-to-eat cereal manufacturers and their television commercials. He claimed that of the 60 cereals he analyzed, 40 were "empty" calories. In a statement to the Senate Subcommittee on the Consumer Choate said that the television commercials stressed sugar, energy, sweetness, chocolate, vigor, frostedness, action, alertness, and prizes. He felt this was a "seduction of the innocent" and thought regulatory measures should be taken to protect children.

Jelliffe (1971) expressed his concern about the responsibility of food advertising, which he believes is a major influence on food selection and emphasizes status and convenience. He pointed out that, in the United States, the nutritional impact of advertisements, especially advertisements for relatively expensive, low-nutrient food for children, has received much consideration and criticism. This is particularly true of advertisements that accompany children's television programs. But the similarities between the possible effects of such advertising on the diets of poor children in the United States and the impact of inappropriate advertising on the nutritional status of infants in developing countries are not often appreciated. Jelliffe believes that advertising has more influence on food selection than health education does.

Tyler (1962), however, believes that advertising is "successful only as a reinforcement of existing mores, customs, and values." She says it does not change the customs and habits of individual children, which are influenced much more by immediate groups such as their peers or their families. Rather, it encourages behavior already sanctioned by the group.

Eating behavior is affected by adjustments children and their families make becuase of the presence of television. Some families eat from trays in the living room in order not to miss a favorite program; some children eat hurriedly in order to rush back to a television show. Many people snack while watching television. TV dinners may have been invented as a response to "tray meals" and busy mothers; however, they are not as popular now as they were when television was still a novelty.

How is food behavior affected as children and youth use mass media for entertainment and as a source of information? Children see on television the stereotyped representations of middle-class family life in family situation comedies, although more ethnic groups are represented on television today. Most children identify themselves with the children in these familiar-seeming situations and accept the ways of living that seem to be approved. This may include what to eat, when to eat it, and how to eat it.

The adult hero — athlete, sheriff, cowboy, detective — is heavily represented in the mass media. Children adore and wish to emulate these characters, and commercial sponsors take advantage of this to stimulate the sale of products such as cereals, candy, pop, and convenience foods. Children respond to the direct urging of their heroes to eat or drink whatever is being advertised.

From television, children also get impressions of what constitutes acceptable adult behavior. Breakfasts of orange juice and coffee, cocktail parties, nightclubs, and coffee breaks are observed by children. As they grow older they tend to acquire the customs, habits, and mores of adults they have observed. However, what children see on television is filtered through the standards and norms of groups — family, peers, church, and school — that they are part of. These groups are influenced by cultural trends, religious values, significant events, and, most of all, the social class to which they belong. Mass media are ineffective when the values they embody conflict with those of the primary groups to which an individual belongs.

The mass media also can be used for educational purposes. Many nutrition educators believe that if they used suitable approaches the mass media institutions (publishers, broadcasters, motion picture producers) could cooperate in a large-scale enterprise to educate American children and youth in nutrition. The nutrition education exemplified in the mass media would need to be demonstrated and favorably considered in nursery schools, boys' clubs, 4-H clubs, Future Farmers of America, scout groups, settlement houses, athletic leagues, neighborhood clubs, summer camps, church groups, and so on.

Family and Income

Directly related to the effects of the mass media on children's food behavior is the influence of the family and the family's income. A child's food habits and practices develop in a small group situation in which each member influences all the others. Not only do parents influence children, but children influence parents as well. And children influence each other too.

Although dad may be master of the house in some matters, it is essentially a mother's world as far as the sanctioning of food behavior is concerned. Physicians, dentists, and contemporaries have peripheral roles, and teachers may be ignored (Litman, Coonery, and Stief 1964). These persons may, however, influence children as a result of their influence on the parents, especially the mother.

Ward and Wackerman (1972) found that highly child-centered mothers bought their children's favorite cereals less frequently than mothers who were less child-centered. Children's attempts to influence purchases may decrease somewhat with age, depending on the type of product; but a mother's yielding to requests increases with the age of the child, which probably reflects her perception of the increased competence of older children to make purchase decisions. The overall percentages of mothers yielding to the requests of 5- to 7-year-olds, 8- to 10-year olds, and 11- to 12-year-olds were 52, 54, and 59 percent, respectively.

One of the cultural behaviors most strongly ingrained in the United States is the pattern of three meals a day. Most parents consider it undesirable for children to eat very much between meals. Because of differences in their schedules, however, it is becoming more and more difficult for all members of a family to sit down together for any meal of the day. This increases between-meal snacking and encourages a trend apparent in school-age children — the tendency to overeat and underexercise, which is resulting in obesity, or an "undue amount of chubbiness" in many children.

Socioeconomic factors that have a major effect on children's diets are income, urbanization, education of the mother, and the number of children in the family (Hendel, Burk, and Lund 1965).

In a study of 302 children 9 to 11 years old, ascorbic acid and vitamin A intake were directly related to income. For the families with higher incomes, major sources of ascorbic acid were citrus juices, tomatoes, and tomato juice. The low-income families obtained ascorbic acid primarily from citrus fruits, potatoes, and apples (Hendel, Burk, and Lund 1965).

Snacks and coffee breaks have become part of our lives. In poor urban or rural families, children may be fed haphazardly for lack of cooking utensils and dishes. But it now appears that the children of more prosperous families, from choice and habit, eat here and there, now and then, too (Lantis 1962a). Children are growing up with the expectation that the family doesn't just stop for gas, it stops for gas and pop; people don't just bowl or skate, they bowl and have a beer or a cup of coffee or a hot dog; children don't wait for a bus, they wait and eat candy bars. Such behavior is closely connected with the development of the vending machine (Lantis 1962b). The child is encouraged on every side, by every conceivable merchandising device, to drink liquids other than water.

It seems that normal Americans will accept food and drink that they may not prefer but that are convenient, inexpensive, and meet minimum standards of cleanliness and palatability. The whole complex business of food production, processing, and marketing is being removed further and further from the consumer's experience. Many children have no idea of the labor and organization required to bring food to them. Therefore, they do not appreciate the intrinsic value of food unless they happen to have been genuinely deprived and hungry.

"According to the 'Law of Engel,' the family spends relatively less on its diet as the income rises" (Van Schaik 1964, p. 229). There is an income level below which people starve. Above that level, however, the amount spent on food does not bear any relation to its nutrient composition (Van Schaik 1964). It has been found that, as the prosperity of families increases and the ratio of wages to prices becomes more favorable, the consumption of animal proteins, fats, and carbohydrates in the form of meat, milk, cheese, eggs, butter, refined flour, and sugar will increase. This may result in a diet that is unbalanced due to an excess of fats and carbohydrates, as is the case in many Western European countries and in North America, and it may lead to a diet high in calories.

Van Schaik (1964), in studying the relationship of family life to food and nutrition, found that children in small families are more apt to be poor or capricious eaters than children in large families. She believes that in small families the mother has too much time to pay attention to the child; she is overly careful, presses the child too much, and is afraid that it does not eat enough. The child responds by refusing to eat. In large families the mother may have little time to pay attention to each child while it is eating; as a result, brothers and sisters help the younger children and do not press them as much as the mother would.

In large families more money is spent on food, but the cost per person is higher for a very small family. Food expenses are also related to the composition of the family. For example, the diet of large children is more expensive than that of small children.

A number of studies indicate that the educational level of the mother is directly correlated with the nutritional adequacy of family diets (Gifft, Washbon, and Harrison 1972).

Physical Needs

Because of the high rate of anabolic activity during childhood, nutritional requirements in proportion to body size are much greater for children than for adults. Childhood is a time of considerable physical activity and, therefore, of greater energy requirements (table 4). Children 7 to 10 years old should have 2,400 kilocalories and those

TABLE 4. NUTRIENT NEEDS OF CHILDREN

Age (years)	7-10
Weight (kg, lb)	30, 66
Height (cm, in)	135, 54
Energy (kcal)[a]	2,400
Protein (g)	36
Fat-soluble vitamins	
Vitamin A activity	
RE[b]	700
I.U.	3,300
Vitamin D (I.U.)	400
Vitamin E activity[c] (I.U.)	10
Water-soluble vitamins	
Ascorbic acid (mg)	40
Folacin[d] (mcg)	300
Niacin[e] (mg)	16
Riboflavin (mg)	1.2
Thiamin (mg)	1.2
Vitamin B_6 (mg)	1.2
Vitamin B_{12} (mcg)	2.0
Minerals	
Calcium (mg)	800
Phosphorus (mg)	800
Iodine (mcg)	110
Iron (mg)	10
Magnesium (mg)	250
Zinc (mg)	10

Source: Data from the National Research Council, *Recommended Dietary Allowances*, 8th ed. (Washington, D.C.: National Academy of Sciences, 1974).

[a]Kilojoules (kj) = 4.2 x kilocalories (kcal).

[b]Retinol equivalents.

[c]Total vitamin E activity estimated to be 80 percent as D-tocopherol and 20 percent other tocopherols.

[d]The folacin allowances refer to dietary sources as determined by *Lactobacillus casei* assay. Pure forms of folacin may be effective in doses less than one-fourth of the Recommended Dietary Allowance.

[e]Although allowances are expressed as niacin, it is recognized that, on the average, 1 mg of niacin is derived from each 60 mg of dietary tryptophan.

engaged in competitive athletics may need more if they are to grow satisfactorily.

To meet the criteria for a good nutritious diet, the pattern of food consumption must (1) permit the individual to achieve the maximum genetic potential for physical and mental development, (2) be conducive to delaying or preventing the onset of degenerative diseases which are so prevalent in America, and (3) be part of satisfying human relationships and contribute to social and personal enjoyment. Individual variation and population variation are major factors in determining the requirements for nutrients at any point in the life cycle.

REFERENCES

The Preschool Child

Altus, W. D. 1966. Birth order and its sequelae. *Science* 151:44.

Ambron, S. 1975. *Child development.* San Francisco: Rhinehart Press.

Appell, C. T. 1963. Television viewing and the preschool child. *Marriage and Family Living* 25:311.

Beyer, N. R., and Morris, P. M. 1974. Food attitudes and snacking patterns of young children. *Journal of Nutrition Education* 6:131.

Caul, J. F. 1951. Sugar as a seasoning. *Sugar Molecule* 5 (2).

Cicirelli, V. G. 1972. The effect of sibling relationship on concept learning of young children taught by child-teachers. *Child Development* 43:282.

Cosper, B. A., and Wakefield, L. M. 1975. Food choices of women: Personal, attitudinal and motivational factors. *Journal of the American Dietetic Association* 66:152.

Dierks, E. C., and Morse, L. M. 1965. Food habits and nutrient intakes of preschool children. *Journal of the American Dietetic Association* 47:292.

Dudley, D. T.; Moore, M. E.; and Sunderlin, E. M. 1960. Children's attitudes toward food. *Journal of Home Economics* 52:678.

Edwards, J. N., and Klemmock, D. L. 1973. Birth order and the conservators of tradition hypothesis. *Journal of Marriage and the Family* 35:619.

Eppright, E. S.; Fox, H. J.; Fryer, B. A.; Lamkin, G. H.; and Vivian, V. M. 1969. The North Central Regional Study of diets of preschool children: 2. Nutrition knowledge and attitudes of mothers. *Journal of Home Economics* 62:327.

Feeney, M. C.; Dodds, M. L.; and Lowenberg, M. E. 1966. The sense of taste of preschool children and their parents. *Journal of the American Dietetic Association* 48:399.

Futrell, M. F.; Kilgore, L. T.; and Windham, F. 1971. Nutritional status of Negro preschool children in Mississippi. *Journal of the American Dietetic Association* 59:224.

Gessell, A.; Halverson, H. M.; Thompson, H.; Ilg, F. L.; Castner, B. M.; Ames, L. B.; and Amatruda, C. S. 1940. *The first five years of life.* New York: Harper and Brothers.

Gibson, J. J., and Gibson, E. J. 1955. Perceptual learning: Differentiation or enrichment? *Psychological Review* 62:32.

Glaser, 1964. Nursery school can influence food acceptance. *Journal of Home Economics* 56:680.

Grissom, E. J. 1957. A critical comparison of food preference of fifteen mothers, fifteen fathers and fifteen of their children in the G. C. Hawley High School community. M.S. thesis, North Carolina College (Durham).

Gutteridge, M. A. 1939. A study of motor achievements of young children. *Archives of Psychology* 34 (244):1.

Hammonds, T. M., and Wunderle, R. E. 1972. Nutrition intervention programs from a market viewpoint. *American Journal of Clinical Nutrition* 25:419.

Holden, P. 1971. How advertising affects food habits. *Food and Nutrition Notes and Reviews* 28:102.

Ireton, C. L., and Guthrie, J. A. 1972. Modification of vegetable-eating behavior in preschool children. *Journal of Nutrition Education* 4:100.

James, R. T. 1961. The influence of parental food attitudes upon food attitudes of children. M.S. thesis, University of Alabama (University).

Jelley, H. M., and Herrmann, R. O. 1973. Understanding the effects of advertising. In *The American consumer,* ed. H. M. Jelley and R. O. Herrmann. New York: McGraw-Hill.

Kerrey, E.; Crispin, S.; Fox, H. M.; and Kies, C. 1968. Nutritional status of preschool children: I. Dietary and biochemical findings. *American Journal of Clinical Nutrition* 21:1274. .

Koch, H. 1956. Children's work attitudes and sibling characteristics. *Child Development* 29:289.

Lackey, C. J. 1974. Family food purchasing: A consumer education program. Ph.D. thesis, University of Tennessee (Knoxville).

Lamkin, G.; Hielscher, M. L.; and James, H. B. 1970. Food purchasing practices of young families. *Journal of Home Economics* 62:598.

Leverton, R. M., and Coggs, M. C. 1951. Food choices of Nebraska children. *Journal of Home Economics* 43:176.

Lewin, K. 1943. Forces behind food habits and methods of change. In *The problem of changing food habits*. National Research Council, Bulletin no. 108. Washington, D. C.: National Academy of Sciences.

Lowenberg, M. E. 1965. Philosophy of nutrition and application in maternal health services. *American Journal of Clinical Nutrition* 16:370.

McNeal, J. U. 1965. An exploratory study of the consumer behavior of children. In *Dimensions of consumer behavior*, ed. J. U. McNeal. New York: Appleton-Century-Crofts.

Manoff, R. K. 1973. Potential uses of mass media in nutrition programs. *Journal of Nutrition Education* 5:125.

Metheny, N. Y.; Hunt, F. E.; Patton, M. B.; and Heye, H. 1962. The diets of preschool children: Nutritional sufficiency findings and family marketing practices. *Journal of Home Economics* 54:297.

Mussen, P. H.; Conger, J. J.; and Kagan, J. 1974. Preschool years. In *Child development and personality*, 4th ed., ed. P. H. Mussen and J. J. Conger. New York: Harper and Row.

National Research Council. 1974. *Recommended Dietary Allowances*. 8th ed. Washington, D.C.: National Academy of Sciences.

Opinion Research Corporation. 1972. *The homemaker's changing attitude toward and her role in family feeding*. Nutley, N. J.: Hoffman-LaRoche.

Phillips, D. E. 1975. Presweetened cereal patterns of older sib families and no older sib families: Child's preference, mother's perception of child's preference and family purchase. Ph.D. thesis, University of Tennessee (Knoxville).

Piaget, J. 1972. Development and learning. In *Readings in child behavior and development*, 3rd ed., ed. C. S. Lavatelli and F. Stendler. New York: Harcourt Brace Jovanovich.

Pinson, C., and Roberto, E. L. 1973. Do attitude changes precede behavior change? *Journal of Advertising Research* 13 (4):33.

Robinson, C. 1973. *Fundamentals of normal nutrition*. New York: Macmillan.

Sanjur, D., and Scoma, A. D. 1971. Food habits of low-income children in northern New York. *Journal of Nutrition Education* 3:85.

Schramm, W.; Lyle, J.; and Parker, E.B. 1961. Television in the lives of our children. In *Studies in American society*, vol. 1, ed. D. L. Phillips. New York: Thomas Y. Crowell.

Sharon, I. M. 1965. Sensory properties of food and their function during feeding. *Food Technology* 19:35.

Sherif, M., and Sherif, C. W. 1969. *Social psychology*. New York: Harper and Row.

Spock, D., and Lowenberg, M. 1966. *Feeding your baby and child*. New York: Pocket Books.

Stone, H., and Pangborn, R. M. 1968. Intercorrelation of the senses. In *Basic principles of sensory evaluation STP 433*. Philadelphia: American Society for Testing and Materials.

Vance, T. F., and Temple, V. M. 1933. The food preferences of preschool children. *Child Development* 4:222.

Wagner, M. G. 1954. Appetites and attitudes: A viewpoint on feeding the young child. *Journal of the American Dietetic Association* 30:329.

Wakefield, L. M., and Merrow, S. B. 1967. Interrelationships between selected nutritional, clinical and sociological measurements of preadolescent children from independent low-income families. *American Journal of Clinical Nutrition* 20:291.

Ward, S. 1972. Children's reactions to commercials. *Journal of Advertising Research* 12 (2):37.

Ward, S., and Wackerman, D. R. 1972. Children's purchase influence attempts and parental yielding. *Journal of Marketing Research* 9:316.

Watson, R. 1973. *Psychology of the child*. New York: Wiley.

Weisberg, S. M. 1974. Food acceptance and flavor requirements in the developing world. *Food Technology* 28 (11):48.

Wells, W. D., and LoScuito, L. A. 1966. Direct observation of purchasing behavior. *Journal of Marketing Research* 3:227.

Wilson, E. D.; Fisher, K. H.; and Fuqua, M. E. 1975. Nutrition of infants and preschool children. In *Principles of Nutrition*, 3rd ed., ed. E. D. Wilson et al. New York: Wiley.

Zee, P.; Walters, T.; and Mitchell, C. 1970. Nutrition and poverty in preschool children. *Journal of the American Medical Association* 213:739.

Six- to Ten-Year-Olds

Alford, B. B., and Tibbets, M. H. 1971. Education increases consumption of vegetables by children. *Journal of Nutrition Education* 3:12.

Anonymous. 1967. School lunch teaches good food habits. *Agricultural Marketing* 12 (10):3.

Anonymous. 1971. Current topics: Feeding and educating children: Child nutrition programs after 25 years. *Journal of Nutrition Education* 3:54.

Anonymous. 1975. News: Action for Children's Television. *Advertising Age* 4 (2):1.

Baker, M. J. 1972. Influence of nutrition education on 4th and 5th graders. *Journal of Nutrition Education* 6:131.

Breckinridge, M. E. 1959. Food attitudes of five- to twelve-year-old children. *Journal of the American Dietetic Association* 35:704.

Choate, R. B. 1970. The seduction of the innocent. Statement made at a hearing of the Subcommittee on the Consumer of the U.S. Senate Commerce Committee, 23 July 1970.

Clancy-Hepburn, K.; Kickey, S. S.; and Neville, G. 1974. Children's behavior response to the food advertisements. *Journal of Nutrition Education* 6:93.

Cohen, S. W. 1973. Wonder Bread decision stalls FTC drive for corrective ads. *Advertising Age* 44 (1):1.

Gifft, H. H.; Washbon, M. B.; and Harrison, G. G. 1972. *Nutrition, behavior, and change.* Englewood Cliffs, N.J.: Prentice-Hall.

Goldberg, M. E., and Gorn, G. J. 1974. Children's reactions to television advertising: An experimental approach. *Journal of Consumer Research* 1 (2):69.

Gussow, J. 1972. Statement made to the Subcommittee on the Consumer of the U.S. Senate Commerce Committee at a hearing on the nutritional content and advertising of dry breakfast cereals, 2 March 1972.

Hawkes, G. R., and Pease, D. 1962. *Behavior and development from 5 to 12.* New York: Harper and Brothers.

Hendel, G. M.; Burk, M. C.; and Lund, L. A. 1965. Socio-economic factors influence children's diets. *Journal of Home Economics* 57:205.

Ilg, F. L. 1948. The child's idea of what and how to eat. *Journal of the American Dietetic Association* 24:658.

Jelliffe, D. B. 1971. Commeriogenic malnutrition. *Food Technology* 25:153.

Lantis, M. 1962a. Cultural factors influencing children's food habits. In *Proceedings of the National Nutrition Education Conference.* Miscellaneous publication no. 913. Washington, D.C.: U.S. Department of Agriculture.

Lantis, M. 1962b. The child consumer — Cultural factors influencing his food choices. *Journal of Home Economics* 54:370.

Litman, T. J.; Coonery, J. P.; and Stief, R. 1964. The views of Minnesota school children on food. *Journal of the American Dietetic Association* 45:433.

McNeal, J. U. 1965. An exploratory study of consumer behavior of children. In *Dimensions of consumer behavior,* ed. J. U. McNeal. New York: Appleton-Century-Crofts.

National Research Council. 1974. *Recommended Dietary Allowances,* 8th ed. Washington, D.C.: National Academy of Sciences.

Robertson, T. S., and Rossiter, J. R. 1974. Children and commercial persuasion: An attribution theory analysis. *Journal of Consumer Research* 1 (1):13.

Robinson, C. H. 1972. *Normal and therapeutic nutrition.* New York: Macmillan.

Todhunter, E. N. 1970. Feeding from a nutritionist's point of view. *American Journal of Public Health* 60:2302.

Tyler, I. K. 1962. The influence of mass media on children's food habits. In *Proceedings of the National Nutrition Education Conference.* Miscellaneous publication no. 913. Washington, D.C.: U.S. Department of Agriculture.

Van Schaik, T. F. 1964. Food and nutrition relative to family life. *Journal of Home Economics* 56:225.

Ward, S. 1972. Children's reaction to commercials. *Journal of Advertising Research* 12 (2):37.
Ward, S., and Wackerman, D. B. 1972. Children's purchase influence attempts and parental yielding. *Journal of Marketing Research* 9:316.
Winick, C.; Williamson, L. G.; and Chuzmir, S. F. 1973. *Children's television commercials.* New York: Praeger.

CHAPTER 6

Food Behavior throughout Life — Preadolescence and Adolescence

PREADOLESCENCE

Growth and Development

The ages of 10 to 14 are sometimes referred to as *preadolescence.* The 14-year-old boy is quite different from the 10-year-old, and same is true for girls. Growth acceleration occurs in boys between the ages of 9 and 15 and in girls between the ages of 8 and 14 (Krogman 1972). Caloric and calcium needs are high during this period (table 5). Acceleration of genital and sex-linked anatomic changes is taking place, and the maturation of the procreative function has great psychological significance. Children 10 to 12 years old are finishing elementary school (the fifth and sixth grades) and are beginning to feel some of the hormonal changes that take place before and during puberty. By age 14 they are confronted with the reality of a changed physical self. The need to shave becomes evident for many boys toward the end of this age range. Most girls will have begun to menstruate by age 14, and some may begin as early as age 10.

The growth spurt of adolescence is the most rapid growth since the first year of life. A child's stomach is often referred to as a "bottomless pit," or it is said that the child has a "hollow leg" that must be filled up. Children this age are eating constantly, and their parents are often irritated because before the dishes are finished they are back in the kitchen asking for more food. During this period of rapid growing children require more food, and since their stomachs are not large enough to hold it all at one time, frequent eating is the answer. Snacking provides many of the nutrients.

Weight

Children's perceptions of their body image develop during this period, and weight problems or severe skin problems can have serious effects on personality development. Weight usually proves to be a more serious problem than acne because acne seems to disappear with time whereas research indicates that losing weight at this age is difficult but that, if it is not lost by age 14, the chances are great that obesity will be a problem throughout life.

TABLE 5. NUTRIENT NEEDS OF ADOLESCENTS

	Male	*Female*
Age (years)	11-14	11-14
Weight (kg, lb)	44, 97	44, 97
Height (cm, in.)	158, 63	155, 62
Energy (cal)[a]	2,800	2,400
Protein (g)	44	44
Fat-soluble vitamins		
Vitamin A activity		
RE[b]	1,000	800
I.U.	5,000	4,000
Vitamin D (I.U.)	400	400
Vitamin E activity[c] (I.U.)	12	12
Water-soluble vitamins		
Ascorbic acid (mg)	45	45
Folacin[d] (mcg)	400	400
Niacin[e] (mg)	18	16
Riboflavin (mg)	1.5	1.3
Thiamin (mg)	1.4	1.2
Vitamin B_6 (mg)	1.6	1.6
Vitamin B_{12} (mcg)	3.0	3.0
Minerals		
Calcium (mg)	1,200	1,200
Phosphorus (mg)	1,200	1,200
Iodine (mcg)	130	115
Iron (mg)	18	18
Magnesium (mg)	350	300
Zinc (mg)	15	15

Source: Data from the National Research Council, *Recommended Dietary Allowances*, 8th ed. (Washington, D.C.: National Academy of Sciences, 1974).

[a]Kilojoules (kj) = 4.2 x kilocalories (kcal).

[b]Retinol equivalents.

[c]Total vitamin E activity estimated to be 80 percent as D-tocopherol and 20 percent other tocopherols.

[d]The folacin allowances refer to dietary sources as determined by *Lactobacillus casei* assay. Pure forms of folacin may be effective in doses less than one-fourth of the Recommended Dietary Allowance.

[e]Although allowances are expressed as niacin, it is recognized that, on the average, 1 mg of niacin is derived from each 60 mg of dietary tryptophan.

Girls 13 and 14 years old, who are obsessed with the desire to become thinner, go on temporary diets to lose weight in spite of the resultant hunger and fatigue. Stunkard (1965) noted that psychological problems may be devastating. It was pointed out by Heald (1971) that teenagers can withstand caloric reduction better when the growth spurt is over than when they are still developing. This may be as early as age 13 for girls but around age 16 for boys (Huenemann 1971). Garn and Clark (1975) found that in the Ten-State Nutrition Survey different proportions of the children were obese in different socioeconomic groupings. Beyond infancy, the percentage defined as "obese" was necessarily less for the poor boys and girls and those below the poverty level. The higher percentages of fat children were more likely to be found among families with moderate incomes. On a study of 13- and 14-year-olds in Israel, the obese children knew more about the nutritive value of food, reported eating less than nonobese children, and ate fewer main meals per day. Similar findings have been reported in the United States. There is no doubt that obesity can be a real problem for the 10- to 14-year-old child in the developed countries. (See chapter 9 for a more complete discussion of obesity.)

Nutrition Education

Jenkins, Stumo, and Voichik (1975) reported that fourth-grade children who viewed "Mulligan Stew," a nutrition education film, increased their knowledge of nutrition. Moreover, the children who saw the film and who reported improved diets also showed the largest increase in nutrition knowledge. Baker (1972) found that nutrition education in the fourth and fifth grades can be effective and that the key is to get the children involved. Von Housen's (1971) program for nutrition education in Nebraska schools encouraged creativity and involvement of all the senses in learning about foods in the fourth, fifth, and sixth grades. Kolasa (1974) reported that many of the women she interviewed said that they had been most interested in learning about foods and cooking around the age of 9 or 10. Perhaps this should be an age when more emphasis is placed on foods and nutrition. Girls commonly become interested in the opposite sex around the age of 12, while boys are more interested in their stomachs until they are 14 or older.

Hinton et al. (1963) studied the eating behavior of girls 12 to 14 years of age in Iowa. Their findings indicated that the girls had better eating behavior and tended to select better diets in winter than in summer. The girls who had the best scores in emotional stability, conformity, adjustment to reality, and family relationships on the Minnesota Counseling Inventory missed fewer meals and had better diets than the other girls.

With maturity and experience, the preadolescent tends to reshuffle priorities affecting food choice. If during preadolescence family relationships are good, the conflicts which characterize adolescence will probably be relatively inconsequential. But if emotional adjustment is poor and family relationships are not healthy, erratic food practices may result. Therefore, it is extremely important that good food behavior be formed during the preadolescent years (Beyer and Morris, 1974).

ADOLESCENCE

Adolescence has been defined in physiological, sociological, and behavioral terms. Krogman (1972) considered the ages of 14 to 18 or 20 as adolescence. Thornburg (1970) referred to adolescence as a period during which the growing person makes the transition from childhood to adulthood. It is not any precise span of years but may be viewed as beginning with signs of puberty and continuing until sexual maturity and maximum physical growth have been achieved. In a similar way, Schoolar (1973) identified adolescence as the stage of life that starts with puberty and ends when independence from the parents has been attained.

From a behavioral perspective, adolescence has been regarded by Sieg (1971) as a period of development in human beings that begins when individuals feel that adult privileges are due them which are not being accorded them, and that ends when society has accorded them the full power and social status of an adult. This definition eliminates certain biological factors as irrelevant, such as puberty, the universality of adolescence, and chronological age. Instead, adolescence is a matter of people's perceptions of their rights. The attempt to attain the power and social status of an adult forms the basis for a person's actions during adolescence. As teenagers move toward independence, their interests, attitudes, and routines change; they try to conform to their conceptions of adult behavior. From the psychological point of view, teenagers are vulnerable to malnutrition because of their need to develop and use their growing sense of independence. They experience an intense need to get away from childhood and the control of their parents, and quite often they use food as one means of expressing their feelings. They may refuse to eat foods that they formerly accepted and liked; to show their objection to criticism or their resentment of advice from parents, they refuse to eat what those in authority say they ought to eat. Bizarre eating practices may result (Edwards 1964).

Coleman (1961) emphasized that the teenagers' subculture has a language all its own and a value system different from that of adults. Reeder (1971) found that the attitudes and values of teenagers were not very different from those of their parents but that the teenagers were more apt to take action. Mead (1972) stated that youth did not want to follow the style of their parents, because they considered it inappropriate to a modern world.

When family relationships are stable, fewer problems with eating behavior develop. For young people who have had unhealthy family relationships and poor emotional adjustment, adolescence seems to be the time when erratic food practices are common —crash diets, crazy fads, violent aversions, and missed meals (Hinton et al. 1963; Bruch 1970). Vegetarian rituals have been widespread among some high school groups (Bowden 1973).

Krogman (1972) said that from a physiological point of view the following changes can be expected to occur in normal adolescents: (1) increases in height and weight, (2) growth in various parts of the body, (3) changes in bone structure, (4) variations in bodily proportions, (5) growth of various internal organs, (6) changes in blood pressure, and (7) external and internal pubertal alterations, usually between the ages of 10 and 15 and earlier in girls than boys (e.g., voice change for boys, changes in the head hair pattern for both boys and girls, onset of menarche and development of the breasts for girls).

In addition to physical growth, adolescents are expected to accomplish certain developmental tasks as they evolve from children into adults. These developmental tasks are defined as "skills, knowledge and functions or attitudes which individuals should acquire within a specific period of their lives" (Thornberg 1970). A person's behavior is ultimately determined by whether or not these tasks are accomplished.

Nutritional Requirements and Food Behavior

All aspects of adolescence—physiological, sociological, and psychological—must be considered in studying the teenager's nutrition and food behavior since they are all interrelated. Because of the rapid physical changes occurring in their bodies, teenagers become particularly vulnerable to malnutrition (Gifft, Washbon, and Harrison 1972). Calorie and protein requirements closely parallel growth rate, and the onset of menarche in girls raises their iron requirement significantly. Furthermore, inefficient use of certain important nutrients, due to the frequency and magnitude of emotional problems, compounds the problem of inadequate nutrition (Stearns 1952). The achievement of independence and the need for solidarity with peers and for individual expression are often expressed in the teenager's choice of words, dress, and music, as well as in the choice of foods and the time and place to eat them (Weiner 1971).

Nutritional problems among the teenage population are similar to those of other population groups in the United States, but they may be accentuated by the high nutritional needs of teenagers (Gifft, Washbon, and Harrison 1972). Problems of underweight and overweight plague a substantial proportion of this group, and complications of pregnancy and the incidence of birth defects among infants of teenage mothers are significant (Everson 1960).

Concern over the nutritional status of teenagers is justified by evidence from several research studies. The Ten-State Nutrition Survey (Robbins 1972) revealed that "children under the age of 17, especially teenagers, had the highest prevalence of nutritional problems." The nutrient needs of teenagers are listed in table 6.

TABLE 6. NUTRIENT NEEDS OF ADOLESCENTS

	Males	Females	Pregnant	Lactating
Age (years)	15-18	15-18		
Weight (kg, lb)	61, 134	54, 119		
Height (cm, in.)	172, 69	162, 65		
Energy (kcal)[a]	3000	2100	+300	+500
Protein (g)	54	48	+30	+20
Fat-soluble vitamins				
Vitamin A activity				
RE[b]	1000	800	1000	1200
I.U.	5000	4000	5000	6000
Vitamin D (I.U.)	400	400	400	400
Vitamin E activity[c] (I.U.)	15	12	15	15
Water-soluble vitamins				
Ascorbic acid (mg)	45	45	60	80
Folacin[d] (mcg)	400	400	800	600
Niacin[e] (mg)	20	14	+2	+4
Riboflavin (mg)	1.8	1.4	+0.3	+0.5
Thiamin (mg)	1.5	1.1	+0.3	+0.3
Vitamin B_6 (mg)	2.0	2.0	2.5	2.5
Vitamin B_{12} (mcg)	3.0	3.0	4.0	4.0
Minerals				
Calcium (mg)	1200	1200	1200	1200
Phosphorus (mg)	1200	1200	1200	1200
Iodine (mcg)	150	115	125	150
Iron (mg)	18	18	18+[f]	18
Magnesium (mg)	400	300	450	450
Zinc (mg)	15	15	20	25

Source: Data from the National Research Council, *Recommended Dietary Allowances*, 8th ed. (Washington, D.C.: National Academy of Sciences, 1974).

[a]Kilojoules (kj) = 4.2 x kilocalories (kcal).

[b]Retinol equivalents.

[c]Total vitamin E activity estimated to be 80 percent as D-tocopherol and 20 percent other tocopherols.

[d]The folacin allowances refer to dietary sources as determined by *Lactobacillus casei* assay. Pure forms of folacin may be effective in doses less than one-fourth of the Recommended Dietary Allowance.

[e]Although allowances are expressed as niacin, it is recognized that, on the average, 1 mg of niacin is derived from each 60 mg of dietary tryptophan.

[f]This increased requirement cannot be met by ordinary diets; therefore, the use of supplemental iron is recommended.

Everson (1960) stated that there is little question that teenagers display limited judgment in choosing food. Several studies that involved determining the nutritional status of this age group revealed dietary shortcomings of several important nutrients. Inadequate quantities of calcium, vitamin A, and ascorbic acid were reported by both Everson (1960) and Schorr, Sanjur, and Erickson (1972), who observed that 21 percent of the teenagers they studied consumed less than two-thirds of the Recommended Dietary Allowance for ascorbic acid, and 44 percent, 69 percent, and 51 percent received less than two-thirds of the Recommended Dietary Allowances for calcium, iron, and vitamin A, respectively. Everson (1960) and Hodges and Krehl (1965) noted that even though the total daily protein intake might appear adequate, poor distribution of protein intake during the day could result in amino acid mixtures that would not support optimal growth. Hodges and Krehl also mentioned high consumption of fats and "empty calories," as did Edwards (1964). The finding of high levels of cholesterol in the blood of a large number of teenagers has increased concern over the diet of this group (Hodges and Krehl 1965). Even though boys are less prone than girls to nutritional inadequacies, owing to the large volume of food they ingest (Schorr, Sanjur, and Erickson 1972), they also consume more fat than girls. An average of 43.5 percent of the total calories consumed by boys in the study by Hodges and Krehl (1965) was in the form of fat, a percentage higher than that recommended by the American Heart Association. Also, the significant correlation found by Hodges and Drehl (1965) between greater height and weight and higher triglyceride concentrations in the blood would prove more problematic for boys than for girls. And finally, frequent between-meal snacks and the consumption of foods high in carbohydrates such as candy, soft drinks, and pastries, have been associated with the development of dental caries among adolescents (Robbins 1972).

Huenemann et al. (1968), in an investigation of teenagers' opinions of their own food practices, asked: "Some people say teenagers don't eat the right foods. Do you agree with the people who say this? Why do you agree or disagree?" About 44 percent of the boys and 48 percent of the girls said they agreed with the statement and about 5 percent were undecided and said that the statement is sometimes right and sometimes wrong. The reasons for disagreeing included such statements as "teenagers eat as well as adults" and "people's views on teenagers' eating habits are inaccurate, prejudiced, or overgeneralized," while others commented that teenagers eat well because "parents provide good guidance." Those who agreed with the statement said that time pressures, peer-group influence, and poor motivation were some of the factors that resulted in their poor food practices. In tests of teenagers' attitudes toward dietary changes needed for reaching the ideal body shape and size, girls seem generally more accepting than boys of dietary modifications.

Dinner was the preferred meal, especially for boys. More girls than boys chose lunch, and breakfast was almost as popular as lunch with the boys, but not so with the girls. At both the ninth- and eleventh-grade levels, the leading reasons given by those who preferred breakfast were its effect in providing energy and relief from hunger. The three leading reasons for choosing lunch in both the ninth and the eleventh grades were the company of friends, the freedom experienced at this meal, and relief from hunger. In the case of dinner, about 70 percent of the ninth graders and eleventh graders who chose this meal as their favorite gave food as the reason—the type, the amount, the method of preparation, and the wide variety offered. Second in frequency, but totaling only 17 percent for boys and 38 percent for girls, were reasons related to the atmosphere at dinner time (leisure, surroundings). Hunger ranked third and the company present was fourth.

Some of the reasons for meal preferences among the teenagers may give an indication of teenage values. It is interesting to note that while ninth-grade boys and girls were alike in mentioning the type of food served as the most frequent reason for their choice, the less frequent reasons of variety in food and company present were mentioned much more often by girls than by boys. By the eleventh grade, environment seemed to have become more important to both sexes and the type of food less so (Huenemann et al. 1968).

Teenagers may skip meals because they do not have the patience to sit down and eat when they are anticipating an event. In interviews with 15- to 17-year-olds, Spindler and Acker (1963) found that every group interviewed expressed the idea that they were often in such a hurry that they did not have time to eat. The amount eaten and the regularity of eating was influenced by time. If a teenager had a school or club activity, a date or a chance to be with friends, meals appeared to be secondary (Spindler and Acker 1963; Spindler 1964).

Leverton (1968) said that teenagers wanted "fast food" and other convenient foods. They were snackers and frequently consumed soft drinks, french fries, and similar items (Ullrich 1972). The snacks they ate with their friends at vending machines, drive-ins, or other places made a beneficial contribution to their daily diet unless the foods were high in calories but low in other nutrients (Spindler 1964; Thomas and Call 1973). Wyman (1972) noted that teenagers may restrict themselves to a few favorite foods or use unusual combinations of foods.

Interest in Food and Nutrition

Orr (1965) found that nutrition rated lowest of all health areas in terms of the expressed health interests of 250 high school seniors. High school students' attitudes toward nutrition education and their knowledge of nutrition were also assessed by Dwyer, Feldman, and Mayer (1970), who found a notable lack of interest among the majority of students tested. Many students commented that nutrition education was "boring" or "old hat" and involved the memorization of useless facts rather than real understanding. Kirk et al. (1975) found that nutrition ranked lowest on the ladder of students' health interests, and Lantagne (1952) found nutrition to be of only "average" interest to 10,000 secondary school students in twenty-six high schools in ten different states. However, when an item analysis of the interest in 300 health topics was made, there were 12 topics related directly or indirectly to food and nutrition that were among the 50 topics of greatest interest to the students. The author concluded that low interest in a health area does not imply that all problems within that area are of little interest to students; rather, in each major health area there may be specific topics in which students are not at all interested and others in which they are very interested. This also seemed to be the case in Orr's study. Again, even though food and nutrition ranked lowest in the health interests of the students, the following were included among the 10 most interesting topics: heart disease, the effects of alcohol on the body, how a human baby develops, the care of the eyes, and skin blemishes in the teen years. These topics certainly can be considered related to food and nutrition. Orr also found that, even though general interest in nutrition was low, causes of overweight and underweight, how glands affect the body's use of food, disorders produced by the lack of vitamins, individual differences in food needs, and the proper cooking of foods were topics that students rated highest in the area of nutrition. Likewise, Dowell (1966) found that secondary students were highly interested in certain topics associated with nutrition, such as fitness, weight control, skin, and eyes, and that they worried most about dental problems, acne, and overweight. Dwyer, Feldman, and Mayer (1960) and

Spindler and Acker (1963) also found among this age group considerable interest in weight problems and skin problems.

Since attitudes often pose blocks to better eating habits, it is important to be aware of prevailing feelings in order to approach nutrition education from a more practical standpoint. Insight into factors that motivate adolescents, pertinent topics for nutrition education, and problem areas through which one might inspire the teenager's interest is essential for planning nutrition education programs. Obviously, programs geared toward meeting the needs of a particular group will be most successful. Kirk et al. (1975), who in an earlier study that found students showed interest in a few nutrition-related topics but had a general lack of interest in the overall area of nutrition, have put their findings to work in a practical manner. They have integrated nutrition instruction into the curriculum of a comprehensive health education program, using appropriate topics in nutrition as the connecting threads between study units. The results of that effort will be available shortly.

The necessity of recognizing and respecting the complexity of the needs and problems that characterize the teenager's world today was stressed by Leverton (1968). Among the reasons she gave for lack of success in encouraging teenagers to adhere to the guidelines prescribed by nutrition educators were (1) too often teenagers have been given the idea that nutrition means eating what you don't like, because it is good for you, rather than eating well because it will help you in what you want to do and become; (2) adolescents are not experiencing the nutritional disaster that adults are telling them will result from poor food habits; (3) food is only one component of the busy lives of teenagers and can receive only a fraction of their attention; and (4) many persons in strategic positions to help them are not knowledgeable about practical nutrition and some are actually misinformed.

Level of Nutrition Knowledge

The teenager's overall lack of interest in nutrition-related topics may be responsible for the apparent low correlation between the amount of effort devoted to nutrition education and the reported measurements of food and nutrition knowledge.

Few studies have been published on the measurement of teenagers' knowledge of food and nutrition. Those that are available are generally limited with regard to geographic location or the percentage of the population tested, or both, and they usually test food and nutrition knowledge along with various other health-related factors. In the study conducted by Dwyer, Feldman, and Mayer (1970), 1,338 students, representing 42 percent of all students in selected grades in five urban high schools in Massachusetts, had a mean score of 55.9 out of a possible score of 100 on a test of nutrition knowledge.

Kirk et al. (1975) found that, even though students at all grade levels received more instruction in the field of nutrition than in any other health-related area, their knowledge of nutrition, as measured by a standardized health behavior inventory, ranked far below their knowledge of all other health areas. Likewise, a national survey of school health education showed that the lowest percentage of correct responses among twelth graders was in the area of nutrition, as compared with eleven other areas of health education (Sliepcevich 1964).

Using a different approach, Dowell (1966) studied the incidence of neglect of nutrition instruction in the secondary schools in relation to nutrition problems encountered in the community, expecting that there would be an inverse relationship between the emphasis on nutrition education and the incidence of nutrition-related problems. Dowell found instead a higher incidence of health problems related to nutrition than had been expected, considering the instruction given.

On a more positive note, Dwyer, Feldman, and Mayer (1970) did find an insignificant but consistent increase in the level of nutrition knowledge from grade to grade, which they attributed to the gathering of more information about nutrition through both formal instruction, in such courses as biology and chemistry and from informal education and experiences outside of school. Schwartz (1975), however, reported that the influence of teenagers' nutrition knowledge on their eating practices seemed to be slight.

Misconceptions about Food and Nutrition

It seems probable that, in addition to low motivation for learning due to lack of interest in food and nutrition, low performance on tests of nutrition knowledge could result from the prevalence among teenagers of misconceptions regarding food and nutrition.

Results of the Tennessee Health Education Project conducted by Kirk et al. (1975), in which low mean nutrition knowledge scores were found on the elementary, junior high, and senior high levels in spite of strong emphasis on nutrition education, prompted the authors' suggestion that possibly the educational program was effectively inculcating *misinformation*. Few attempts have been made to distinguish between wrong answers resulting from lack of information and wrong answers due to misinformation, even though wrong answers on nutrition tests may well indicate that students are misinformed rather than uninformed (Dwyer, Feldman, and Mayer 1970).

Wang (1971) defined a *misconception* as "a belief commonly held as true but which is not in accord with scientific evidence"; misconceptions "include fallacies, fads, and half-truths." Wrong learning or misinformation as well as inadequate learning or insufficient information can give rise to misconceptions (Heflin and Pangle 1966).

According to Gifft, Washbon, and Harrison (1972), teenagers are, in general, psychologically and socially prone to nutritional problems. Their need to express independence is often reflected in the adoption of eating patterns calculated to test adult restrictions. Fad diets and peculiar notions about the positive and negative attributes of foods are perpetuated by the all-important peer group. Fads and cult practices such as Zen macrobiotic diets appeal to the teenager's need for independence and identity. Concern over the rapid physiological changes occurring in their bodies often causes teenagers to manipulate their diet in an attempt to influence their physical appearance. When such changes in diet are based on erroneous beliefs or misinformation, they are undesirable, at the least, and sometimes dangerous.

Nutrition concepts are open to various interpretations, and misinformation abounds. Teenagers, along with the vast majority of the American public, are bombarded with nutrition information and misinformation from a variety of sources (Bruch 1970; Henderson 1974; New and Priest 1967; Rynearson 1974; Sipple 1964). Possibly more misconceptions and half-truths are still believed by the American public about nutrition than about any other area of health. Kilander et al. (1975) concluded from the results of a thirty-three-item multiple-choice test that nearly one-half of the 5,000 subjects, a majority of whom were high school graduates and 30 percent of whom were college graduates, lacked sufficient knowledge to choose adequate diets for themselves.

A high prevalence of misconceptions regarding food and nutrition has been found among children, students in junior and senior high school, 4-H youths, university students, college graduates, and low-income Negro and white urban families.

Misconceptions relating to health, especially in the area of nutrition, are common among children and youth. Seven out of ten girls in the tenth grade believed that any food that does not smell or taste spoiled is safe to eat. Three out of four fifth- and sixth-grade pupils and more than half of a group of tenth-grade girls believed that taking vitamin pills guaranteed good health, and one-half of the tenth-grade girls believed vitamins in pills are better than vitamins in natural foods. The belief that hot food is more nutritious than cold was held by one out of three college students (Sutton 1962).

Williams (1956) developed an instrument to measure high school students' misconceptions about health. A study done with ninth, tenth, eleventh, and twelfth graders in North Carolina showed that they had a great many, most of which had to do with nutrition and personal and environmental health. Ninth graders had more misconceptions about nutrition than students in the other three grades.

In a study of the prevalence of nutrition misconceptions among college freshmen prior to instruction in nutrition (Osman 1967), the mean number of misconceptions about nutrition was 30.90 out of 144 and the mean "don't know" score was 33.84, resulting in a total of 64 statements out of 144 which the students could not answer correctly. Boys subscribed to more misconceptions and had more "don't know" responses than did girls, although the differences were not significant.

Heflin and Pangle (1966) administered the Dearborn Health Knowledge Test to 243 Peabody College students in a required health education course. A substantial number of students exhibited misconceptions on six out of the fifteen questions related to nutrition and diet. Likewise Adams (1959), who studied the health misconceptions of college freshmen at the University of Oregon, found the greatest percentage of misconceptions to be in the area of foods and nutrition and to be held by males. Females believed 43 percent of the nineteen nutrition misconceptions whereas males believed 49 percent.

In a study by McCarthy and Sabry (1973), first-year students at a Canadian university subscribed to a substantial number of nutrition misconceptions. The mean misconception score on a seventy-item questionnaire to which students could answer "true," "false," or "don't know" was 18.6, the mean correct answer score was 37.8, and the mean "don't know" response was 13.6. The sex of the student made little difference in either the misconception or the correct answer score, nor were misconception scores related to whether a student's background was rural or urban or to the number of years the student has been in a 4-H club.

On the basis of information obtained through studies of the prevalence of misconceptions about food and nutrition, it can be surmised that the percentage of misconceptions varies according to the categories of topics covered in the survey. McCarthy and Sabry (1973) found a high number of misconceptions regarding environmental factors (food additives, pesticide residues, food processing, and food enrichment) and fewer misconceptions regarding special "health" foods, soil depletion, chemical fertilizers, and insecticides.

It also has been observed that, for some population groups, formal training in home economics or related areas may lower misconception scores and increase correct responses on tests designed to measure food and nutrition knowledge and misconceptions. In Wilson and Lamb's (1968) study of 119 women belonging to three different women's organizations, women with backgrounds in home economics did not have as many misconceptions about food as did their peers with higher education in academic disciplines other than home economics. In general, however, college graduates accepted more false beliefs about food than did women who were not college graduates. The investigators concluded that education in home economics at the college level contributes to correct beliefs about food. Likewise, Bremer and Weatherholtz (1975) found that adults with formal training in nutrition and biochemistry were more skeptical of the value of "organic" and "health" foods than those without such training.

McCarthy and Sabry (1973) found that home economics education in secondary school appeared to be related to lower misconception scores and higher correct answer scores among first-year Canadian university students. However, Singleton (1974) observed that high school home economics instruction was unrelated to the soundness of the dietary practices of pregnant teenagers. A study by Harrison and Irwin (1964) showed that a large percentage of junior high students subscribed to a number of harmful misconceptions about health, many in the area of food and nutrition, regardless of their metropolitan area, sex, or grade level or the number of semesters of health instruction they had had. Moreover, in a study conducted by Baker, Frank, and Pangle (1964), it appeared that the recency of health instruction bore no relation to the number of misconceptions held by the subjects and did not reduce the prevalence of their misconceptions. In this study, which measured misconceptions related to food and nutrition along with ten other health areas, students with no previous health instruction tended to have no more misconceptions than those who had already had some health instruction. Williams (1956), however, noted a slight but progressive decline in misconceptions about nutrition as the pupils moved from the ninth to the twelth grade.

The ability of 4-H youth to distinguish nutrition misconceptions from facts was found by Wang (1971) to be similar to that of low-income homemakers, which was poor compared with middle-income homemakers. She attributed the differences in knowledge of nutrition to the differences in level of education and concomitant greater varieties of experience. Similarly, according to Jalso, Burns, and Rivers (1965), the respondents to a questionnaire on beliefs about food who were classified as food "faddists" had less formal education and less nutrition education than did "non-faddists" and were concentrated in the older age and lower income groups. Also, in a study of 310 low-income, urban black heads of households, Cornely, Bigman, and Watts (1963) found education to be more closely related to the rejection of folk beliefs than age, previous residence, or number of children in specific age categories. It was concluded that low-income families have insufficient information about the essentials of an adequate diet and that they retain faith in a number of erroneous folk beliefs concerning food and nutrition.

It seems that certain populations may be more open to misinformation than others. In a study conducted to determine whether faddist beliefs and practices are associated with age and educational level, there was a positive correlation between educational level and scores for both nutritional practices and opinions; but as age increased, scores for both opinions and practices decreased (Jalso, Burns, and Rivers 1965).

Dwyer, Feldman, and Mayer (1970) noted a surprising discrepancy between the level of knowledge and the areas of interest in food and nutrition of the teenage girls they studied. The areas of greatest interest to the girls, as expressed on a five-question open-ended questionnaire, were the very ones they knew least about. The investigators attributed this inconsistency to the fact that, of all nutritional topics, weight control and energy balance are probably those about which misinformation is most abundant and most publicized. It may be that the girls absorbed more information on those subjects because they were interested in them and because information (including misinformation) was readily available from many sources. Exposure to more sources of information may also account for Wilson and Lamb's (1968) finding more misconceptions about nutrition among the women who were college graduates than among those who were not.

The evidence, then, is contradictory regarding the relationship between prevalence of misconceptions and degree of education. It seems that, in one instance, training in home economics decreased the number of false beliefs about food. It also appears, however, that, while general education and an interest in specific topics related to food and nutrition result in greater exposure to information on the subject, much of that information may be erroneous. It seems plausible that the general characteristics of certain population groups (for example, the aged and adolescents) contribute to their gullibility where food and nutrition misinformation is concerned.

The Effect of Misinformation on Nutrition-related Behavior

It is important to consider the effect that common misinformation about nutrition and food has on the food behavior of various population groups, since knowledge of scientifically correct information often has relatively little effect on a person's behavior. While people do realize scientific knowledge, they also pay attention to symbolic relationships, and their emotions may override reason, rigorous logic, and scientific knowledge.

Although it is important to gear nutrition education programs to teenagers' values and interests, it is equally important to recognize that a teenager's methods of realizing values and satisfying interests are often based on erroneous information. For instance, health ranked first in a study conducted to determine the values influencing the food choices of teenage boys (McElroy and Taylor 1966), but the layman's notion of what is healthful or good to eat is often based on unfounded beliefs rather than on scientific evidence (Dwyer, Feldman, and Mayer 1970). Litman, Cooney, and Stief (1964) studied 1,039 subjects between the ages of 10 and 22 and found that their preferences for such foods as milk, meat, eggs, spinach, fruits, and fruit juices were indeed based on health- and nutrition-related rationale. An evaluation of the students' responses revealed, however, that only 60 percent of their reasons could be adjudged nutritionally accurate. Furthermore, there seemed to be considerable reliance on erroneous information. Dwyer, Feldman, and Mayer (1970, p. 65) maintained that

> teaching based on overcoming deeply entrenched mistaken notions about nutrition based on incorrect information and replacing it with correct concepts is a more difficult task than teaching the correct concept to a totally naive subject. Those who have misconceptions are often less responsive and attentive pupils since they believe they already possess the correct information.

Sources of Information on Food and Nutrition

If misinformation is such a critical factor in determining the food behavior of teenagers, it would seem essential to determine how, where, and why they receive information about food and nutrition. A review of the available literature reveals that few studies have been conducted to identify the sources of teenagers' information on nutrition.

Jalso, Burns, and Rivers (1965) studied the nutritional opinions and practices of 101 subjects representing a wide range of age, income, and formal education. They found that subjects classified as faddists read more nutrition books of questionable validity than books considered reliable by nutritionists. Magazines and newspapers were the main sources of nutrition information for both faddists and nonfaddists, whereas radio and television were not major sources of information from either group. It is not possible, however, to generalize the results of this study to the teenage population, because differences among age groups were not determined in the investigation.

In a study of the nutritional knowledge, attitudes, and practices of Canadian public health nurses (Schwartz 1976), nurses who had received nutrition instruction and information from a nursing instructor during their training program achieved significantly lower scores in tests of nutritional knowledge and practices than nurses who were taught by a nutritionist or a dietitian. Schwartz concluded that it should not be assumed that all sources of nutrition education contribute to the improvement of the knowledge, attitudes, and practices of public health nurses.

A somewhat dated, but nevertheless disturbing, review conducted by a government committee, in which selected public-school textbooks were reviewed for the scientific accuracy of their health information, revealed that nutrition ranked high in the percentage of errors reported and that the errors increased with the age of the book (Committee on Health Content Textbooks 1953).

Interest in the subject matter is an important prerequisite to learning. Bremer and Weatherholtz (1975) studied the nutritional attitudes of 670 people in a university community and found that those who indicated the greatest interest in nutrition had the best scores on factual questions on nutrition and expressed the greatest confidence in the relationship between diet and health. Shipmen and McCannon (1964) found that people were more interested in topics that had personal relevance for them and were more apt to seek out information on such topics.

Understanding the changing food habits, food beliefs, and food practices of preadolescents and adolescents is a difficult task. The teenager's concern about acne or overweight or underweight or time affects food behavior but may be short-lived. Rather than investing time and resources in dealing with such specific concerns, food and nutrition professionals must direct their skills toward providing information that will help the teenager form a life-time food pattern that will ensure adequate nutrition.

REFERENCES

Preadolescence

Baker, M. 1972. Influence of nutrition education on fourth and fifth graders. *Journal of Nutrition Education* 4:55.

Beyer, N. R., and Morris, P. M. 1974. Food attitudes and snacking pattern of young children. *Journal of Nutrition Education* 6:131.

Garn, S., and Clark, D. 1975. Nutrition, growth, development and maturation: Findings from the Ten-State Nutrition Survey of 1968-1970. *Pediatrics* 56:306.

Heald, F. 1971. Health status of youth. In *Proceedings of the National Nutrition Education Conference.* Miscellaneous publication no. 1254. Washington, D.C.: U.S. Department of Agriculture, April 1973.

Hinton, M. A.; Eppright, E. S.; Chadderdon, J.; and Wolins, L. 1963. Eating behavior and dietary intake of girls 12 to 14 years old. *Journal of the American Dietetic Association* 43:223.

Huenemann, R. 1971., A review of teenage nutrition in the United States. In *Proceedings of the National Nutrition Education Conference.* Miscellaneous publication no. 1254. Washington, D.C.: U.S. Department of Agriculture, April 1973.

Jenkins, S.; Stumo, M.; and Voichik, J. 1975. Evaluation of the nutrition film series "Mulligan Stew." *Journal of Nutrition Education* 7:17.

Kaufmann, N.; Poxnanski, R.; and Guggenheim, K. 1975. Eating habits and opinions of teenagers on nutrition and obesity. *Journal of the American Dietetic Association* 66:264.

Kolasa, K. 1974. Foodways of selected mothers and their adult daughters in upper east Tennessee. Ph.D. thesis, University of Tennessee (Knoxville).

Krogman, W. 1972. *Child growth.* Ann Arbor: University of Michigan Press.

Stunkard, A. 1965. Psychological factors in the development of obesity. Presented at the 49th Annual Meeting of the Federation of American Societies for Experimental Biology, 14-16 April.

Van Schaik, T. F. 1964. Food and nutrition relative to family life. *Journal of Home Economics* 56:225.

Von Housen, A. A. 1971. Food—Life depends on it. *Journal of Nutrtiion Education* 3:61.

Adolescence

Adams, S. L. 1959. Health misconceptions among students enrolled in freshmen health classes at the University of Oregon. M.S. thesis, University of Oregon (Eugene).

Baker, B.; Frank, J.; and Pangle, R. 1964. A new approach in determining health misconceptions. *Journal of School Health* 34:300.

Bowden, N. J. 1973. Food patterns and food needs of adolescents. *Journal of School Health* 43:165.

Bremer, M., and Weatherholtz, W. M. 1975. Nutrition attitudes in a university community. *Journal of Nutrition Education* 7:60.

Bruch, H. 1970. The allure of food cults and nutritional quackery. *Journal of the American Dietetic Association* 57:316.

Buchan, J. W. 1972. *America's health: Fallacies, beliefs, practices.* DHEW publication no. (FDA) 75-2017. Washington, D.C.: Government Printing Office.

Carruth, B. R., and Foree, S. B. 1971. Cartoon approach to nutrition education. *Journal of Nutrition Education* 3:57.

Coleman, J. S. 1961. The adolescent society: The social life of the teenager and its impact on education. Free Press of Glencoe. New York.

Committee on Health Content Textbooks. 1953. Accuracy of health content of school textbooks. *American Journal of Public Health* 43:128.

Cornely, P. B.; Bigman, S. K.; and Watts, D. D. 1963. Nutritional beliefs among a low-income urban population. *Journal of the American Dietetic Association* 42:131.

Dowell, L. J. 1966. A study of selected health education implications. *Research Quarterly* 37:23.

Dwyer, J. T.; Feldman, J. J.; and Mayer, J. 1970. Nutritional literacy of high school students. *Journal of Nutrition Education* 2:59.

Edwards, C. H. 1964. Nutrition survey of 6200 teenage youth. *Journal of the American Dietetic Association* 45:543.

Erhard, D. 1971. Nutrition education for the "now" generation. *Journal of Nutrition Education* 3:135.

Everson, G. J. 1960. Bases for concern about teenagers' diets. *Journal of the American Dietetic Association* 36:17.

Fusillo, A. 1974. Food shoppers' beliefs: Myths and realities. DHEW publication no. (FDA) 75-2017. Washington, D.C.: Government Printing Office.

Gifft, H. H.; Washbon, M. B.; and Harrison, G. G. 1972. *Nutrition, behavior, and change.* Englewood Cliffs, N.J.: Prentice-Hall.

Harrison, P. E., and Irwin, L. W. 1964. Certain harmful health misconceptions of junior high school students attending public schools in metropolitan areas. *Research Quarterly* 35:491.

Heflin, B., and Pangle, R. 1966. Health misconceptions of college students. *Journal of the American College Health Association* 14:154.

Henderson, L. M. 1974. Programs to combat nutritional quackery. *Nutrition Reviews* 32 (supplement 1):67.

Hinton, M. A.; Eppright, E. S.; Chadderdon, H.; and Wolins, L. 1963. Eating behavior and dietary intake of girls 12 to 14 years old. *Journal of the American Dietetic Association* 43:223.

Hodges, R. E., and Krehl, W. A. 1965. Nutritional status of teenagers in Iowa. *American Journal of Clinical Nutrition* 17:200.

Huenemann, R. L.; Shapiro, L. R.; Hampton, M. C.; and Mitchell, B. W. 1968. Food and eating practices of teenagers. *Journal of the American Dietetic Association* 53:17.

Huntsinger, P. 1971. The status of health instruction in the public schools of Tennessee. Ph.D thesis, University of Tennessee (Knoxville).

Jalso, S. B.; Burns, M. M.; and Rivers, J. M. 1965. Nutritional beliefs and practices. *Journal of the American Dietetic Association* 47:263.

Kilander, R. H.; Hamrick, M.; and McAfee, D. C. 1975. Nutrition in health instruction: The Tennessee Health Education Project. *Journal of Nutrition Education* 7:68.

Kirk, R. H.; Hamrick, M.; and McAfee, D. C. 1975. Nutrition in health instruction—The Tennessee Health Education Project. *Journal of Nutrition Education* 7:68.

Kolasa, K. M. 1974. Foodways of selected mothers and their adult daughters in upper east Tennessee. Ph.D. thesis, University of Tennessee (Knoxville).

Krogman, W. M. 1972. *Child growth.* Ann Arbor: University of Michigan Press.

Lantagne, J. E. 1952. Health interests of 10,000 secondary school students. *Research Quarterly* 23:330.

Leverton, R. M. 1968. The paradox of teenage nutrition. *Journal of the American Dietetic Association* 53:13.

Litman, T. J.; Cooney, J. P.; and Stief, R. 1964. The views of Minnesota school children on food. *Journal of the American Dietetic Association* 45:433.

McCarthy, M. E., and Sabry, J. H. 1973. Canadian university students' nutrition misconceptions. *Journal of Nutrition Education* 5:193.

McElroy, J., and Taylor, B. 1966. Adolescents' values in selection of food. *Journal of Home Economics* 58:651.

Mead, M. 1972. Youth and culture. In *Youth: Problems and approaches,* ed. S. J. Shamsie. Philadelphia: Lea and Febiger.

National Research Council. 1974. *Recommended Dietary Allowances.* 8th ed. Washington, D.C.: National Academy of Sciences.

New, P. K., and Priest, R. P. 1967. Food and thought: A sociological study of food cultists. *Journal of the American Dietetic Association* 51:13.

Orr, O. P. 1965. An evaluation of health interests and health needs as basic premises in selecting health content in secondary schools of Knoxville, Tennessee. Ph.D. thesis, University of Tennessee (Knoxville).

Osman, J. D. 1967. Nutrition misconceptions of college subjects. M.S. thesis, University of Maryland (College Park).

Reeder, W. W. 1971. The attitudes, values and life styles of youth. In *Proceedings of the National Nutrition Education Conference.* Miscellaneous publication no. 1254. Washington, D.C.: U.S. Department of Agriculture, April 1973.

Reynolds, W. J. 1960. A determination of the prevalence of certain harmful health misconceptions among high school coaches and physical educators in Massachusetts. M.S. thesis, Boston University.

Robbins, C. E. 1972. Ten-State Nutrition Survey: Educational implications. *Journal of Nutrition Education* 4:157.

Rynearson, E. B. 1974. Americans love hogwash. *Nutrition Reviews* 32 (supplement 1):1.

Schoolar, J. C. 1973. *Current issues in adolescent psychiatry.* New York: Brunner-Mazel.

Schorr, B. C.; Sanjur, D.; and Erickson, E. C. 1972. Teen-age food habits. *Journal of the American Dietetic Association* 61:415.

Schwartz, N. E. 1975. Nutritional knowledge, attitudes and practices of high school graduates. *Journal of the American Dietetic Association* 66:28.

Schwartz, N. E. 1976. Nutrition knowledge, attitudes and practices of Canadian public health nurses. *Journal of Nutrition Education* 8:28.

Shipman, J. A., and McCannon, N. R. 1964. Urbanites must be approached through recognized information sources. *Journal of Home Economics* 56:744.

Sieg, A. 1971. Why adolescence occurs. *Adolescence* 6:337.

Singleton, N. C. 1974. Adequacy of the diets of pregnant teenagers: Educational, nutritional, and socioeconomic factors. Ph.D. thesis, Louisiana State University (Baton Rouge).

Sipple, H. L. 1964. Combatting nutrition misinformation through coordinated programs. *American Journal of Public Health* 54:823.

Sliepcevich, E. M. 1964. *School health education study: Summary report of a nationwide study of health instruction in the public schools.* School Health Education Study. Washington, D.C.: U.S. Department of Health, Education and Welfare.

Spindler, E. B. 1964. Better diets for teenagers. *Nursing Outlook* 12 (2):32.

Spindler, E. B., and Acker, G. 1963. Teen-agers tell us about their nutrition. *Journal of the American Dietetic Association* 43:228.

Stearns, G. 1952. Nutritional health of infants, children and adolescents. In *Proceedings of the National Food and Nutrition Institution,* Agricultural Handbook no. 56. Washington, D.C.: U.S. Department of Agriculture.

Stevenson, E. H. 1965. Nutrition nonsense. In *Yearbook of agriculture, 1965.* Washington, D.C.: Government Printing Office.

Sutton, W. C. 1962. Misconceptions about health among children and youth. *Journal of School Health* 32:347.

Swedish Nutrition Foundation. 1969. *Food cultism and quackery.* Eighth symposium of the Swedish Nutrition Foundation, Uppsala.

Thomas, J. A., and Call, D. L. 1973. Eating between meals: A nutrition problem among teenagers? *Nutrition Reviews* 31:137.

Thornburg, H. 1970. Adolescence: Reinterpretation. *Adolescence* 5:463.

Ullrich, J. D. 1972. Nutrition Education Conference: Youth nutrition-community. *Journal of Nutrition Education* 4:7.

Walker, M. A. 1975. Homemakers' food and nutrition knowledge—Implications for nutrition education. *Nutrition Program News,* May-June, p. 1.

Wang, V. L. 1971. Food information of homemakers and 4-H youths. *Journal of the American Dietetic Association* 58:215.

Weiner, I. B. 1971. The generation gap—Fact or fancy? *Adolescence* 6:155.

Williams, L. M. 1956. Critical study of some health misconceptions held by 9th, 10th, 11th and 12th grade pupils in Eastman High School, Enfeld, North Carolina. M.S. thesis, North Carolina College (Durham).

Wilson, M. M., and Lamb, M. W. 1968. Food beliefs as related to ecological factors in women. *Journal of Home Economics* 69 (2):115.

Wyman, J. R. 1972. Teenagers and food: Their eating habits. *Food and Nutrition* 2 (1):3.

Food Behavior throughout Life — The Adult Years

YOUNG FAMILIES

Parents of young children range in age from teenagers to adults in their middle thirties or older. The family's surroundings, its composition (number of members, age, sex, race, etc.), the schedules of the various members, the success of the parents in their careers, and the relations between family members all affect the family's food behavior (Van Schaik 1964). The nutrient needs of adults under age 50 are given in tables 7 and 8.

Societal expectations of young married couples and the developmental tasks they need to accomplish are (1) learning to live with a partner, (2) starting a family, (3) rearing children, (4) managing a home, (5) getting started in an occupation, (6) taking on civic responsibility, and (7) finding a congenial group of friends. Successful achievement of these tasks leads to a more stable family life (Kaluger and Kaluger 1974).

Each partner brings to a family a set of values modified by his or her development in a particular family, in a particular place in that family, and in a particular social group (Bott 1971). The new family is an amalgamation of the traits of the original families modified to suit the needs of the new family. The family is the cultural link between generations. During meals the child is taught table manners—how to eat, sit, speak, and so forth. Through this and the table talk, the family transmits its culture to the child and lays the basis for the child's future food behavior.

The family can have a positive or a negative effect on food patterns. The inability of parents to educate their children in food behavior essential for good health may result in unbalanced nutrition in later years. If parents use food of high caloric value to show love for or to reward or punish their children, the results may be decayed teeth, a poor appetite, and a diet rich in "empty calories" and poor in animal protein, minerals, and vitamins. The children's physical growth may be impaired and they may become obese.

One reason for the tenacity of food habits is their association with family. The family meal is one of the most important influences on a family's morale and sense of unity. The roles of close relative, father, brother, sister, and grandmother are clearly

TABLE 7. NUTRIENT NEEDS OF ADULTS (AGES 19-22)

	Males	Females	Pregnant	Lactating
Age (years)	19-22	19-22		
Weight (kg, lb)	67, 147	58, 128		
Height (cm, in.)	172, 69	162, 65		
Energy (kcal)[a]	3000	2100	+300	+500
Protein (g)	54	46	+30	+20
Fat-soluble vitamins				
Vitamin A activity				
RE[b]	1000	800	1000	1200
I.U.	5000	4000	5000	6000
Vitamin D (I.U.)	400	400	400	400
Vitamin E activity[c] (I.U.)	15	12	15	15
Water-soluble vitamins				
Ascorbic acid (mg)	45	45	60	80
Folacin[d] (mcg)	400	400	800	600
Niacin[e] (mg)	20	14	+2	+4
Riboflavin (mg)	1.8	1.4	+0.3	+0.5
Thiamin (mg)	1.5	1.1	+0.3	+0.3
Vitamin B_6 (mg)	2.0	2.0	2.5	2.5
Vitamin B_{12} (mcg)	3.0	3.0	4.0	4.0
Minerals				
Calcium (mg)	800	800	1200	1200
Phosphorus (mg)	800	800	1200	1200
Iodine (mcg)	140	100	125	150
Iron (mg)	10	18	18+[f]	18
Magnesium (mg)	350	300	450	450
Zinc (mg)	15	15	20	25

Source: Data from the National Research Council, *Recommended Dietary Allowances*, 8th ed. (Washington, D.C.: National Academy of Sciences, 1974).

[a]Kilojoules (kj) = 4.2 x kilocalories (kcal).

[b]Retinol equivalents.

[c]Total vitamin E activity estimated to be 80 percent as D-tocopherol and 20 percent other tocopherols.

[d]The folacin allowances refer to dietary sources as determined by *Lactobacillus casei* assay. Pure forms of folacin may be effective in doses less than one-fourth of the Recommended Dietary Allowance.

[e]Although allowances are expressed as niacin, it is recognized that, on the average, 1 mg of niacin is derived from each 60 mg of dietary tryptophan.

[f]This increased requirement cannot be met by ordinary diets; therefore, the use of supplemental iron is recommended.

TABLE 8. NUTRIENT NEEDS OF ADULTS (AGES 23-50)

	Males	Females	Pregnant	Lactating
Age (years)	23-50	23-50		
Weight (kg, lb)	70, 154	58, 128		
Height (cm, in.)	172, 69	162, 65		
Energy (kcal)[a]	2700	2000	+300	+500
Protein (g)	56	46	+30	+20
Fat-soluble vitamins				
Vitamin A activity				
RE[b]	1000	800	1000	1200
I.U.	5000	4000	5000	6000
Vitamin D (I.U.)			400	400
Vitamin E activity[c] (I.U.)	15	12	15	15
Water-soluble vitamins				
Ascorbic acid (mg)	45	45	60	80
Folacin[d] (mcg)	400	400	800	600
Niacin[e] (mg)	18	13	+2	+4
Riboflavin (mg)	1.6	1.2	+0.3	+0.5
Thiamin (mg)	1.4	1.0	+0.3	+0.3
Vitamin B_6 (mg)	2.0	2.0	2.5	2.5
Vitamin B_{12} (mcg)	3.0	3.0	4.0	4.0
Minerals				
Calcium (mg)	800	800	1200	1200
Phosphorus (mg)	800	800	1200	1200
Iodine (mcg)	130	100	125	150
Iron (mg)	10	10	18+[f]	18
Magnesium (mg)	350	300	450	450
Zinc (mg)	15	15	20	25

Source: Data from the National Research Council, *Recommended Dietary Allowances*, 8th ed. (Washington, D.C.: National Academy of Sciences, 1974).

[a]Kilojoules (kj) = 4.2 x kilocalories (kcal).

[b]Retinol equivalents.

[c]Total vitamin E activity estimated to be 80 percent as D-tocopherol and 20 percent other tocopherols.

[d]The folacin allowances refer to dietary sources as determined by *Lactobacillus casei* assay. Pure forms of folacin may be effective in doses less than one-fourth of the Recommended Dietary Allowance.

[e]Although allowances are expressed as niacin, it is recognized that, on the average, 1 mg of niacin is derived from each 60 mg of dietary tryptophan.

[f]This increased requirement cannot be met by ordinary diets; therefore, the use of supplemental iron is recommended.

illustrated for the child as the family eats together. Certain foods eaten early in life become associated with feelings about the family and thereby acquire the power to trigger a flood of childhood memories. In some societies it is considered very important that the family eat together as a unit.

Lowenberg (1974) believes that a young child does not form fixed habits but may be "patterned" by adults to eat certain foods and not others. Lowenberg's research showed that foods the father did not like, and which the mother therefore did not serve, were not familiar and would not be eaten by the child.

Cross, Herrman, and Warland (1975) found that a major concern of young families was the need to economize. Seventy-five percent of those sampled set a mental limit on the amount of money they would spend when shopping for food and most looked for bargains and specials. Saving time was not as important for them as for the other 25 percent, because most were full-time homemakers and the need to economize was more important. Ilkeda (1975) reported that the greatest expressed need of low-income homemakers in California was for education in food preparation, and the sub-category in which they most needed help was shopping for food.

Although much food and nutrition education material is aimed at homemakers, two studies found that the husband exerted the greatest influence on food-buying practices and, therefore, on the food available to the family. Cosper and Wakefield (1975), in a study in Kansas, found that, of all factors studied, the husband exerted the strongest influence on the food-buying practices of most of the women, and the husband was noted as the most influential family member. Yetley (1974) studied personal and spouse factors that influenced the eating behavior of young husbands and wives. She concluded that, of four goals studied, maintaining or improving the quality of their diet was ranked lowest by both husband and wife. She also found that the husband's nutrition knowledge exerted a positive effect on the variety of "nutritious" food consumed by the wife but the wife's knowledge of nutrition did not affect the husband's eating behavior. Husbands ranked health goals as less important than either economic or social goals. Wives ranked economic goals as more important than health, and social goals as least important.

In the Marketplace

Young adults with a higher-than-average income, occupational status, and education are generally considered to be "innovators," and "early adopters" (Rogers 1972). Their food expenditure patterns are therefore indicative of future buying trends.

A study conducted in Atlanta, Georgia, showed that as a household's income increased, the consumption of breakfast cereals increased in an almost linear manner (Raunikar, Purcell, and Elrod 1966). Burk (1969), in Minnesota, found that for upper-income families a larger percentage of the income was spent on cereals and cereal products when the head of the household was under 45 years old and the youngest child under 6 years old than when the head of the household was over 45 and/or the children were older. Upper-income families with lower social positions spent relatively more for cereals than did upper-income families with higher social status.

Although each status group has its own marketing leaders, women in higher status groups can afford to socialize more, which increases their potential for market leadership (Lazarsfeld 1965). In Lazarsfeld's study, women between 25 and 44 years old with two or more children were the most likely to become market leaders, and women with the experience of making purchases for a family seemed to be more influential than women with no children.

Nutrition Knowledge

Jalso, Burns, and Rivers (1965), in their study of food faddism, found that as age increased, the validity of nutritional opinions and practices decreased. The age factor in this study could have been confounded by the educational level of the subjects. Their education, not with reference to the number of years completed but in terms of the information available when they were in school, might have influenced their beliefs about food and nutrition.

The educational level of the mother has been related to the nutritional quality of the meals she serves her family, her knowledge of food and nutrition, and her awareness of the importance of good food practices. In the North Central Regional Study of preschool children's nutritional status, the educational level of the mother influenced diet quality more than income did (Eppright et al. 1970).

Morse, Clayton, and Eosgrone (1967) interviewed 237 mothers of students in the seventh, eighth, and ninth grades about nutrition and diet. They concluded that the more education the mother had had, the better her knowledge of food and nutrition was. A nutrition course was directly beneficial. Jalso, Burns, and Rivers (1965) also found that, as education increased, the validity of nutritional opinions and practices increased. And Pearson (1969) noted that the mistaken ideas women had concerning food and nutrition usually involved the relative amounts of certain nutrients in specific foods and the amounts of various nutrients needed by people of different ages, not general ideas of what is "good" or "bad" for people.

According to Young, Beresford, and Waldner (1956), a homemaker's age was less important than her knowledge of food and nutrition in determining food practices, although young homemakers did a somewhat better job of feeding their families than older homemakers. Food practices were better at the higher educational levels and were positively correlated with knowledge.

When knowledge of food and nutrition was measured by having mothers name nutrients and/or state the functions of nutrients, Emmons and Hayes (1973) found that the women frequently could not give a valid reason for using specific foods. Their food practices were not based on understanding, but on habit and custom. In fact, they served a greater variety than they mentioned, and thus, in general, their food practices were superior to the knowledge they exhibited.

Some studies indicate that increased knowledge means a greater probability that a homemaker will serve her family a balanced diet (Gassie and Jones 1972). However, as has been noted, other studies show the father's knowledge to be more influential in this regard (Yetley 1974).

THE MIDDLE YEARS

At this stage of the life cycle, the age of children in a family can range from infancy to the late twenties. Most family members are likely to be engaged in a variety of activities. In the early middle years, both the father and the mother may be employed and both may be active in civic, professional, and child-related activities and recreational events. Children are involved in school and in activities with their peers. All of this means varied schedules. Meals may be skipped or eaten at erratic times. It is difficult for families to have even one meal a day together, although many families do manage this. The early middle years are quite different from the late middle years (Diekelmann and Galloway 1975).

Adults in the family are striving for advancement in their professions and often are under stress. In a study by Hayes and Stinnett (1971), approximately 51 percent of the subjects felt this to be the happiest period of their lives. The children's welfare was their greatest worry. They believed that the advantage to this stage of life was the higher income. Single adults also are striving and may miss family support at this time.

The central concept for the early middle years is maximum responsibility to others, that is, children, spouse, older relatives, and the community (Kahn and Castairs 1965). Success is likely to peak during this period (Winick 1971). Reduction of physical vitality is usually so slight that it is barely recognized until age 45 or older. (Bodily functions diminish at a rate of approximately 5 percent annually after age 30.) Some visible evidence of aging may be observed as body fat deposits shift deeper into the skin, resulting in wrinkles (women have thinner skin than men and wrinkle earlier), and the effects of exposure to sunlight and weather may begin to appear during this part of life (Milne and Milne 1968).

During the late middle years (ages 50 to 60) problems may arise concerning self-concept. Adults realize that some of the ambitions fixed earlier in life have not been, and may never be, fulfilled, and they begin to recognize the assets and liabilities in all aspects of personality. Life seems to be set in a pattern from which the future can be predicted and plans made for achieving long-range goals during the late middle years (Pikunas and Albrecht 1961). Also, there may be less family responsibility: children are choosing mates and are independent. Some older parents may need help from the homemaker, but other women who have been homemakers may be finding that there is too much free time. Food preparation is not the satisfying, creative adventure it once was, for there is no one to appreciate it.

The nutrient needs of adults during the late middle years are shown in table 9. Wohl and Goodhart (1968) pointed out that the two decades from 20 to 40 are the period during which nutrition has maximum impact on the prevention of disease in the 40- to 60-year bracket. The ability to digest and absorb fat decreases with age. A maximum of 30 percent total calories derived from fat, predominantly unsaturated, is advised by most health experts (Chaney and Ross 1971; Hoover 1974).

Women may still be using birth control pills during some of this period and may need more folic acid. Major diseases associated with food intake at this age are anemia, osteoporosis, and obesity (Winick 1975). Weight, too, is a problem for women. Curtis and Bradfield (1971) found that the obese women they studied spent more than one-half their time sleeping and sitting. They also noted that 25 percent of the total calories these women ingested came from snacks.

Several writers have pointed out health problems and discussed possible nutritional modification of our food supply (Clause 1973; Altschul 1974; Hoover 1974; Bowen, Reid, and Moshy 1974). They propose helping to prevent cardiac diseases by using more vegetable proteins, formulating food lower in saturated fat, cholesterol, and salt, and producing meat products with less saturated fat. Most of the literature about the middle years is concerned with the prevention and causes of atherosclerosis. Kennel (1971), in a review of the Framingham Study, listed high blood pressure, overweight, cigarette smoking, lack of exercise, and liberal intake of sucrose as the causes of atherosclerosis in the United States.

Much more needs to be known about food behavior and its relationship to lifestyle during this period of high expectations of self, family, and society. Both men and women are affected, and stress seems to be equally present for single persons and those with families.

TABLE 9. NUTRIENT NEEDS OF ADULTS (AGE 51+)

	Males	Females
Age (years)	51+	51+
Weight (kg, lb)	70, 154	58, 128
Height (cm, in.)	172, 69	162, 65
Energy (kcal)[a]	2400	1800
Protein (g)	56	46
Fat-soluble vitamins		
Vitamin A activity		
RE[b]	1000	800
I.U.	5000	4000
Vitamin D (I.U.)		
Vitamin E activity[c] (I.U.)	15	12
Water-soluble vitamins		
Ascorbic acid (mg)	45	45
Folacin[d] (mcg)	400	400
Niacin[e] (mg)	16	12
Riboflavin (mg)	1.5	1.1
Thiamin (mg)	1.2	1.0
Vitamin B_6 (mg)	2.0	2.0
Vitamin B_{12} (mcg)	3.0	3.0
Minerals		
Calcium (mg)	800	800
Phosphorus (mg)	800	800
Iodine (mcg)	110	80
Iron (mg)	10	10
Magnesium (mg)	350	300
Zinc (mg)	15	15

Source: Data from the National Research Council, *Recommended Dietary Allowances*, 8th ed. (Washington, D.C.: National Academy of Sciences, 1974).

[a]Kilojoules (kj) = 4.2 x kilocalories (kcal).

[b]Retinol equivalents.

[c]Total vitamin E activity estimated to be 80 percent as D-tocopherol and 20 percent other tocopherols.

[d]The folacin allowances refer to dietary sources as determined by *Lactobacillus casei* assay. Pure forms of folacin may be effective in doses less than one-fourth of the Recommended Dietary Allowance.

[e]Although allowances are expressed as niacin, it is recognized that, on the average, 1 mg of niacin is derived from each 60 mg of dietary tryptophan.

THE ELDERLY

Generalizations describing the food behavior of elderly Americans abound. Testimony at the 1969 Senate hearings on Nutrition and Human Needs that focused on the dietary practices of the elderly was, for the most part, anecdotal. Since striking differences in food behavior exist among individuals and groups of all ages throughout the United States, it might be assumed that the food behavior of elderly Americans also varies widely. And yet, casual observation in hospitals, nursing homes, and other institutions in the United States will show the trays for senior citizens similarly laden with gelatin desserts, hot cereal, warm milk, mushy and chopped foods, and liquids.

Only a few years ago there were few research reports describing the foods elderly Americans regularly consume. However, with the implementation of the Title VII senior nutrition program (see chapter 13), reports have been published on the attitudes of the elderly toward food and nutrition, their knowledge of nutrition, their food patterns and general food behavior, and the effect of these factors on their health. Boykin (1975) asked that "soul foods" be provided for some older Americans. The significance of a lifetime of food preferences and food behavior should not be overlooked by food and nutrition professionals developing food programs for the elderly.

The elderly American, the senior citizen, the aged, the older American—how is this group defined? Dietary studies investigating the nutritional status of Americans of age 55 and up have referred to people that age as elderly. Other studies have classified the elderly as those who have reached their sixty-fifth birthday. However, since the Title VII senior nutrition program includes anyone 60 years old or older, the term senior citizen will be used here to mean someone who is 60 or more years old.

It will become clear that, in terms of food behavior and nutritional status, age 60 has no specific meaning. Changes in food behavior that are related to aging occur at individual rates, although some trends will be indicated.

Healthy Elderly Persons Living Independently

Until recently, studies reporting the nutrient intakes of elderly Americans presented little or none of the data that had been collected from food histories, dietary recalls, records of food eaten, menus, plate waste, or actual observation of food consumption (Steinkemp, Cohen, and Walsh 1965; Swanson 1964; Justice, Howe, and Clark 1974; Joering 1971). Rather, such data were translated into nutrient intake values, using the United States Department of Agriculture's Agricultural Handbook No. 8 or similar sources. Sometimes recommendations for changing the food behavior of the elderly were made without adequately describing their actual food behavior. On the other hand, Guthrie, Black, and Madden (1972) studied the relationship of age, education, income, medical restrictions, size of household, general dental health, and nutrient intake among the elderly of rural Pennsylvania and recommended modifications or enrichment of foods traditionally eaten by them.

The question remains—what do the elderly eat? How are the foods packaged, marketed, advertised, prepared, and stored? LeBovit (1965) reported data from a 1957 survey of food consumption, grouping the foods older people frequently consumed. These food groups are: milk; meat, poultry, and fish; eggs; vegetables and fruits; grain products; sugar and sweets; and fat and oil. But the groups provide few clues to help the community food and nutrition professional understand the food behavior of the elderly.

A review of the literature indicates that many of the elderly eat poorly balanced meals consisting of foods that require little preparation (Rao 1973). Reference is continually made to the idea that the elderly fall prey to food fads, especially those that promise renewed vigor and youth or cures for arthritis or disease. While some writers maintain that most older persons do not seek novelty and variety in foods, since it is the "familiar"—the remembered—that gives the most enjoyment (Howell and Loeb 1969), others disagree. Dichter (1972) pointed out that not all elderly persons are infirm nor do they all have denture or digestive difficulties. He suggested that there are some who like to experience unusual and new tastes in foods.

Several researchers have attempted to describe the foods eaten by healthy older persons who do not live in institutions. Jordan et al. (1954) found that yellow and green leafy vegetables were frequently omitted from the diet. In general, starch and sweets were not consumed in large amounts. The older men and women whom Lyons and Trulson studied (1956) did not eat many yellow or green leafy vegetables either, and less than half of them consumed adequate quantities of milk or cheese. Half of the women interviewed ate four eggs per week. Davidson et al. (1962) found that middle-class elderly subjects avoided fried foods. An analysis of data collected for the 1965 Survey of Food Intake of Individuals in the North Central Region (Pao 1971) indicated that vegetables and citrus fruits were lacking in the diet and that dairy products were used sparingly. The survey also showed that cereal products were generously used.

Several other researchers have found that the diets of elderly Americans do not meet the Recommended Dietary Allowances for iron, vitamins A and C, calcium, and protein (Fry, Fox, and Linkswiler 1963; Brin, Schartzberg, and Arthur-Davies 1964; Pao and Burk 1972; Emerson 1964). Emerson attributed the low nutrient levels to the omission of yellow and green vegetables, citrus fruits, and milk from the diet.

A few attempts at reporting meal patterns of elderly Americans have been made. Pao (1971) noted that men ate more substantial breakfasts than women. Eggs or meat, cereal with eggs or meat or both, and cereal were consumed by 30 percent, 20 percent, and 29 percent of the men, respectively. Those same main items were consumed by 25 percent, 5 percent, and 35 percent of the women, respectively. These older people, who resided in the North Central region, also consumed midday and evening meals that were similar in content, although one meal was more substantial in quantity. White potatoes and bread were generally included in these meals. A beverage, usually coffee, was drunk at all three meals. Participants who included snacks in their daily intake most often did so in the evening. Coffee was reported frequently as a snack item. Women listed cake, cookies, pies, fruit, milk, and ice cream, and men listed milk, fruit, cake, cookies, pie, bread, and ice cream, in decreasing order of preferred snack foods.

Case studies demonstrating the low nutrient intakes of senior citizens participating in nutrition programs in the North Central region were presented by Wruble (1976). The profile of Mr. M., who received three home-delivered meals a week, showed the following daily food pattern. Breakfast included toast and coffee. Three days a week he received a home-delivered lunch of meat, potatoes, vegetable, fruit, milk, and dessert. On days when no meal was delivered, Mr. M. ate a sandwich for lunch. His dinner consisted of macaroni or eggs or leftover food from the home-delivered meal. Occasionally neighbors brought him a casserole.

Mr. C. attended a congregate meal about three times a week. He reported that he usually ate cookies and drank coffee in the morning. If he attended the meal provided by the senior nutrition program, he got a lunch of meat, fruits and vegetables, bread and butter, milk, and dessert. If he stayed home for lunch, he prepared warm potatoes and bread and butter. While he rarely ate an evening meal, every night before bed he consumed twenty-four saltine crackers broken into a bowl of milk.

Are there typical meal patterns? We still know too little about the food behavior of older Americans to say.

The impact of social participation on the food behavior of all segments of society is interesting to observe. Clancy (1975) studied the food behavior of forty-seven elderly persons, forty-one women and six men, all of whom lived independently. These persons followed the typical pattern of three meals a day; yet their diets were low in calcium and vitamins A and C. A further look at their diet patterns showed that 40 percent drank milk and ate fresh fruit once a day, 50 percent drank orange juice once a day, and 50 percent reported never drinking soda or beer or eating cupcakes, pretzels, potato chips, or popcorn. About one-fourth of the sample ate cookies daily or cake several times a week.

Limited food and nutrition data were collected in a Michigan health survey (Beck 1974). The survey showed that the food intake of those studied was not related to their age, living situation, or income or to whether they lived in a rural or urban area, rented or owned their homes, or were employed. The respondents in the survey were asked what foods they regularly consumed. Almost all of them ate bread and cereal and drank coffee or tea or another beverage. More than half said they consumed green and other vegetables, fruit or juice, and milk. About one-third had eggs and soup regularly. Only a very few respondents reported eating meat or fish regularly.

Although none of the studies indicates that ethnic food behaviors and food preferences are followed, one can assume, from the data for the food behavior of other age groups, that traditional ethnic foods are eaten by the elderly. The studies also do not indicate whether the foods consumed by persons 60 years old are the same foods consumed by persons of 70, 80, and 90 years of age. Again, it can be assumed that there is a wide variation in the kinds of foods actually consumed by the older American population. The studies cited here suggest that the elderly drink little milk and eat few yellow and green vegetables, only a limited quantity of citrus fruits, and limited servings of meat, poultry, and fish. Such a description of what the elderly do *not* eat leaves the impression that they subsist largely on potatoes, bread, sweets, and beverages such as coffee and tea. If this in fact describes the diet of the elderly American, *it has not been documented.* The question remains—What do healthy, independently-living Americans over the age of 60 eat? Community nutrition and food professionals need to know so that programs aimed at elderly Americans can be as effective as possible.

Institutionalized Elderly Persons

Reports on food served in institutions for the elderly are, for the most part, observational in nature. Reports describing foods that can be served easily to the elderly can be found in trade journals. There are, however, a few reports that describe the food behavior of institutionalized senior citizens. Brogdon and Alford (1973) studied the preferences of twenty-one elderly women and five elderly men residing in a ambulatory care facility. In general, fruits, cereals, and eggs were well liked. Dairy products and meats were the least-liked foods served, and few vegetables were eaten.

Meal Patterns

It generally is believed that senior citizens enjoy breakfast more than any other meal of the day. Studies that describe food behavior sometimes include a description of the meal pattern. Jordan et al. (1954) found that almost all of the elderly persons they interviewed in the state of New York ate three meals a day. Forty percent of the respondents had the large meal of the day at noon. Lyons and Trulson (1956) also found that most of the elderly in the Boston area who were interviewed ate three meals a day. More men than women, however, followed that pattern. More recently, Clancy (1975) interviewed forty-one independently-living women and six men. In general, almost all of the subjects ate breakfast four to five times a week. Forty-two of the respondents reported preparing their own lunch, and three said they usually ate lunch at a restaurant. While forty-three of these elderly people regularly ate dinner, fewer than half of them ate snacks after dinner.

Research data, then, suggest that elderly persons eat two or three meals a day. Some community food and nutrition professionals have observed that participants in the senior nutrition programs make the lunch their sole meal for the day. No data to support this observation have been reported.

Changes in Food Behavior

Just as it is difficult to describe the foods that elderly Americans actually consume, it is difficult to document changes in the food pattern that are beneficial or detrimental to the well-being of the aged person. While many people believe that food behavior is static or very difficult to modify, many elderly persons changing their life-style also change their food behavior (Gifft, Washbon, and Harrison 1972). Foods that take a long time to prepare, that require manual dexterity to prepare or eat, or that are difficult to chew are thought to be eliminated from the diet (Pao and Hill 1974). There is paucity of data to either support or refute these generalizations.

Howell and Loeb (1969) suggested that elderly people tend to follow the dietary patterns of the community in which they live. Todhunter, House, and Vander Zwaag (1974) studied the food attitudes and beliefs, the eating patterns, and the nutritional adequacy of the diets of noninstitutionalized elderly persons residing in middle Tennessee. While most white males and females and black females felt no foods were prohibited in the diet of an elderly person, most black males living in that community identified foods that an older person should not eat.

Some nutritionists, dietitians, and food psychologists believe that people should continue eating foods they know about and have learned to eat. Furthermore, they think change in food behavior should be initiated only for a good reason. Several studies describing the effect of changing food behavior on nutrient adequacy have been completed.

The dietary practices of women from 40 to 75 years of age were studied by Ohlson and coworkers in 1948 (Ohlson et al. 1950). In general, the food selections were made in accordance with traditional food patterns. Reduction of caloric intake with age was associated with reduced consumption of protein foods. In general, the data suggested that some of the chronic ill health reported by women might be related to changes in their food patterns (i.e., to reduced quantity and lower quality of foods eaten).

The eating habits of educated, middle-class persons from 50 to 79 years of age were studied and changes in their consumption of milk, eggs, meat, and fish were noted by Davidson et al. (1962). About one-fourth of the subjects increased their consumption of milk because it was available and they developed a preference for it, and about the same number decreased their consumption of milk because of a change in health or life-style. A small number of subjects changed from whole to skim milk. While some subjects in their sixties increased their consumption of eggs because eggs are easy to prepare and come in single serving portions, others ate fewer eggs because they believed that eggs are not healthful. Little change was reported in meat consumption, although some subjects decreased their intake of meat because of diminished appetite or a belief that meat was "not good for the aging." About one-third of the elderly interviewed decreased their consumption of fish because it was unavailable or difficult to prepare.

Swanson (1964) analyzed the adequacy of the diets of a group of Iowa women 30 to 90 years old. In general, the caloric value of the diet did not change substantially until the subjects reached the age of 70. A decline in protein intake was manifested earlier, at age 65. It appeared that, generally, the older women maintained their traditional diet but limited the quantities of food they ingested. The quantities of sweets and desserts eaten seemed to remain fairly constant throughout life, but the consumption of meat, fish, and poultry declined. A survey of elderly Californians also indicated that food patterns changed little but that caloric intakes were reduced significantly at age 75 (Steinkamp, Cohen, and Walsh 1965). Schlenker (1975) found that urban elderly women decreased their caloric intake and it did not result in poor nutrition, and Wruble (1976) found that rural elderly persons decreased their total food intake too.

Several researchers have indicated that, in general, the elderly follow a traditional food pattern until medical or social reasons force dietary changes (Jordon et al. 1954; LeBovit 1965; Todhunter, House, and Vander Zwaag 1974; Wruble 1976). While the data presented by Davidson et al. (1962), Guggenheim and Margulec (1965), and Schlenker (1975) indicate that people who eat alone change their food behavior (with significant effects on their nutritional status), Batata et al. (1967) concluded that the diet of the older person living alone was no more likely to be deficient than the diets of those living with companions.

Loneliness and health are cited often as reasons for changes in the food behavior of the elderly. Living arrangements can be either a cause or an effect of loneliness and health. To discover how changes in food behavior are related to living arrangements, age, and health, Clarke and Wakefield (1975) compared elderly persons living independently with those living in nursing homes. In general, neither type of residence, independent home or nursing home, ensured that the elderly person would have an adequate diet. The data did indicate, however, that the more individuals changed their traditional eating patterns the lower their nutritional scores were. Changes in food patterns made by those living in the nursing homes correlated negatively with nutritional scores. It appeared that the nursing home residents had changed their food behavior in many ways, while the elderly who lived independently had made only a few changes in their food behavior.

Rountree and Tinklin (1975) also studied the effect of living arrangements on food practices. Elderly persons over 60 years of age who resided in a modern, high-rise apartment complex for senior citizens were interviewed about their food beliefs and food practices, and so were elderly persons who did not live in the complex. While there were some differences in the frequency of planning meals, the adequacy of food storage space, the type of grocery store selected, and the degree of participation in senior meals programs, in general the food-purchasing, preparation, and consumption practices of the two groups were similar. It can thus be assumed that moving into a high-rise complex does not require the changes in food behavior that occur when an elderly person moves to a nursing home.

Living arrangements may change the traditional diet of older Americans by affecting their ability to prepare meals. A large proportion of the elderly people in Michigan who lived with someone other than their spouse needed help or were unable to prepare meals (Beck 1974). About 40 percent of the respondents in that Michigan health survey indicated that they had a vision problem. It is assumed that vision problems affect the ability both to prepare food and to benefit from nutrition education materials; however, no studies have been reported that investigate those variables. Pastalan (1971) suggested that the elderly experience sensory deterioration which results in a reduction of the "home range"—the complex of familiar objects and people distributed in space with meaningful functions and relationships. Pastalan further suggested that the housing environment of the elderly should be planned so that space is organized to stimulate people by making orientation easy and giving them a feeling of mastery over their environment. The relationship between nutrition and changes in food behavior because of housing environment has had only limited study.

The Social Role of Food

The purposes of eating for the elderly were described by Howell and Loeb (1969). Eating is remembering; eating is life-giving; eating is relating to other people. Weinberg (1972) said that food is a medium of socialization. He viewed food as a symbol for the elderly of behavioral patterns and interpersonal relationships. Food can thus become a symbol of security or of rejection for older Americans.

Skillman, Hemwi, and May (1960) noted that the incidence of undernutrition in the total elderly population is small but that overnutrition (obesity) is a problem. Of the 200 outpatients they studied in Ohio, 68 percent were overweight by more than 10 percent of their ideal body weight. Increased food consumption to compensate for reduced participation in social activity was seen as a possible cause. About 8 percent of the sample were underweight. Some of the people in this group had withdrawn from society and found it difficult to obtain and prepare food.

Weinberg (1972), also observed that as the elderly lose friends and relatives they seek replacements. Some find substitute pleasure in eating and others enjoy complaining about food. Weinberg suggested that young Americans build unhappy perceptions of old age and later those beliefs lead to self-depreciation and denial.

Howell and Loeb (1969) speculated that eating in isolation may encourage depressing reminiscences. Other feelings too are often played out in relation to food and eating. Some of these behaviors include withdrawing from people by rejecting food, expressing a domineering character through demands related to food, being overly fussy in selecting food, and showing indecisiveness in relation to food.

Some recommendations have been made for encouraging anxious, depressed, suspicious, and confused elderly persons to eat. The anxious person demands frequent assurance that everything is all right. The depressed individual tends not to eat as a result of feelings of hopelessness. The suspicious person questions the safety of the food and the motives of those who prepare and serve it. The confused older person may no longer recognize even simple aspects of food behavior and will require explanations of mealtime, food, drink, and all eating procedures.

Troll (1971) classified elderly people living alone as either isolates or desolates. Isolates live alone and like it; desolates live alone and do not like it. The attitude of people toward their living arrangements affects their food behavior. Troll warned that life in old age is merely a continuation of past ways of living and therefore it would be a mistake to adopt fixed rules about diets and eating practices for older people.

Howell and Loeb (1969) said that interference in an elderly person's food choices may place stress on the person's self-perception. A couple who have lived together for their entire adult lives have most likely reinforced each other's food habits and attitudes. If one spouse dies and the other is placed in an institution or goes to live with the children, changes in food behavior may prove detrimental to health or morale. Sherwood (1973) indicated that social isolation correlates positively with poor nutritional status. It seems clear that food and eating do indeed serve social functions for the aged.

Nutritional Status

Many health professionals recognize that the elderly are particularly vulnerable to nutritional problems (Rao 1973; Anderson 1968). These problems may be the result of inadequate diet or of altered nutrient requirements caused by physiological changes or diseases that accompany aging. With the exceptions of the Ten-State Nutrition Survey and the Health and Nutrition Examination Survey, most studies have been conducted with small numbers of subjects. Only a brief account of the information available on the nutritional status of the elderly will be presented here.

Although some studies report that the caloric intake of Americans over 65 years of age exceeds two-thirds of the Recommended Dietary Allowances (Fry, Fox, and Linkswiler 1963), most studies show that the elderly consume less than the standards (Guthrie, Black, and Madden 1972; U.S. Department of Health, Education and Welfare 1972, 1974). Obesity is a factor often associated with premature death, but only limited data are available to describe the incidence of obesity and underweight in the aged American population.

Most surveys indicate that most elderly Americans have sufficient protein intakes (Justice, Howe, and Clark 1974; Todhunter, House, and Vander Zwaag 1974; Fry, Fox, and Linkswiler 1963). Hematocrit and hemoglobin values recorded in the Ten-State Nutrition Survey showed that many of the elderly had low or deficient values. Several researchers have reported low dietary intakes of iron among the elderly (Justice, Howe, and Clark 1974; Todhunter, House, and Vander Zwaag 1974; Guthrie, Black, and Madden 1972). Low dietary intakes of vitamin A have been reported in almost all studies of the elderly, including the Ten-State Nutrition Survey and the Health and Nutrition Examination Survey. Reports on the adequacy of vitamin C in the diet vary widely. While generous intakes may be reported in one study, inability to meet two-thirds of the Recommended Dietary Allowances is reported in other studies. Thiamin was one of the nutrients most frequently consumed in amounts below the Recommended Dietary Allowances by subjects receiving meals through senior nutrition programs or home-delivered meals programs (Joering 1971). While mean intakes reported in the Ten-State Nutrition Survey were higher than standards, intakes were below standards in other studies (Todhunter, House, and Vander Zwaag 1974; Guthrie, Black, and Madden 1972). Riboflavin, too, has been reported as insufficient in the diets of the elderly (Justice, Howe, and Clark 1974; Joering 1971; Todhunter, House, and Vander Zwaag 1974; Guthrie, Black, and Madden 1972).

The relationship between osteoporosis, a prevalent disease in the elderly, and dietary intake of calcium is unclear. However, the Ten-State Nutrition Survey indicated that about 35 percent of persons over 60 years of age consume less than 400 milligrams of calcium a day. While several researchers have noted low calcium intakes among the elderly (Todhunter, House, and Vander Zwaag 1974; Guthrie, Black, and Madden 1972; Fry, Fox, and Linkswiler 1963), Joering (1971) found that participating in meal programs increased the calcium intake of elderly persons.

Sensory Activity

The sense of taste and smell are less acute in later life. Is this statement more than a popular belief? The research on taste sensitivity and aging is inconclusive. It is known that the number of taste buds decreases with age, but it is unclear to what degree the functioning of the taste buds is impaired. Some studies report a decline in taste sensitivity in the elderly (Nizel 1974; Richter and Campbell 1940; Cooper, Bilash, and Zubek 1959; Hughes 1969), while other studies report no significant differences between the gross taste perceptions of young adults and those of elderly people (Aubek 1959; Cohen and Gitman 1959; Byrd and Gertman 1959; Fischer 1971).

Odor, too, is an important attribute of food. Fortunato (1958) and Catalano (Fortunato and Catalano 1958) studied the degeneration of olfactory sensitivity in elderly persons and found greater degeneration in males than in females for those 80 years old or older. More recent studies have demonstrated that persons 60 to 69 years old require greater molecular concentrations of substances (other than water) to meet their olfaction thresholds than younger people do, and persons 70 to 82 years old need higher concentrations than 60- to 69-year-olds (Kimbrell and Furchtgott 1963; Hinchcliff 1962).

The texture of food affects its acceptability. It is often said that elderly people with no teeth or poorly fitted dentures must modify their food behavior. There has been little data presented to support this common belief. LeBovit and Baker (1965) found few elderly persons who had changed their food behavior because of their dentition. Anderson (1971) studied the eating patterns of men before and after the insertion of dentures and observed that, although their eating patterns were modified for a short time, after they had worn the dentures for a few months, the men were able to eat crisp raw vegetables. The subjects' consumption of bread decreased, but no change was observed in their consumption of milk, protein foods, green and yellow vegetables, citrus fruits, and other fruits and vegetables. Schlenker (1975) noted that the lack of teeth in elderly women did not interfere with obtaining adequate nutrition.

Recommendations

A variety of factors have been identified that contribute to unsatisfactory food behavior. Rao (1973) listed some problems that must be addressed if the nutritional status of the elderly is to be improved: limited income, loneliness and decreased appetite, decreased activity and increased fatigue, social isolation (especially in urban areas), lack of family support, food fads, alcoholism, chronic invalidism, poor dental health, and mental disturbances. Rao recommended that food for the elderly be acceptable and appetizing; readily available and inexpensive; easily stored, prepared, masticated, and digested; and highly nutritious. Other workers have suggested that nutrition education should be provided for the elderly. Elwood (1975) noted that retired persons were concerned about cholesterol, weight, foods related to disease conditions, dietary supplements, and food composition.

Some researchers have made recommendations for the diet of the aged person. Schlenker and coworkers (1973) thought that the amount of fat in the diet should be reduced. Theuer (1971) felt that milk would be a good food to emphasize in the diets of the elderly because it is a liquid and would meet calcium and vitamin D needs. Generally, a diet low in calories and fat but high in protein has been recommended for the elderly. They are encouraged to include adequate amounts of fluids and roughage, or fiber, in their diet and also foods that are good sources of iron, calcium, and vitamins A and C. Table 10 summarizes some of the information gathered by researchers on the changes associated with aging.

TABLE 10. CHANGES ASSOCIATED WITH AGE

Researcher	60-64 years	65-69 years	70-74 years	75-79 years	80-84 years	85+ years
Olhson et al. (1950)	Need 1600 to 1800 kcal/day		Some need only 1500 kcal/day			
Gillum and Morgan (1955)				Hemoglobin levels decrease		
Davidson et al. (1962)	Decreased egg intake for health reasons		Increased egg intake because of easy preparation			
Morgan (1962)	Rise in serum levels of vitamin and carotene					
	Need 66 g of protein		Need 59 g of protein			
	Women's cholesterol higher than men's					
Swanson (1964)	Decreases in calorie and protein intake similar		Calorie intake decreases			
	28% more than 20% overweight		9% of calories from meat, fish, poultry; 22% from bread and cereal			

Researcher	60-64 years	65-69 years	70-74 years	75-79 years	80-84 years	85+ years
LeBovit (1965)				Dietary adequacy declines		
Steinkamp et al. (1965)	Women's mean calorie intake is 1600 kcal/day					
	Men's mean calorie intake is less than 2200 kcal/day			Calorie intake decreases		
	Mean weight loss of 20 lb					
Dibble et al. (1967)			Have 5.6 chronic conditions			
			Less overweight; decreased skin fold			
Lutwak (1969)		30% of population may have fractures				
USDHEW (1972) Ten-State Nutrition Survey	Decreased milk and vitamin C intake		Plateaus	Men decrease calcium, vitamin A, riboflavin, ascorbic acid intake		

TABLE 10—*Continued*

Researcher	60-64 years	65-69 years	70-74 years	75-79 years	80-84 years	85+ years
Pao and Hill (1974)	Women eat more vitamin C food than men Men increase intake of vitamin A foods			Women decrease calcium, iron, riboflavin, ascorbic intake Meat intake plateaus Men eat more vitamin C food than women Use many vitamin supplements; snack less		
USDHEW (1974) HANES 1971-72		Periodontal disease in 90% of population				

REFERENCES

Young Families

Bott, E. 1971. *Family and social network: Roles, norms and external relationships.* 2nd ed. New York: Free Press.

Burk, M. C. 1969. *Food expenditures by upper income families.* Technical Bulletin 269. St. Paul: University of Minnesota Agricultural Experiment Station.

Committee on Nutrition. 1964. Factors affecting food intake. *Pediatrics* 33:135.

Cosper, B., and Wakefield, L. 1975. Food choices of women: Personal, attitudinal and motivational factors. *Journal of the American Dietetic Association* 66:152.

Cross, B.; Herrman, R.; and Warland, R. 1975. Effect of family cycle stage on concerns about food selections. *Journal of the American Dietetic Association* 67:131.

Ellis, E. 1973. The family: Nutrition and consumer problems. In *U.S. nutrition policies in the seventies,* ed. J. Mayer, San Francisco: W. H. Freeman.

Emmons, L., and Hayes, M. 1973. Nutrition knowledge of mothers and children. *Journal of Nutrition Education* 5:134.

Eppright, E.; Fox, H.; Fryer, B.; Lamkin, G.; and Vivian, V. 1970. The North Central Regional Study of diets of preschool children: 2. Nutrition knowledge and attitudes of mothers. *Journal of Home Economics* 62:327.

Gassie, E., and Jones, J. 1972. Sustained behavioral change. *Journal of Nutrition Education* 4:19.

Ilkeda, J. 1975. Expressed information needs of low-income homemakers. *Journal of Nutrition Education* 7:104.

Jalso, S.; Burns, M.; and Rivers, J. 1965. Nutritional beliefs and practices. *Journal of the American Dietetic Association* 47:263.

Kaluger, G., and Kaluger, M. F. 1974. Early adulthood. In *Human development: The span of life,* pp. 238-261. St. Louis: Mosby.

Lazarsfeld, P. 1965. Who are the marketing leaders? In *Dimensions of consumer behavior,* ed. J. McNeal. New York: Appelton-Century-Crofts.

Lowenberg, M. E. 1974. The development of food patterns. *Journal of the American Dietetic Association* 65:263.

Morse, E.; Clayton, M.; and Eosgrone, L. 1967. Mothers' nutrition knowledge. *Journal of Home Economics* 59:667.

National Research Council. 1974. *Recommended Dietary Allowances.* 8th ed. Washington, D.C.: National Academy of Sciences.

Pearson, J. M. 1969. Interrelationships of home environment and industrial employment: Education and homemakers' food and nutrition knowledge and attitudes. M.S. thesis, Iowa State University (Ames).

Raunikar, R.; Purcell, J.; and Elrod, J. 1966. *Consumption and expenditure analysis for bakery and cereal products in Atlanta, Georgia.* Technical Bulletin 54. Atlanta: Georgia Agricultural Experiment Station.

Rogers, E. 1972. *Diffusions of innovations.* New York: Free Press of Glencoe.

Van Schaik, T. F. 1964. Food and nutrition relative to family life. *Journal of Home Economics* 56:225.

Wilson, M., and Lamb, M. 1968. Food beliefs and ecological factors in women. *Journal of Home Economics* 60:115.

Yetley, E. 1974. A causal model analysis of food behavior. Ph.D. thesis, Iowa State University (Ames).

Young, C.; Berresford, K.; and Waldner, B. 1956. What the homemaker knows about nutrition: III. Relation of knowledge to practice. *Journal of the American Dietetic Association* 32:321.

The Middle Years

Altschul, A. 1974. Vegetable proteins in prudent diet foods. *Food Technology* 28 (1):24.

Bowen, R. E.; Reid, E. J.; and Moshy, R. J. 1974. Formulating foods for the cardiac-concerned. *Food Technology* 28 (1):22.

Chaney; M., and Ross, M. 1971. *Nutrition.* Boston: Houghton Mifflin.

Clause, A. 1973. Improving the nutrition quality of food. *Food Technology* 27 (6):36.

Curtis, D., and Bradfield, R. 1971. Long-term energy intake and expenditure of obese housewives. *American Journal of Clinical Nutrition* 24:1410.

Diekelmann, N., and Galloway, K. 1975. The middle years: A time of change. *American Journal of Nursing* 75:994.

Hayes, M., and Stinnett, M. 1971. Life satisfaction of middle-aged husbands and wives. *Journal of Home Economics* 63:659.

Hoover, S. R. 1974. Decreasing the saturated fatty acid content of animal products. *Food Technology* 28 (1):22.

Kahn, J., and Carstairs, G. 1965. *Human growth.* New York: Pergamon Press.

Kennel, W. B. 1971. The disease of living. *Nutrition Today* 6 (3):2.

Milne, M., and Milne, L. J. 1968. *The ages of life.* Harcourt, Brace and World.

National Research Council. 1974. *Recommended Dietary Allowances.* 8th ed. Washington, D.C.: National Academy of Sciences.

Pikunas, J., and Albrecht, E. 1961. *Psychology of human development.* New York: McGraw-Hill.

Winick, M. 1975. Nutritional disorders of American women. *Nutrition Today* 10 (5 and 6).

Wohl, M., and Goodhart, R. 1968. *Modern nutrition in health and disease.* 4th ed. Philadelphia: Lea and Febiger.

The Elderly

General

Aubek, J. P. 1959. Intellectual and sensory processes in the aged: A terminal report. *Canadian Medical Services Journal* 15:731.

Barnett, C. H., and Cobbold, A. F. 1968. Effects of age upon the mobility of human finger joints. *Annals of the Rheumatic Diseases* 27:175.

Beck, A. 1974. *Survey of the aging in Michigan.* Lansing: Michigan Office of Services to the Aging.

Bloom, M. 1972. Measurement of the socio-economic status of the aged: New thoughts on an old subject. *Gerontologist* 12:375.

Emerson, M. 1964. Pasadena Health Happenings: Department of Public Health. Cited in R. C. Steinkamp, N. L. Cohen, and H. E. Walsh, 1965, Resurvey of an aging population—Fourteen-year follow up, *Journal of the American Dietetic Association* 46:103.

Gifft, H. H.; Wasbon, M. B.; and Harrison, G. G. 1972. *Nutrition, behavior, and change.* Englewood Cliffs, N.J.: Prentice-Hall.

Guggenheim, K., and Margulec, I. 1965. Factors in the nutrition of elderly people living alone or as couples and receiving community assistance. *Journal of the American Geriatrics Society* 13:561.

Howell, S. C., and Loeb, M. B. 1969. *Nutrition and aging: A monograph for practitioners.* St. Louis: The Gerontological Society.

Moss, M. S.; Gottesman, L. E.; and Rosenkaimer, D. P. 1974. Some considerations in developing a questionnaire to assess needs of the aged in community. Presented at the 27th Annual Scientific Meeting of the Gerontological Society, Portland, Oregon.

Pao, E., and Burk, M. 1972. Some alternatives in appraising modern urban nutritional problems. *Proceedings of the 9th International Congress on Nutrition* 4:32.

Schiffman, S. 1977. Food recognition by elderly. *Journal of Gerontology* 32:586.

Shock, N. W. 1970. Physiologic aspects of aging. *Journal of the American Dietetic Association* 56:491.

U.S. Department of Health, Education and Welfare. 1972. *Ten-State Nutrition Survey, 1968-1970: Part III. Clinical, anthropometry and dental; Part IV. Biochemical; Part V. Dietary.* Washington, D.C.: Government Printing Office.

U.S. Department of Health, Education and Welfare. 1974. *Preliminary findings of the first Health and Nutrition Examination Survey, United States, 1971-1972: Dietary intake and biochemical findings.* Washington, D.C.: Government Printing Office.

Walton, W. G. 1967. Visual problems of the institutionalized aged. *American Journal of Optometry* 44:319.

Anderson, E. L. 1971. Eating patterns before and after dentures. *Journal of the American Dietetic Association* 58:421.

Boykin, L. S. 1975. Soul foods for some older Americans. *Journal of the American Geriatrics Society* 23:380.

Brogdon, H. G., and Alford, B. B. 1973. Food preferences in relation to dietary intake and adequacy in a nursing home population. *Gerontologist* 13 (3, part 1):355.

Burkhart, A., and Lachance, P. 1976. Food for the elderly. Cook College *Bulletin*. New Brunswick, N.J.: Rutgers University.

Campbell, V. A., and Dodds, M. L. 1967. Collecting dietary information from groups of older people. *Journal of the American Dietetic Association* 51:29.

Clancy, K. L. 1975. Preliminary observations on media use and food habits of the elderly. *Gerontologist* 15:529.

Clark, M., and Wakefield, L. M. 1975. Food choices of institutionalized vs. independent-living elderly. *Journal of the American Dietetic Association* 66:600.

Davidson, C. S.; Livermore, J.; Anderson, P.; and Kaufman, S. 1962. The nutrition of a group of apparently healthy aging persons. *American Journal of Clinical Nutrition* 10:191.

Dichter, E. 1972. 3rd agers—The new hedonists. *Food Product Development* 6 (4):31.

Elwood, T. W. 1975. Nutritional concerns of the elderly. *Journal of Nutrition Education* 7:50.

Guthrie, H. A.; Black, K.; and Madden, J. P. 1972. Nutritional practices of elderly citizens in rural Pennsylvania. *Gerontologist* 12:330.

Harrill, I.; Erbes, C.; and Schwartz, C. 1976. Observations on food acceptance by elderly women. *Gerontologist* 16:349.

Hendricksen, B., and Cate, H. D. 1971. Nutrient content of food served vs. food eaten in nursing homes. *Journal of the American Dietetic Association* 59:126.

Joering, E. 1971. Nutrient contribution of a meals program for senior citizens. *Journal of the American Dietetic Association* 59:129.

Jordan, M.; Kepes, M.; Hayes, R. B.; and Hammond, W. 1954. Dietary habits of persons living alone. *Geriatrics* 9:230.

Kelley, L.; Ohlson, M. A.; and Harper, L. J. 1957. Food selection and well being of aging women. *Journal of the American Dietetic Association* 33:466.

LeBovit, C. D. 1965. The foods of older persons living at home. *Journal of the American Dietetic Association* 46:285.

LeBovit, C. D., and Baker, D. A. 1965. *Food consumption and dietary levels of older households in Rochester, New York.* Home Economics Research Report no. 25. Washington, D.C.: U.S. Department of Agriculture, Agricultural Research Service.

Lyons, J. S., and Trulson, M. F. 1956. Food practices of older people living at home. *Journal of Gerontology* 11:66.

McKain, W. C.; Stockwell, E. G.; and Weir, J. R. 1958. *Campaigns to increase the meat consumption of older persons.* Bulletin 344. Storrs: University of Connecticut Agricultural Experiment Station.

Morgan, A. F. 1962. Nutrition of the aging. *Gerontologist* 2:77.

Ohlson, M. A.; Jackson, L.; Boek, J.; Cederquist, D.; Brewer, W. D.; and Brown, E. 1950. Nutrition and dietary habits of aging women. *American Journal of Public Health* 40:1101.

Pao, E. M. 1971. Food patterns of the elderly. *Family Economics Review* 62-5 (December):16. (Agricultural Research Service)

Pao, E. M., and Hill, M. M. 1974. Diets of the elderly, nutrition labeling, and nutrition education. *Journal of Nutrition Education* 6:96.

Pastalan, L. A. 1971. How the elderly negotiate their environment. Presented at Environment for the Aged, San Juan, Puerto Rico.

Rao, D. B. 1973. Problems of nutrition in the aged. *Journal of the American Geriatrics Society* 22:362.

Rountree, J. L., and Tinklin, G. L. 1975. Food beliefs and practices of selected senior citizens. *Gerontologist* 15:537.

Sherman, E. M., and Brittan, M. R. 1973. Contemporary food gatherers: A study of food shopping habits of an elderly urban population. *Gerontologist* 13:358.

Sherwood, S. 1973. Sociology of food and eating: Implications for action for the elderly. *American Journal of Clinical Nutrition* 26:1108.

Skillman, T. J.; Hemwi, G. J.; and May, C. 1960. Nutrition in the aged. *Geriatrics* 15:464.

Todhunter, E. N.; House, F.; and Vander Zwaag, R. 1974. *Food acceptance and food attitudes of the elderly as a basis for planning nutrition programs.* Nashville: Tennessee Commission on Aging.

Troll, L. E. 1971. Eating and aging. *Journal of the American Dietetic Association* 59:456.

Wruble, C. 1976. Changes in food behavior with age. M.S. thesis, Michigan State University (East Lansing).

Nutritional Status

Anderson, W. F. 1968. Unanswered questions in the nutrition of elderly people. *Proceedings of the Nutrition Society* 27:185.

Batata, M.; Spary, G. H.; Bolton, F. G.; Higgins, G.; and Wollner, L. 1967. Blood and bone marrow changes in elderly patients with special reference to folic acid, vitamin B_{12}, iron, and ascorbic acid. *British Medical Journal* 2:667.

Brin, M.; Schwartzberg, S. H.; and Arthur-Davies, I. 1964. A vitamin evaluation program as applied to ten elderly residents in a community home for the aged. *Journal of the American Geriatrics Society* 12:493.

Dibble, M. V.; Brin, M.; Theile, V. F.; Peel, A.; Chen, N.; and McMullen, E. 1967. Evaluation of the nutritional status of elderly subjects, with a comparison between fall and spring. *Journal of the American Geriatrics Society* 15:1031.

Fry, P. C.; Fox, H. M.; and Linkswiler. 1963. Nutrient intakes of healthy older women. *Journal of the American Dietetic Association* 42:218.

Gillum, H. L., and Morgan, A. F. 1955. Nutritional status of the aging: I. Hemoglobin levels, packed cell volumes and sedimentation rates of 577 normal men and women over 50 years of age. *Journal of Nutrition* 55:265.

Gillum, H. L.; Morgan, A. F.; and Sailer, F. 1955. Nutritional status of the aging: V. Vitamin A and carotene. *Journal of Nutrition* 55:655.

Jowsey, J.; Riggs, B. L.; Kelly, P. J.; and Hoffman, D. L. 1972. Effect of combined therapy with sodium flouride, vitamin D and calcium in osteroporosis. *American Journal of Medicine* 53:43.

Justice, C. L.; Howe, J. M.; and Clark, H. E. 1974. Dietary intakes and nutritional status of elderly patients. *Journal of the American Dietetic Association* 65:639.

Lutwak, L. J. 1969. Symposium on osteoporosis: Nutritional aspects of osteroporosis. *Journal of the American Geriatrics Society* 17:115.

Nizel, A. E. 1974. The role of nutrition in the oral health of the aging patients. Presented at the Food Writer's Conference of the National Dairy Council, 3-4 June 1974, Chicago.

Schlenker, E. D. 1975. Nutritional status of older women. Ph.D. thesis, Michigan State University (East Lansing).

Schlenker, E. D.; Feurig, J. S.; Stone, L. H.; Ohlson, M. A.; and Mickelson, O. 1973. Nutrition and health of older people. *American Journal of Clinical Nutrition* 26:1111.

Steinkamp, R. C.; Cohen, N. L.; and Walsh, H. E. 1965. Resurvey of an aging population—Fourteen-year follow-up. *Journal of the American Dietetic Assocaition* 46:103.

Swanson, P. 1964. Adequacy in old age: II. Nutrition education program for the aging. *Journal of Home Economics* 56:728.

Theuer, R. C. 1971. Nutrition and old age: A review. *Journal of Dairy Science* 54:627.

Walker, A. R. P. 1972. The human requirement of calcium: Should low intakes be supplemented? *American Journal of Clinical Nutrition* 25:518.

Weinberg, J. 1972. Psychologic implications of the nutritional needs of the elderly. *Journal of the American Dietetic Association* 60:293.

Sensory Acuity

Byrd, E., and Gertman, S. 1959. Taste sensitivity in aging persons. *Geriatrics* 14:381.

Cohen, T., and Gitman, L. 1959. Oral complaints and taste perception in the aged. *Journal of Gerontology* 14:294.

Cooper, R. M.; Bilash, I.; and Zubek, J. P. 1959. The effect of age on taste sensitivity. *Journal of Gerontology* 14:56.

Fischer, R., and Kaplan, A. R. 1971. Letter to the editor. *Gerontologia Clinica* 12:314.

Fortunato, V. 1958. Ofattonelle varie eta. In *Olfatto e sue correlazioni,* ed. V. Fortunato and P. Niccolini, p. 519. Catania: Tipografia dell 'Universita.'

Fortunato, V., and Catalano, G. B. 1958. La struttura dell 'aparato olfattivo nell'uomo. In *Olfatto e sue correlazioni,* ed. V. Fortunato and P. Niccolini, p. 5. Catania: Tipografia dell'Universita.'

Hinchcliffe, R. 1962. Aging and sensory thresholds. *Journal of Gerontology* 17:45.

Hughes, G. 1969. Changes in taste sensitivity with advancing age. *Gerontologia Clinica* 11:224.

Kelly, J. E.; VanKirk, L. E.; and Garst, C. 1967. *Total loss of teeth in adults: U.S. 1960-1962.* National Center for Health Statistics, PHS publication 1000, series 11, no. 27. Washington, D.C.: Government Printing Office.

Kimbrell, G., and Furchtgott, E. 1963. The effect of aging on olfactory threshold. *Journal of Gerontology* 18:364.

Richter, C. P., and Campbell, K. H. 1940. Sucrose taste thresholds of rats and humans. *American Journal of Physiology* 128:291.

Szczesniak, A. S., and Kohn, E. L. 1971. Consumer awareness of and attitudes to food texture. *Journal of Texture Studies* 2:280.

Tilgner, D. J., and Barylko-Pikielna, N. 1959. Threshold and minimum sensitivity of the taste sense. *Acta Physiologica Polonica* 10:741.

	CHAPTER
Impairments as Modifiers of Food Behavior	**8**

Many people have impairments—physical or mental or both—that affect their food behavior. Persons who are born with an impairment or who become impaired early in life may have their food behavior affected from the beginning. Those who become impaired later in life may need to modify their food behavior. The discussion in this chapter will focus on the development of food behavior in children with specific impairments.

PHYSICAL IMPAIRMENTS

Physical impairments include blindness, deafness, and limitations of body movements and functions.

Blindness

The number of blind persons in the United States is estimated at 450,000. Less than 10 percent of the blind population are children and approximately 50 percent are over 65 years old. There are more blind males than females.

Blindness can be caused in a number of ways: by infectious diseases, by eye injuries, by diseases that affect the eye, and by diseases of the eye itself.

Some infectious diseases that may result in blindness are trachoma (an eye infection that can cause scar tissue to develop on the eye), onchocerciasis (an infestation of a parasitic worm), opthalmia neonatorum (inflammation of the eyes of newborn infants that occurs during birth), and syphilis (a veneral disease that develops in three stages). Trachoma has been especially troublesome among American Indians in the West. Other diseases that cause blindness, though less frequently, are leprosy (a chronic disease primarily affecting the skin, mucous membranes, and nervous system), tuberculosis (a disease primarily affecting the respiratory system), meningitis (inflammation of the membranes lining the central nervous system), measles, diptheria (an acute infectious disease associated with an inflammation of the throat), and scarlet fever (an

This chapter was written by Dr. Kitty R. Coffey and Dr. Carolyn Lackey specially for this book.

acute infectious disease associated with high fever, sore throat, and red rash). A wide variety of physical and chemical eye injuries from industrial, domestic, playground, and other accidents also can cause blindness.

Diseases affecting the eye include diabetes, arteriosclerosis (a thickening and hardening of the arteries), diseases of the central nervous system, nephritis or Bright's disease (inflammation of the kidneys), and anemia. In some cases dietary intake may contribute to the development of the disease, and in others, diet modification is part of the treatment.

Diseases of the eye itself may also lead to blindness. Some of these diseases may be caused by nutritional deficiency; for example, a vitamin A deficiency can lead to xeropthalmia (a type of dry conjunctivitis) and keratomalacia (softening of the cornea). Cataracts (opacity of the lens), which are prevalent in older people, and glaucoma (hardening of the eye from intraocular pressure upon the optic nerve) are two more eye diseases that can cause blindness.

The blind person is handicapped in a wide range of activities and functions—in written and visual communication, in recreational activities, and in a host of routine daily tasks and activities. Eating is one such activity. Although quite simple for the sighted person, it can cause an array of frustrations, humiliations, and possible nutritional problems for the blind person. One need only consider the countless ways vision is used by a sighted person during a regular meal to begin to appreciate the implications of blindness in eating. Vision is used to locate the various foods and the utensils for eating them, to determine what utensils are appropriate for each food and whether any of the food requires cutting or breaking into small pieces, and to coordinate all of the fine movements involved in the mechanics of eating. For the person with no sight, trying to determine the contents of a dish, cutting meat into appropriate-sized pieces, and getting peas onto a fork can become frustrating tasks indeed. While no studies compare the nutritional status of sighted and nonsighted people, professionals working with blind persons reported that many of them limit their intake to a small variety of foods they can comfortably manipulate. Extra care may be needed to ensure that blind persons receive adequate nutrients in their diet. Although some of these difficulties can never be totally overcome, much can be done to help make mealtime an enjoyable and nutritious experience for the blind person, rather than a frustrating, awkward one.

During the transition from breast-feeding or bottle-feeding to more solid foods, the seeing infant relies on sight to know when the parent is preparing to feed, what the food is, and when the food is approaching the mouth. The parent of a blind child must emphasize the use of the child's other senses, such as touch and hearing, to help orient the infant during feeding. The child should be given the security of knowing what will happen, so that the unpleasant sensation of being surprised by something unknown and unexpected can be avoided. This can be accomplished by putting the child's hands on the cup or spoon as it is drawn toward the mouth, by giving the child time to smell or feel whatever is on the spoon or in the cup, and by giving verbal reassurances. As the child grows accustomed to the feeding process, less effort will be required to communicate the situation.

Touching and feeling the food is often especially important for a blind child; it gives the child a familiarity with the feeding process that is difficult to achieve otherwise. Picking food up and bringing it to the mouth teaches the child the motions that will eventually be required in learning to eat with a spoon. Blind children should be encouraged to use a spoon, although their readiness for it may be somewhat later than that of sighted children. Learning to eat with a spoon can be made easier by serving the food from a deep bowl rather than a flat plate and by using a lightweight spoon so the child can better sense how much food, if any, is on the spoon. The handle should be short and wide so it can fit entirely within the child's fist.

Each new eating technique should be introduced slowly to minimize the child's feelings of unfamiliarity. Furthermore, a new food should not be introduced simultaneously with a new feeding technique or instrument.

After mastering eating with a spoon, perhaps sometime during the third year, the child should be encouraged to use a fork. Again, it should be lightweight. In the beginning, only foods that are relatively easy to handle with a fork should be served and they should be served on a small plate. Having the child use a piece of bread to push the food onto the fork is sometimes helpful. As the child becomes more adept with the fork, other foods should be introduced.

Teaching the blind youngster to use a knife should be left until considerably good hand coordination has been acquired and the child is quite comfortable using a fork. In cutting meat the fork is held in the left hand to find the meat on the plate and to secure it, preferably by the left side. The prongs of the fork can be used as guides for the knife blade in cutting the meat. After cutting, the knife can be used to feel whether the piece of meat remaining on the fork is small enough to eat, and the piece is then eaten or recut. Cutting meat is one of the more difficult eating tasks that confront blind persons and many prefer to have their meat cut for them.

A child that has learned to eat independently can be greatly aided in two ways. First, the child should be informed what food is being served, so that smelling the food closely or feeling it for identity will not be necessary. Second, the table setting should be as consistent as possible from meal to meal to minimize the amount of searching or reteaching needed. The location of the various foods on the plate is often described as if the plate were the face of a clock. If vegetables are consistently placed at "three o'clock," meat at "twelve," and so forth, the need for reexplanation at each meal can be further reduced. The simple practice of putting salt or pepper in the hand first and using sugar cubes can greatly facilitate the seasoning of food. Describing the content and location of the meal and the place setting and trying to maintain some consistency can be helpful to the blind person throughout adult life.

When a blind child desires to help prepare the food, encouragement should be given. There are many tasks such as setting the table, washing vegetables, and husking corn that will give the child satisfaction. As for all children, mealtime for the blind child should be an enjoyable, relaxed experience. Too much pressure to learn conventional eating patterns and table manners can result in the child's becoming anxious and fussy about eating, and that may affect nutritional status. Comparisons with sighted children should also be avoided. Although more time and patience may be required to teach a blind child to eat independently, the eventual accomplishment of that goal is very satisfying.

Special utensils and cooking equipment can help blind persons in preparing meals. There are special saucepans and pot drainers, knives with slicing guides, clocks with removable covers, and mechanical and switch timers. Cookbooks are available in large type and braille and on records and tape cassettes. Some cookbooks printed in large type are *Simple Cooking for the Epicure* by J. H. Campbell and G. Kameron (Keith Jennison Large Type Books, Franklin Watts, Inc.), *Cooking with Betty Crocker Mixes* (General Mills, Inc., Minneapolis), and *Food at Your Fingertips* (American Printing House for the Blind, Louisville). Large type and braille cookbooks are available from the Campbell Soup Company, Campbell Place, Camden, NJ 08101. *Cooking without Looking* by E. Tipps (American Printing House for the Blind, Louisville, 1959) is available in both large type and braille. Information on services for the blind can be obtained from the American Foundation for the Blind, 15 West Sixteenth Street, New York, NY 10011.

Deafness and Impaired Hearing

Types of hearing loss are classified as *deafness,* a hearing loss of at least 80 decibels; *impaired hearing,* a hearing loss of 20 to 80 decibels; or *distorted hearing,* an impairment resulting not from loss of auditory sensitivity but from damage to the central nervous system.

Approximately 5 percent of school-age children have some hearing impairment and about 10 percent of the adult population have some hearing loss. It is estimated that the incidence of severely handicapping hearing loss is about 5 percent in the total population. Hearing impairment may be conductive, receptive, transmissive, or perceptive. If the hearing loss occurs before birth or before age 3, the child may not learn to talk and communication is a problem. One of the important aspects of eating behavior in deaf children is the development of mouth movements, such as sucking, that can eventually facilitate the process of learning to speak. Garton and Bass (1974) found that deaf children did not know the names of many of the foods they were eating in the school cafeteria. The foods were not labeled and the children pointed to the food they wished placed on their plates. Efforts need to be made to communicate to deaf children the information normally transmitted verbally about food. Deafness in old age presents other problems. Many people are ashamed of being deaf and try to stay out of situations where they must respond to others. Companionship while eating may be limited.

Limitations of Body Movements

The inability to perform properly the functions of eating because of problems with sucking, swallowing, chewing, lip closure, and tongue control will influence a person's behavior. There may be dentofacial handicaps such as underdeveloped lower jaw, facial asymmetry, or protruding teeth, malformations which disturb the functions of speech, chewing, swallowing, or sucking. Congenital cleft lip and cleft palate and other facial clefts pose problems in feeding the infant. Missing or paralyzed limbs and immobility as a result of birth defects or of accidents later in life influence food behavior. Recognizing the psychological and sociological, as well as the physiological, needs for food and helping the individual to meet those needs is a challenge for the community food and nutrition professional. Special feeding techniques and equipment have been developed by the health department of Los Angeles, California, by the University of Tennessee Child Development Center, and by others. These include spoons with bent handles, padded handles, or handles with a strap attached for better grasping and also handles in animal forms, for motivation.

Feeding Procedure. The handicapped child should be encouraged to help in whatever way possible in the preparation of the meal—washing hands and face, setting the table or individual place setting, and serving the food. If the child requires assistance in serving the food, the server should explain what is happening, express enthusiasm about the meal, and encourage the child to do whatever is possible. A severely handicapped child may need to be spoon-fed. A small amount of food should be placed in the center of the lips, which should then close over the food. Closing the lips may need to be done manually by the feeder. The swallowing reflex should follow, but it may need to be stimulated by rubbing or lightly pinching the child's throat. This process should be repeated until the food has been eaten. (Any dripped food should be wiped from the patient's mouth as necessary.) This method, although slow and laborious, is preferable to the usual method of putting large quantities of food or liquid into the handicapped person's mouth and hoping that the person will swallow some portion of it.

Handicapped children should be encouraged to eat a wide variety of foods to help ensure that adequate nutrients are ingested. Because some textures are harder to manage than others, chewy or crispy foods should be introduced when the child is very hungry.

Chronic conditions caused by disability and aging may also affect food and nutrient intake. Adults often need assistance in meal preparation. Klinger (1978) has discussed the basic techniques and findings for meal preparation by the disabled. Great care and planning are needed to make sure handicapped persons receive adequate nutrition from their meals.

Some conditions, such as cerebral palsy, can put a person at nutritional risk, and then special care must be given to planning food and nutrition behavior. The constant movement of cerebral palsy patients creates an increased need for calories, while the lack of neuromuscular control may make eating and drinking very difficult (Barret 1972).

Children with cerebral palsy, as well as other physically handicapped children, should be seated in an arrangement that offers full support of the trunk, head, and feet. It is best if the table is at the level of the child's elbows. In order to gain some independence in the feeding process, the child should be encouraged to drink with a straw. The sucking reflex can be stimulated by massaging the child's cheeks and by dipping the straw into the liquid before placing it in the child's mouth. The child's lips may have to be held around the straw in the beginning. Learning the motions necessary for straw drinking will also meliorate breathing control and lip and tongue function. Chewing may be taught by placing a piece of meat between the child's molars on one side and then passively moving the jaw up and down until the child understands the idea and can initiate the motion.

Physically handicapped patients who can balance their heads, sit, and raise a hand to the mouth may be able to learn self-feeding. This should be initiated by introducing the hand-to-mouth pattern with finger foods such as crackers or pieces of candy. After this pattern has been well established, spoon training should begin. The spoon should be modified so the handle is easier for the child to grasp and bent so the spoon is close to the mouth when it is raised to mouth level. The dish should be deep and held in place by a suction cup or plate holder. Sticky foods such as mashed potatoes, custard, and applesauce are best for training.

Because children with cerebral palsy generally have a low intake of protein and iron and consume fewer calories than are recommended for children their age (Barret 1972), care should be taken to give them high-calorie foods that contain these nutrients. Milk puddings, custards, eggnogs, and milk shakes can serve this purpose. In food prepared for severely physically handicapped patients such as those with cerebral palsy, dry powdered milk can be added to meat loaf, and in cooked cereals and puddings, evaporated milk substituted for the same quantity of whole milk will increase the food value of the diet.

The need for trained nurses, dietitians, and other professionals who can help the handicapped is great. The attitude of these professionals toward severely handicapped persons, especially, is an important element in any health care program. Any feelings of repulsion must be overcome if the goals of better health and nutrition, improved speech, and greater independence are to be realized.

MENTAL IMPAIRMENTS

Mental Retardation

Mental retardation is defined by the American Association on Mental Deficiency as significantly subaverage general intellectual functioning existing concurrently with defects in adaptive behavior and manifested during the development period (Grossman 1973). Numerous systems of classification for degress of mental retardation have been used (Grossman 1973; Browning 1974; Begab and Richardson 1975). The legal-administrative classifications are found in the laws of most states and regulate eligibility for services for the mentally retarded. From an educational standpoint, the mentally retarded have been classified as (1) educable, (2) trainable, and (3) custodial (those who are entirely dependent on others to live).

The American Association on Mental Deficiency has developed more extensive systems that classify the individual according to intellectual level and adaptive behavior. A positive relationship exists between adaptive behavior and intelligence. The degree of impairment may be identified as mild, moderate, severe, or profound (Grossman 1973). The ultimate goal of habilitation is to have each mentally retarded person functioning at his or her maximum level of ability. This includes achieving maximum independence with regard to feeding.

The number of mentally retarded persons in a population is usually estimated at 3 percent. There are an estimated 6 million retarded individuals in the United States, with 2.5 million of these being under 20 years of age (U.S. Department of Health, Education and Welfare 1972a). The number of public institutions for the mentally retarded increased by 76 percent between 1960 and 1970, from 108 to 190. The cost to society of institutionalizing mentally retarded persons is rising. In 1970 the total operating and maintenance costs of public institutions was $871 million, representing a threefold increase over 1960 (U.S. Department of Health, Education and Welfare 1972a, 1972b).

Nutritional services to the mentally retarded include maternal and infant care projects with emphasis on preventive health care and clinics for the detection and early treatment of inborn errors of metabolism. Treatment programs for the mentally retarded which involve food and nutrition professionals include:

1. Small residential facilities associated with hospitals to demonstrate how intensive care of severely damaged children can help develop skills in self-care such as self-feeding.
2. Comprehensive treatment centers for the multiply handicapped retarded child in hospital pediatric departments which also serve as centers for personnel training.
3. Expanded services in day training centers, institutions, and other group care programs for young retarded persons.
4. Expanded clinic facilities for the observation of children in a group setting so that group approaches and techniques can be used in diagnosis and treatment.
5. Short-term and long-term training programs for personnel serving the mentally retarded (Egan 1969; Springer 1971).

In addition, twenty-two federal departments and agencies have programs related to mental retardation (President's Committee on Mental Retardation 1972).

Foodways of the Mentally Retarded. The availability of food to the mentally retarded is determined by two important factors: (1) the supply of food provided by parent, guardian, or institution and (2) the feeding skills of the mentally retarded individual.

The assurance of an adequate supply of food for mentally retarded persons in institutions is provided in the *Standards for Residential Facilities for the Mentally Retarded* published by the Accreditation Council for Facilities for the Mentally Retarded of the Joint Commission on Accreditation of Hospitals (1971). Assurance of adequate food for persons served by community agencies for the mentally retarded is provided by a similar document established by the same group (1973). The supply of food available to mentally retarded persons who are not institutionalized depends mainly upon the socioeconomic and educational level of the parents or the guardian, but it may be supplemented by any number of state or federal programs or by local philanthropy.

The inability to feed themselves limits the supply and consistency of food available to the mentally retarded. Self-feeding is one of the activities of daily living in the habilitation or rehabilitation process. When persons become able to feed themselves, they are starting on the road to independence. The food and nutrition professional must plan and work with nurses, psychologists, speech pathologists, and special educators, as well as with occupational therapists in teaching mentally retarded individuals to feed themselves. The primary technique used in the acquisition phase of feeding skill training is manual guidance. Intensive training has been shown to be effective even with profoundly retarded individuals (Colwell, Richards, and McCarver 1973). The "mini-meal," using controlled correctional procedures and the simple-to-complex rules, has been effective in teaching feeding skills to the mentally retarded (Azrin and Armstrong 1973). The adaptation of feeding equipment to individual needs can make feeding skills easier to learn (Dittman 1959; Smith 1971; Gertenrich 1970; Springer 1971; Hallas, Fraser, and MacGillivary 1974).

After food has been made more readily available by the acquisition of feeding skills, there follows (or accompanies) the motivation phase, which encourages acceptance of the food. The most important technique used in the motivation phase is removal of the person from the meal (called "time-out") when errors are made. Food is often used as a reward in training based upon operant procedures that make use of tangible positive reinforcers. As the training progresses, the tangible rewards are gradually replaced by praise. Candy, cookies, and soda pop have been used for reinforcers (Colwell, Richards, and McCarver 1973; Hollis 1973).

Some mentally retarded persons may have difficulty chewing or swallowing or sucking and may therefore be unable to eat solid food; others, while able to chew, swallow, and suck, may depend on someone else to feed them. Close supervision is needed, and trained personnel are cautioned to be aware of possible strangulation in feeding (Hille and Reeves 1964; Smith 1971; Wallace 1972). The nutritional care of such persons may require that the selection, consistency, and methods of preparation of foods be modified and special feeding equipment employed to make the food acceptable to them (Hille and Reeves 1964). A special feeding technique has been reported to be effective for feeding chronic regurgitators (Ball et al. 1974).

A safe food supply is assured for mentally retarded persons living in institutions approved by the Joint Commission on Accreditation of Hospitals (Accreditation Council for Facilities for the Mentally Retarded 1971, 1973). In cases of inborn errors of metabolism, various state and federal agencies provide dietary treatment plans as a safety measure to prevent mental retardation and, in some instances, to improve the behavior of mentally retarded persons with previously untreated inborn metabolic errors.

The nutritive quality of the diet of mentally retarded persons who are institutionalized is protected in part by the Joint Commission on Accreditation of Hospitals (Accreditation Council for Facilities for the Mentally Retarded 1971, 1973). Few studies are available on the food intake patterns of the mentally retarded, and most of the work that has been done has involved children. Hammar and Barnard (1966), in a study of forty-four noninstitutionalized retarded adolescents, found that their diets differed little from the diets of their normal contemporaries; however, the parents of many of the retarded adolescents used food, particularly candy and desserts, as a reward for good behavior. The diets generally were high in carbohydrates and low or marginal in iron and ascorbic acid. Two of the adolescents were obese.

Culley and Middleton (1969) studied the caloric requirements of mentally retarded children with and without motor dysfunction. Children whose motor disfunction was severe enough to make them nonambulatory required approximately 75 percent as many calories as ambulatory children of comparable height (caloric needs were expressed in terms of body height instead of age).

An estimated 500,000 children in our country are afflicted with cerebral palsy (Wallace 1972). Hammond, Lewis, and Johnson (1966) evaluated the diets of children with cerebral palsy and found that intakes of milk, vegetables of all types, meat, and eggs were low but citrus fruits and whole grain cereals were eaten frequently. One-half of the subjects' diets met the 1958 National Research Council's Recommended Dietary Allowances.

Coffey and Crawford (1971) reported on the food intake patterns of 116 mentally retarded children at the University of Tennessee Affiliated Child Development Center. Approximately 25 percent had diets below the 1968 Recommended Daily Allowance. Nutrients most often lacking were iron and calcium and vitamins A and C. Twenty-eight percent of the retarded children were underweight; 8 percent were overweight or obese. Forty-seven percent of the patients had poor food behaviors, including multiple food dislikes, skimping on or skipping meat, irregular meal patterns, eating in unpleasant surroundings at mealtime, and overstuffing and/or having to be force fed. Bizarre food habits such as eating inedible material (e.g., paper, match heads, hand lotion) or eating salt by the handful, butter by the stick, sugar by the bowl, or raw meats were observed in 11 percent of the mentally retarded children. Delayed development of feeding skills was found in 36 percent of the children. Mechanical feeding difficulties, such as problems with sucking, swallowing, or chewing, were present in 45 percent of the children.

Gouge and Ekvall (1975) more recently reported on the diets of patients at the University Affiliated Cincinnati Centers for Developmental Disorders. Primary nutritional and feeding problems were (1) low ascorbic acid and iron intakes, (2) lack of a daily flouride source, (3) protein intake of borderline quality, and (4) mechanical and postnatal feeding problems. Nineteen percent of the children had problems feeding themselves and 33 percent had difficulty sucking, chewing, or swallowing. The incidence of mechanical feeding difficulties and problems with feeding skills was considerably lower than reported by Coffey and Crawford (1971): 19 percent versus 36 percent for feeding skills and 33 percent versus 45 percent for mechanical feeding difficulties. In both studies, the more severe the retardation, the more prevalent the feeding problems.

Mental Illness

Food can be an important element in the treatment of emotionally disturbed persons. Anorexia nervosa, an emotional disturbance in which a person refuses to eat and starves to death, is an example of how food is involved with emotional well-being. Neimeyer (1971) discussed the need for dietitians to use judgment, decision, and careful evaluation of behavior to determine the ability and willingness of disturbed persons to assume responsibility for their own diets after treatment. Wilkinson et al. (1971) conducted food and nutrition classes for mentally disturbed women in Nebraska. The classes provided opportunities for social interaction and enhancement of self-esteem as well as for learning the principles of nutrition and meal management.

Food intake and nutrition are important factors in the prevention and treatment of mental retardation and mental illness. To date, relatively few studies have dealt with the foodways of the mentally retarded and the emotionally ill. An interdisciplinary team approach is advocated to assure a readily available, safe, acceptable, and nutritious diet to the mentally retarded, mentally ill, and multiple handicapped.

REFERENCES

Physical Impairments

American Foundation for the Blind. 1972a. *For young readers: Talking books.* New York: American Foundation for the Blind.

American Foundation for the Blind. 1972b. *Talking books adult catalog.* New York: American Foundation for the Blind.

American Foundation for the Blind. 1974. *A step-by-step guide to personal management for blind persons.* New York: American Foundation for the Blind.

American Public Health Association. 1955. *Service for children with dentofacial handicaps.* New York: American Public Health Association.

Anonymous 1970. We can do it. *Plant and Business Food Management,* September, p. 26.

Anonymous. 1971. Current comment: Nutrition and eating problems of the elderly. *Journal of the American Dietetic Association* 58:43.

Aronovitz, R., and Conroy, C. W. 1969. Effectiveness of the automatic toothbrush for handicapped persons. *American Journal of Physical Medicine* 48 (4):193.

Atkinson, M. 1949. Meniere's syndrome. *Archives of Otolaryngology* 50:564.

Clark, L., ed. 1973. *International catalog of aids and appliances for blind and visually impaired persons.* New York: American Foundation for the Blind.

Encyclopaedia Britannica. 1973. Deaf and hard of hearing, Training and welfare of: and Deafness and impaired hearing. Vol. 7. Chicago: William Benton.

Encyclopaedia Britannica. 1973. Blindness; and Blind, Training and welfare of. Vol. 3. Chicago: William Benton.

Encyclopaedia Britannica. 1974. *Micropaedia,* vol. 2. Blindness. Chicago: William Benton.

Encyclopaedia Britannica. 1974. *Micropaedia,* vol. 13. Nutrition and diet, Human. Chicago: Helen H. Benton.

Freyberger, P. E. 1971. Comparative methods in teaching cooking to the congenitally vs. the adventitiously blind adult. *The New Out Look for the Blind,* May. (American Foundation for the Blind)

Fritchie, L. Undated. *A step-by-step guide to food preparation for blind persons.* Reno: University of Nevada Press.

Garton, N. B., and Bass, M. A. 1974. Food preferences and nutrition knowledge of deaf children. *Journal of Nutrition Education* 6:60.

Gertenrich, R. L. 1970. A simple adaptable drinking device for mental retardates lacking arm-hand control (pilot project). *Mental Retardation* 8 (3):51.

May, E. E.; Waggoner, N. R.; and Boettke, E. M. 1966. *Homemaking for the handicapped.* New York: Dodd, Mead.

On Your Own Newsletter. University: University of Alabama, Continuing Education in Home Economics.

Smith, M. A. H., ed. 1971. *Feeding the handicapped child.* Memphis: University of Tennessee Child Development Center.

U.S. Department of Health, Education and Welfare, 1973. *Feeding the child with a handicap.* Washington, D.C.: Government Printing Office.

U.S. Department of Health, Education and Welfare/The Industrial Home for the Blind. 1958. *Rehabilitation of deaf-blind persons,* vol. 1. Washington, D.C.: Booklin. (The Industrial Home for the Blind)

Wilson, E. D.; Fisher, K. H.; and Fuqua, M. E. 1975. *Principles of nutrition.* New York: Wiley.

Yost, A. C.; Schroeder, S. L.; and Rainey, C. 1977. *Home economics rehabilitation: A selected, annotated bibliography.* Columbia: University of Missouri, College of Home Economics.

Mental Impairments

Accreditation Council for Facilities for the Mentally Retarded. 1971. *Standards for residential facilities for the mentally retarded.* Chicago: Joint Commission on Accreditation of Hospitals.

Accreditation Council for Facilities for the Mentally Retarded. 1973. *Standards for community agencies serving persons with mental retardation and other developmental disabilities.* Chicago: Joint Commission on Accreditation of Hospitals.

Azrin, N. H., and Armstrong, P. M. 1973. The "mini-meal"—A method of teaching eating skills to the profoundly retarded. *Mental Retardation* 11 (1):9.

Ball, T. S.; Hendricksen, H.; and Clayton, J. 1974. A special feeding technique for chronic regurgitation. *American Journal of Mental Deficiency* 78:486.

Barret, J. 1972. Improving the nutrition of the handicapped child: The role of the LP/VN. *Journal of Practical Nursing,* August, p. 22.

Begab, M. J., and Richardson, S. A. 1975. *The mentally retarded and society: A social science perspective.* Baltimore: University Park Press.

Browning, P. L. 1974. *Mental retardation.* Springfield, Ill.: Charles C. Thomas.

Coffey, K. R., and Crawford, J. 1971. Nutrition problems commonly encountered in the developmentally handicapped. In *Feeding the handicapped child,* ed. M. A. H. Smith. Memphis: University of Tennessee Child Development Center.

Colwell, C. N.; Richards, E.; McCarver, R. B.; and Ellis, N. R. 1973. Evaluation of self-help habit training of the profoundly retarded. *Mental Retardation* 11 (3):14.

Culley, W. J., and Middleton, T. O. 1969. Caloric requirements of mentally retarded children with and without motor dysfunction. *Journal of Pediatrics* 75:380.

Dittman, L. L. 1959. *The mentally retarded child at home—A manual for parents.* Washington, D.C.: U.S. Department of Health, Education and Welfare, Social and Rehabilitation Service, Children's Bureau.

Egan, M. C. 1969. Combating malnutrition through maternal and child health programs. *Children* 16 (2):67.

Gertenrich, R. L. 1970. A simple, adaptable drinking device for mental retardates lacking arm-hand control (pilot project). *Mental Retardation* 8 (3):51.

Gouge, A. L., and Ekvall, S. W. 1975. Diets of handicapped children: Physical, psychological, and socioeconomic correlations. *American Journal of Mental Deficiency* 80:149.

Grossman, H. J. 1973. *Manual on terminology and classification in mental retardation.* Special Publication Series no. 2. Washington, D.C.: American Association on Mental Deficiency.

Hallas, C. H.; Fraser, W. I.; and MacGillivary, R. C. 1974. *The care and training of the mentally handicapped.* Baltimore: Williams and Wilkins.

Hammar, S. L., and Barnard, K. E. 1966. The mentally retarded adolescent: A review of the characteristics and problems of 44 non-institutionalized adolescent retardates. *Pediatrics* 38:845.

Hammond, M. I.; Lewis, M. N.; and Johnson, E. W. 1966. A nutritional study of cerebral palsied children. *Journal of the American Dietetic Association* 49:196.

Hille, H. M., and Reeves, M. 1964. The battle against mental retardation: The dietitian's share. *Hospitals* 38 (22):101.

Hollis, J. H. 1973. "Superstition": The effects of independence and contingent events on free operant responses in retarded children. *American Journal of Mental Deficiency* 77:585.

Klinger, J. L. 1978. *Mealtime manual for people with disabilities and the aging.* Camden, N.J.: Institute of Rehabilitation Medicine and the Campbell Soup Company.

Niemeyer, K. A. 1971. Nutrition education is behavioral change. *Journal of Nutrition Education* 3:32.

President's Committee on Mental Retardation. 1972. *Federal Programs for the retarded.* Washington, D.C.: President's Committee on Mental Retardation.

Smith, M. A. H., ed. 1971. *Feeding the handicapped child.* Memphis: University of Tennessee Child Development Center.

Springer, N. S. 1971. *Nutrition and mental retardation: An annotated bibliography.* Ann Arbor: University of Michigan, Institute for the Study of Mental Retardation.

U.S. Department of Health, Education and Welfare. 1972a. *Mental retardation activities.* Office of Mental Retardation Coordination. Washington, D.C.: Government Printing Office.

U.S. Department of Health, Education and Welfare. 1972b. *Mental retardation source book for D.H.E.W.* Office of Mental Retardation Coordination, DHEW publication no. (OS) 73-81. Washington, D.C.: Government Printing Office.

Wallace, H. M. 1972. Nutrition and handicapped children. *Journal of the American Dietetic Association* 61:127.

Wilkinson, M.; Kerry, E.; Ganshorn, R.; and Kies, C. 1971. Food and nutrition education for mentally disturbed women. *Journal of Nutrition Education* 3:14.

CHAPTER 9

Food Behavior and Obesity

Obesity, defined as the excessive accumulation of body fat, has been identified as the "major public health problem confronting the United States and other affluent nations" (Bray 1974, p. 423) as well as the most frequent nutritional disturbance of childhood (Winick 1974). Although national statistics for the prevalence of incidence of juvenile obesity are not available, 12 to 20 percent of the preadult population is estimated to be obese, and the percentage is expected to increase (Seltzer and Mayer 1970).

Obesity in childhood tends to persist, with approximately 80 percent of obese children becoming obese adults (Mobbs 1970). Moreover, obesity which develops in childhood or adolescence is more difficult to treat and may cause more severe personality and psychological problems than obesity that develops in adulthood (Bruch 1973a). The last trimester of pregnancy, the first 3 years of life, and adolescence may be the most critical periods in determining whether a person will be obese (Winick 1974).

The 1973 New York City Conference on Childhood Obesity, sponsored by the Institute of Human Nutrition of the College of Physicians and Surgeons of Columbia University identified childhood obesity as a very dangerous form of obesity and a significant health hazard. The conference urged that the medical and nutritional communities and concerned parents throughout the United States institute the necessary programs "to study and eradicate what is perhaps the greatest 'nutritional danger' in our country today" (Winick 1974, 1975).

Despite the magnitude of the problem and the long history of research in this area, little undisputed knowledge has been accumulated regarding the etiology and treatment of obesity. The etiology of a small number of cases was attributed by Schachter (1971a) to genetic factors or to injury to the hypothalamus, hormonal imbalance, or other metabolic abnormalities. More recently, the fat cell theory has suggested that there are two types of obesity: hyperplastic, wherein a person has too many fat cells (characteristic of early or childhood onset obesity), and hypertrophic,

This chapter was written by Dr. Kitty R. Coffey specially for this book.

wherein a person has excessive large fat cells (characteristic of late or adult onset obesity) (Hirsch and Knittle 1970). It appears, however, that most obesity, whether of adult or juvenile onset, can be attributed not to abnormal metabolism but to food habits maladjusted to the person's metabolic needs; that is, obese persons eat more food than they need or they fail to reduce their food intake to match lowered metabolic requirements (Winick 1974).

With regard to the etiological classification of obesity, Van Itallie and Campbell (1972, p. 386) presented the following tentative groupings of forms of obesity according to mechanism.

I. Regulatory obesity (no primary metabolic abnormality)
   A. Psychologic
      1. Non-neurotic overeating (orientation toward "external" and sensory cues relating to the eating process)
      2. Overeating associated with neurosis
   B. Physiologic
      1. Increased energy intake (brain damage)
      2. Decreased energy output (sedentary existence)
II. Metabolic obesity
   A. Enzymatic (? certain forms of genetic obesity)
   B. Hormonal (hyperadrenocorticism)
   C. Neurologic (? certain forms of lipodystrophy)
III. "Constitutional" obesity
   A. Fat cell hyperplasia

The etiology of obesity is not yet clear; the interrelationships between the metabolic and regulatory factors affecting energy balance are extremely intricate. Recognizing the complexity of the etiological factors in obesity, Van Itallie and Campbell (1972) recommended a multidisciplinary approach to the problem, involving methodologies drawn from both the metabolic and the behavioral sciences.

The term *obesity* does not refer to weight, relative weight, or personal overweight. An overweight muscular person may be lean, whereas an underweight, slightly built person may be overly fat. Obesity is defined in terms of fatness rather than body weight, and it is measured as fat (Garn 1972).

Data from the Ten-State Nutrition Survey indicated that the commonly used criterion of 20 percent overweight for adults was not an appropriate definition for obesity in infants and children (Garn and Clark 1975; Garn, Clark, and Guire 1975). Garn (1972) recommended as a definition of adolescent obesity the upper 15 percent of fatness (i.e., above the 85th percentile as measured by skin fold thickness).

THE OBESE ADOLESCENT

Obese adolescents can be described in terms of their social, physical, and psychological characteristics as well as their behavior in regard to food and activity. Care must be taken not to overgeneralize, however, for obese adolescents, like all human beings, exhibit many individual differences.

Physical Characteristics

There are several physical characteristics that differentiate the obese from the nonobese adolescent. For example, obese boys and girls are taller than their lean peers from at least the second year of life and tend to have advanced bone age. Since epiphysical closure takes place earlier than normal, owing to the advanced bone age, the obese adolescent is not excessively tall as an adult. Nevertheless, because skeletal development is advanced in obese adolescents, they exhibit greater skeletal mass than their nonobese peers (Garn and Clark 1975). Other physical characteristics of obese adolescents are early menarche (Hammar et al. 1972), elevated hemoglobin levels and hematrocrit values (Garn and Clark 1975), increased fat-free weight (Garn, Clark, and Guire 1975), and increased size and number of fat cells (Winick 1974). Physical complications of adolescent obesity include suspected hypogenitalism (male genitalia appear small due to surrounding adipose tissue), suspected gynecomastia (male mammary glands appear to be excessively developed due to adipose tissue), cutaneous striae (streaks or lines on the skin caused by stretching), and high blood pressure. Various orthopedic problems that may occur are genu valgum (a deformity in which the knees are abnormally close together and the space between the ankles is increased, also known as knock knee), coxa vara (a deformity of the hip in which the angle formed by the axis of the head and neck of the femur and the axis of its shaft is materially decreased), and slipped femoral epiphysis (a dislocation of the epiphysis of the head of the femur) (Jones 1972).

Stunkard et al. (1972), in a study of the triceps skin folds of 3,344 white schoolchildren 5 to 18 years old, found obesity to be more prevalent in girls of lower social class than in girls of higher social class. By the time they were 6 years old, 29 percent of the girls of lower social class were obese, as opposed to 3 percent of the upper-class girls. This class-associated difference continued through age 18, falling to a minimum at 12 years of age, when 13 percent of the lower-class girls and 9 percent of the upper-class girls were obese. Less dramatic, though similar, trends were found among males of the divergent social classes.

By adulthood a strong inverse relationship exists between socioeconomic status and obesity. Goldblatt, Moore, and Stunkard (1965) and Moore, Stunkard, and Stole (1962) reported that obesity was six times more prevalent among women of lower socioeconomic status than among women of higher socioeconomic status. They found an inverse relationship between obesity and parental socioeconomic status. Furthermore, upwardly mobile females were less obese than were downwardly mobile females. Finally, the longer a woman's family has been in this country, the less likely she was to be obese. Similar but less marked trends were observed in men.

The work of Garn and Clark (1974, 1975), however, contradicts that of Stunkard et al. (1972). When Garn's definition of obesity (above the 85th percentile in fatness) was applied to the Ten-State Nutrition Survey data as a whole, the proporation of obese children varied with the different socioeconomic groups. In general, beyond infancy and into adolescence the obese were the more affluent and the lean were those below the poverty level within each ethnic and racial group for which there were sufficient subjects for comparison. This generalization was applicable to males of all ages, with some expections among younger children, and to females through early adolescence (Garn and Clark 1974, 1975). When Garn and Clark (1975) separated the super-obese (the upper 5 percent in fatness) from the others, however, those individuals were not primarily middle-income as were the simply obese. Thus, perhaps the discrepancy in findings of Stunkard et al. (1972) and Garn and Clark (1974, 1975) is partly attributable to differences in their criteria for defining obesity.

Regardless of age or socioeconomic group, females exhibit more surface fatness at all ages, beginning in childhood, than do males. Adolescence for females, both rich and poor, is a period of increasing surface adiposity. As adolescence progresses, however, females of lower socioeconomic status become fatter, whereas those of higher socioeconomic status become leaner (Garn, Clark, and Guire 1975).

Psychological Characteristics

Obese adolescents, especially girls, exhibit a number of social and psychological problems. Obese juveniles are the victims of intense prejudice and often come from psychologically disturbed families. Moreover, developmentally obese adolescents manifest emotional disturbances, perhaps the most important of which is the feeling of not being in control of their own sensations and actions (e.g., lacking awareness of hunger). In their families, obese adolescents appear to occupy a unique position: they are often the focus of parental conflicts, a source of embarrassment, or a sibling scapegoat. In addition, their families often fail to recognize them as individuals or to allow them to express themselves (Bruch 1971, 1973b; Hammar et al. 1972).

Monello and Mayer (1963) found that obese girls tended to be passive, to have an obsessive concern with self-image, to expect rejection, and to progressively withdraw—traits strikingly similar to those exhibited by ethnic and racial minority groups that are victims of intense prejudice. Bullen et al. (1963) noted that obese girls had significantly fewer dates and were in fewer non-sports organizations and groups both in and outside of school than were nonobese girls. Furthermore, obese girls participated less actively in the groups of which they were members than did nonobese girls.

Obese adolescents of both sexes are often characterized by depression, low self-esteem, social isolation, and defective body-image development (Hammar et al. 1972). Body image, the physical aspects of one's self-concept, consistently appears as a personality problem among obese juveniles (Stunkard and Burt 1967; Stunkard and Mendelson 1967; Lerner and Gellert 1969; Nathan and Pisula 1970; Nathan 1973). Negative evaluations of body size or shape may develop during a relatively short period of time in childhood and adolescence, but persons becoming obese during their adult years seem not to make negative evaluations, regardless of their body size (Stunkard and Burt 1967). Body image appears to be formed between the ages of 8 and 14, with little change after age 14 (Faterson and Witkin 1970).

Patterns of Activity and Food Behavior

Excessive energy intake and reduced energy expenditure are the two major environmental causes of obesity in children (Garn and Clark 1975; Garn, Clark, and Ullman 1975). Mayer (1975) proposed the latter as the more important variable, based upon studies of obese adolescents in summer camps. Other investigators have demonstrated a relationship between physical inactivity and obesity (Duddleston and Bennion 1970; Hammar et al. 1972; Johnson, Mastropaolo, and Wharton 1972). Obese adolescents are less physically active and more interested in sedentary pursuits than are their nonobese counterparts, and they appear to exert themselves less vigorously when they do engage in physical activity (Johnson, Burke, and Mayer 1956; Stefanik, Heald, and Mayer 1959; Bullen et al. 1963; Bullen, Reed, and Mayer 1964; Huenemann, Shapiro, Hampton, and Mitchell 1966; Huenemann et al. 1967; Huenemann et al. 1974; Hammar et al. 1972). Longitudinal investigation of adolescents suggests that the obese consume fewer calories than the nonobese and tend to be physically inactive (Hampton et al. 1966; Huenemann, Hampton, Shapiro, and Behnke 1966; Huenemann, Shapiro, Hampton, and Mitchell 1966, 1968; Huenemann et al. 1967; Huenemann et al. 1974). Work by Bradfield, Paulos, and Grossman (1971) supports those findings.

Several workers have reported the food preferences and food habits of obese adolescents. Perhaps the most interesting finding was that the obese adolescents ate no more, and perhaps ate less, than nonobese adolescents (Johnson, Burke, and Mayer 1956; Stefanik, Heald, and Mayer 1959; Huenemann, Hampton, Shapiro, and Behnke 1966; Huenemann, Shapiro, Hampton, and Mitchell 1966, 1968; Huenemann et al.

1974; Bradfield, Paulos, and Grossman 1971; Hammar et al. 1972). (Heald [1975] has questioned the reliability of studies indicating that obese adolescents eat less than their nonobese peers and suggests that, as a "defense mechanism," the obese subjects may have underreported their food intakes.) The obese boys and girls were breakfast skippers; but obese boys snacked more than boys who were not obese, and obese girls the same or less than other girls (Bullen et al. 1963; Huenemann, Hampton, Shapiro, and Behnke 1966; Huenemann, Shapiro, Hampton, and Mitchell 1966, 1968; Huenemann et al. 1974). Obese boys and girls ate smaller amounts of dairy products, vegetables, and fruits than did the nonobese subjects (Huenemann, Hampton, Shapiro, and Behnke 1966; Huenemann, Shapiro, Hampton, and Mitchell 1966, 1968; Huenemann et al. 1974). Obese girls reported more dieting and eating sprees than did nonobese girls, and they attributed their obesity to food (Bullen et al. 1963).

In studies of the food choices and eating rates of adults, Gates, Huenemann, and Brand (1975) observed that, compared to nonobese persons, the obese subjects chose larger quantities of food and selected more foods from the high-calorie, low-nutrient group than from the protective food group (i.e., milk, meat, fruits and vegetables, cereals). The obese adults took more bites (Gaul, Craighead, and Mahoney 1975), spent less time chewing (Gaul, Craighead, and Mahoney 1975; Wagner and Hewitt 1975), and generally ate faster (Hill and McCutcheon 1975) than the adults who were not obese.

Weinseir (1976) noted that leaner population groups emphasized vegetables, fruits, and starches in their diets, whereas fatter population groups emphasized meats, sweets, and fats. The relative caloric densities of those food groups are shown in table 11. The foods of higher caloric density can be eaten faster and have less bulk, or residue, than the foods of lower caloric density.

TABLE 11. RELATIVE CALORIC DENSITIES OF FOOD GROUPS

Food Group	Density (kcal/oz)
Vegetables	5-10
Fruits	15
Starches	50
Meats	75
Sweets	150
Fats/Oils	170-270

Data from R. Weinseir, Nutritional considerations in the treatment of obesity (paper presented at the Child Nutrition Workshop, 30 November 1976, in Birmingham, Ala.).

Several workers have established that obese persons eat more high-preference food and less low-preference food than do nonobese individuals (Hashim and Van Itallie 1965; Goldman, Jaffa, and Schachter 1968; Nisbett 1968b; Schachter 1971b; Price and Grinker 1973; Hill and McCutcheon 1975). Closely associated with the preference hypothesis has been the popular idea that people become obese by overindulging in high-preference sweets or carbohydrates (Grinker, Price, and Greenwood 1976). In studies of sucrose sensitivity in obese adults, Grinker, Hirsch, and Smith (1972) reported no difference in the thresholds of obese subjects and subjects of normal weight. The sucrose thresholds of obese persons were not affected by their age at the onset of obesity. Pangborn and Simone (1958) indicated that, among 12,505 persons participating in a consumer survey, no significant difference in preferences for apricots, pears, peaches, and vanilla ice cream (foods of differing sugar content) could be attributed to variation in body size.

Only a few studies have been done on children's taste preferences for sucrose. Grinker, Price, and Greenwood (1976) used the method of paired comparisons to study the preferences of normal-weight and obese children 8 to 10 years old for sucrose solutions of 1.95 to 19.5 percent. They found that the preferences of the obese children were inversely related to sucrose concentration. Using hedonic ratings, they studied the taste preferences of obese children ages 8 to 11 for Kool-Aid solutions sweetened with sucaryl (ranging from 1.0 to 2.5 times the manufacturer's recommended sweetness). And they also obtained hedonic ratings and sweetness magnitude estimates for cherry Kool-Aid solutions sweetened with sucaryl (0, 0.5, 1.0, and 2.0 times the manufacturer's recommended sweetness, corresponding to sucrose solutions of 5.60 to 27.38 percent) from ninety obese adolescent girls and seven boys at a summer camp in North Carolina and from fourteen obese adolescent girls at a camp in California. The children's preferences for Kool-Aid were related to the degree of overweight, with the more overweight children having a lower preference for the sweeter Kool-Aid solutions. Based on their findings, Grinker, Price, and Greenwood suggested that a preference for the sweet foods is unlikely to be a major factor in the establishment and maintenance of the obese state. This is contrary to the popular reasoning that the obese have a "sweet tooth" (Nordsiek 1972).

In the past decade nonneurotic overeating, the result of orientation toward external rather than internal cues related to eating, has been studied rather extensively in adults. Topics of investigation include the effects of food deprivation, time, work involvement, cue prominence, and taste sensitivity on eating behavior as associated with differences in body weight. (See Schachter, Goldman, and Gordon 1968; McKenna 1972; Goldman, Jaffa, and Schachter 1968; Schachter and Gross 1968; Nisbett and Gurwitz 1970; Schachter 1971a; Nisbett 1968a, 1968b; Kozlowski and Schachter 1975; Hashim and Van Itallie 1965; Grinker, Hirsch, and Smith 1972; Grinker 1975.) Relatively little work, however, except for that of Grinker, Price, and Greenwood (1976), has been done on the external and sensory cues that affect food behavior in children.

Knowledge of the Relationship between Food and Activity

Huenemann, Shapiro, Hampton, and Mitchell (1966) and Huenemann et al. (1974) reported that, in general, obese adolescents have a reasonably good knowledge of dietary needs and of the causes of obesity, although popular misconceptions do exist. Dwyer, Feldman, and Mayer (1967), in a study of 446 high school girls, found that the girls had little knowledge of the relatiohship of kilocalories to food and activity; however, girls who dieted or who were obese had a better understanding than the others.

Obese adolescents, in their belief that food is primarily responsible for their obesity, lack knowledge regarding the relationship of exercise to weight and fail to recognize their disinclination to exercise (Bullen et al. 1963; Bullen, Reed, and Mayer 1964). The attitudes of obese persons toward exercise and physical activity are reflected in their being less physically active and more interested in sedentary pursuits than nonobese persons are (Johnson, Burke, and Mayer 1956; Stefanik, Heald, and Mayer 1959; Bullen et al. 1963; Bullen, Reed, and Mayer 1964; Huenemann, Shapiro, Hampton, and Mitchell 1966, 1967; Huenemann et al. 1974; Hammar et al. 1972).

Wooley (1972) and Wooley, Wooley, and Dunham (1972) investigated perceived caloric values of food in relation to hunger. Wooley obtained evidence that both obese and nonobese subjects ate significantly less and reported a greater feeling of satiety after drinking a 200-kilocalorie milk shake designed to appear high in calories than after drinking a 600-kilocalorie milk shake designed to appear low in calories. Wooley et al. observed that their seven obese and seven nonobese subjects demonstrated almost no ability to identify liquid meals of disguised caloric content as either high or low calorie; moreover, the subjects reported hunger in relation to their beliefs about the caloric value of the food they had consumed rather than its actual caloric content.

MODIFICATION OF FOOD BEHAVIOR

Historically, most treatment programs for obesity that have been reported in the medical literature have proved relatively ineffective. Anyone who has dealt with obese patients is depressingly aware of the failure of any one treatment to lead to significant and sustained weight loss in all but a small number of cases. The difficulty of treating obesity effectively seems an overwhelming problem independent of the mode of therapy.

In a 1959 review of the medical management of obesity for the previous 30 years, Stunkard and McLaren-Hume reported that all programs were equally ineffective in their treatment of obesity. Attrition rates in the programs reviewed ranged from 20 to 80 percent. Only 25 percent of those who stayed in therapy lost 9 kilograms (20 pounds), and only 5 percent lost as much as 18 kilograms (40 pounds). Stunkard 1958, p. 79) concluded: "Most obese persons will not stay in treatment for obesity. Of those who stay in treatment most will not lose weight and of those who do lose weight, most will regain it." Until recently, this summary of the results of outpatient treatment for obesity was unchallenged.

In 1970, Wollersheim reviewed the relevant literature and concluded that, although from a physiological standpoint obesity may result from multiple etiologies, overeating was the only behavioral or personality characteristic consistently distinguishing the obese from the nonobese. In the great majority of cases, successful weight reduction was dependent upon reducing the positive energy balance that resulted from the consumption of more kilocalories than were expended.

Although hundreds of papers have been published on the treatment of obesity, only recently have researchers begun to look at systematically modifying the patterns of eating behavior in obese persons. In the past 10 years, attempts to apply behavior modification to the treatment of obesity have resulted in some of the most successful programs reported in the literature (Levitz 1973).

Behavior modification is relatively new. Only in the past 30 years have experimentally derived, scientific concepts been used to change maladaptive patterns of behavior in a systematic fashion. The field of behavior therapy represents an extension of the basic research on animal learning done by I. P. Pavlov and B. F. Skinner to problems in human behavior. The current interest in behavior modification and the evidence of its effectiveness in the control of several conditions have rendered inevitable its application to the problems of overeating and obesity. To date, behavior modification or behavior therapy have been used successfully to deal with problems as diverse as anorexia nervosa, childhood autism, chronic pain, depression, hysteria, phobias, poor study habits, stuttering, alcoholism, and mental retardation (Pomerleau, Bass, and Crown 1975).

The behavioral approach emphasizes relating measurable activity (responses) to antecedent and subsequent environmental events (stimuli). Two of the concepts growing out of this approach, contingency management and stimulus control, have proved particularly productive (Pomerleau, Bass, and Crown 1975).

According to Levitz (1973, pp. 22-23), in behavior therapy "the focus of attention is on observable behavior and observable behavior change." "Efforts are made to measure precisely the target behavior and to assess the degree of change that occurs.... The most distinctive characteristic of behavior therapy is that it attempts to abstract effective clinical techniques from general psychologic principles, primarily from research in human learning and social psychology." It may be administered by "psychotherapists, teachers, psychiatric nurses, or hospital aides" or by self-management by the client. "Behavior therapy, as applied to obesity, is characterized by: (a) determination of observable eating and activity habit patterns; (b) measurement of the target behaviors before and during treatment; (c) a series of techniques abstracted from psychologic research in learning; and (d) an educational approach to the development of self-management." Levitz found it "significant that behavior therapists' interest in obesity was stimulated by the reliable and observable measure of therapeutic success it provided as much as by the medical and social problem it represented.

Programs for the Behavioral Treatment of Obesity

In general, behavioral treatment of obesity has progressed from the use of a limited number of techniques for a short time to procedures using multiple techniques and involving baseline, treatment, and follow-up phases. The effectiveness of treatment has appeared to increase correspondingly.

Of the early attempts to treat obesity by behavioral means, the work of Ferster, Nurnberger, and Levitt (1962) has been most influential, even though their methodology has been assessed as only moderately successful. They reported a modal weight loss of 10 pounds, with a range of 5 to 20 pounds, for the 10 patients in their study (Penick et al. 1971). Their study provided the conceptual basis for the more clinically sophisticated approach that followed. The developments that grew out of their work included (1) the use of stimulus-control and analysis to determine the variables controlling overeating, (2) the specification and subsequent disruption of the reinforcers maintaining overeating, (3) the development of new reinforcers for behaviors that could serve as alternatives to overeating, and (4) the identification of the "ultimate aversive consequences" of overeating, to provide a rationale and motivation for attempting behavior change.

Stuart (1967) adapted the self-control approach of Ferster, Nurnberger, and Levitt to a small group setting in order to provide social reinforcement, and he devised several innovations with regard to stimulus control. Stuart (1971) further described the program of behavioral control of overeating as a three-dimensional program for the treatment of obesity, involving (1) control over the eating environment, (2) development of an individualized dietary program, and (3) development of an individualized aerobic exercise program based, in most cases, upon walking.

In 1972, Stuart, a social worker, and Davis, a dietitian, published their program for behavioral control of obesity, a book entitled *Slim Chance in a Fat World*. Their approach involved a calorically restricted diet, exercise, and behavioral management of the environment for both eating and exercising. The behavioral management included the elimination or suppression of factors leading to problematic eating (e.g., arranging to eat in only one room and keeping food out of sight) as well as the strengthening of factors leading to appropriate food behavior (e.g., making low-calorie food as attractive as possible). In essence, Stuart and Davis's program was an effort to manipulate antecedent, response, and consequent variables in the manner conducive to behavior change. Exercise was managed in much the same way as diet. A recent addition to the behavior modification programs is James M. Ferguson's *Learning to Eat: Behavior*

Modification for Weight Control (1975). Ferguson's program is designed to be used by the lay public and has both a leader's manual and a student's manual. The program was treated and revised at the Stanford Eating Disorders Clinic in the Department of Psychiatry and Behavioral Sciences at Stanford Medical School. Ferguson used many standard techniques, such as keeping a daily food diary and eating in a designated place. In addition, he included a number of innovative forms of feedback, such as the eating place record, which provides useful information about the extent to which a person is achieving the goal of confining all eating to the designated place, and the behavioral analysis form, which depicts progress made in cutting down on snacking and confining eating to mealtimes.

Results of Behavioral Treatment Programs for Obesity

Stuart (1967) reported the weight losses of eight female patients over a 1-year period (ten patients began treatment but two did not finish). Those were the best results to that date in the outpatient treatment of obesity. Three patients (30 percent of the original sample of ten) lost nearly 40 pounds, and five patients (50 percent of the original sample) lost more than 30 pounds. The average weight loss was 12.6 pounds for the 12 weeks of active treatment and 25.2 pounds for the 40 weeks of follow-up, giving a total average weight loss of 37.8 pounds over a 12-month period.

Subsequently, Stuart (1971) extended his behavioral treatment to additional groups with comparable success, using the patients as their own controls in what is known as a *crossover design*. He divided the six moderately obese female subjects, ranging in age from 27 to 41 years old, into two groups of three. During a preliminary 5-week period, the subjects kept careful records of their weight and their food intake. Group 1 then participated in treatment sessions of approximately 40 minutes twice a week for about 15 weeks. Meanwhile, group 2 was given diet-planning materials and an exercise program, both of which also were offered to group 1. The women in group 1 lost an average of 15 pounds, whereas those in group 2 (the control group) gained an average of 5 pounds. At the end of the 15 weeks, group 1 continued with the program on its own while group 2 received 15 weeks of the same treatment group 1 had received (group therapy plus diet planning and a program of exercise). Under these circumstances, those in group 1 lost an additional 10 pounds, but at a slightly lower rate than when they were in active treatment. Subjects in group 2, on the other hand, who had gained weight during the preceding 15 weeks, lost 15 pounds, as had those in group 1 under the same conditions. Both groups continued to lose without further treatment during the subsequent 12 weeks.

In a series of formal, controlled comparisons, Penick et al. (1971) duplicated Stuart's 1971 work and demonstrated that a behavioral approach to weight reduction was more effective with severely obese patients than traditional group therapy. Fifteen patients (eleven females and four males), ranging in age from 21 to 61 years old, were seen for weekly group sessions lasting about 2 hours each for 3 months. A group of seventeen persons (thirteen females and four males), ranging in age from 15 to 61 years old was used as control. The control group's losses were comparable to those reported in the medical literature. None lost 30 pounds, but 24 percent lost more than 20 pounds. By contrast, 13 percent of the group undergoing behavior modification lost more than 40 pounds, 33 percent lost more than 30 pounds, and 53 percent lost more than 20 pounds. Although the differences between the behavior modification and control groups' losses over 20 and 40 pounds were not statistically significant, the difference for weight losses over 30 pounds was significant. Furthermore, those who had lost weight during active treatment continued to lose weight during the follow-up period of 6 months.

Harmatz and Lapuc (1968) reported on the application of behavior modification principles to the treatment of obesity among long-term schizophrenic patients in a Veterans' Administration hospital. Seven men, matched for degree of overweight, were assigned to each of three treatment groups: (1) behavior modification, (2) group therapy, and (3) diet only. Treatment was carried out over a 6-week period with a 4-week follow-up. Behavior modification involved a penalty schedule requiring forfeiture of part of a $5.00 weekly allowance for failure to lose weight during the previous week. Weight loss carried no reward other than assuring the patient of his regular allowance. Group therapy sessions were held once each week for 1 hour. At the sessions the patients were weighed and received encouraging comments for weight losses, and the reasons for losses and gains were discussed. Patients in these two groups lost significantly more weight during the 6-week period than those whose only treatment was diet. The behavior modification subjects, however, lost significantly more weight during the 4-week follow-up than did the group therapy subjects.

Harris (1969) reported a well-controlled study which used behavioral techniques to control eating in mildly overweight college students. Two groups each consisting of three male and five female students, received treatment and were compared with a control group of eight students. In order not to discourage them and thereby bias the results, the control subjects were told that they could not enter treatment at once, because of a conflict in schedules, but that they would receive treatment later. Treatment sessions were held twice weekly for the first 2 months and then on a more irregular basis for the next 2 to 3 months. The mean weight loss for the experimental groups was 10.5 pounds as compared with a weight gain of 3.6 pounds for the control group, a difference that was highly significant (P = 0.001). Although the results for the groups receiving treatment were clearly far superior to those for the control group, they were not as good as others reported in the literature; only 21 percent of Harris's subjects lost 20 pounds and none lost as much as 40 pounds. A major reason for these results was that Harris's subjects were less obese than subjects studied by other investigators.

Wollersheim (1970), in an elaborate study, attempted to disentangle the contributions of various techniques by establishing the following experimental conditions: (1) "focal" behavior treatment, (2) nonspecific therapy, (3) social pressure, and (4) control groups of persons promised treatment but not yet receiving it. The study thus contained three treatment groups (1, 2, and 3) and three control groups (2, 3, and 4) for the behavior modification group (group 1). Subjects were mildly (10 percent overweight female college students. Four therapists treated groups of five subjects under each of the three treatment conditions. A course of treatment consisted of ten sessions extending over a 3-month period. At the end of treatment and after an 8-week follow-up, the results for the behavior modification group were superior not only to those for the controls receiving no treatment but also to those for the other two treatment groups. The social pressure group had participated in 20-minute sessions based on TOPS (Take Off Pounds Sensibly). The purpose of the group receiving nonspecific therapy was to control for the effects of group treatment that resulted from such nonspecific factors as increased attention, expectation of relief, and presentation of a treatment rationale and meaningful "ritual."

Hagen (1974), following up the work of Wollersheim, accepted Wollersheim's finding that behavior modification was the most effective method for the treatment of obesity. He turned his attention to determining whether the results obtained were due only to the specific behavioral techniques used or were dependent also upon the personal influence of the therapist. He constructed an experimental design similar to Wollersheim's, using the following groups: (1) group behavior therapy, eighteen subjects,

(2) bibliotherapy (therapy from a written manual), eighteen subjects, (3) group behavior therapy and bibliotherapy combined, eighteen subjects, and (4) treatment promised but not yet received, thirty-five subjects.

The eighty-nine subjects in Hagen's study were mildly (10 percent) overweight female college students who were assigned randomly to one of the four experimental groups in such a way that the groups were comparable with respect to the obesity of their members. Three therapists treated six subjects each in the group therapy and combined therapy conditions. Ten treatment sessions were held over a 3-month period. The greatest weight loss occurred in the combined therapy group, whose members lost an average of 15 pounds during treatment and gained 2 pounds during the 4-week follow-up period. However, the difference in weight loss between the combined therapy group and the other two treatment groups was not statistically significant. There was a significant difference (P = 0.01) between the combined therapy group's weight loss and that of the group not receiving treatment. Thus, Hagen's work showed that it was possible to treat obesity effectively by using a written manual that embodied behavioral therapy principles. Moveover, this treatment apparently was as effective as one that involved therapists.

Self-help Groups. Because both behavior modification and self-help groups showed some notable success, Jordan and Levitz (1973) conducted a pilot study to evaluate the feasibility of combining these two approaches. The initial behavior modification programs had been successful, but the number of patients treated was small and the ratio of therapists to patients high. At a time when there were not enough professional therapists to meet treatment demands, the training of nonprofessionals to conduct therapy seemed a logical approach to relieving this shortage. Jordan and Levitz trained a formerly very obese executive in the basic principles of behavior therapy and made him the leader of a group of seven obese men and women. The use of typical TOPS social pressure for the first 12 weeks resulted in an average weight loss of 3 pounds. During the next 12 weeks the use of behavior modification techniques resulted in an average weight loss of 10 pounds among the seven obese subjects.

Levitz and Stunkard (1974) followed Jordan and Levitz's 1973 pilot study with an investigation of sixteen TOPS chapters with a total of 234 members. The members received one of four treatments: (1) behavior modification conducted by a professional therapist, (2) behavior modification conducted by the TOPS leader, (3) nutrition education conducted by the TOPS leader, and (4) continuation of the usual TOPS program. During the 3-month treatment period, behavior modification produced significantly lower attrition rates and significantly greater weight losses than did the alternative treatment methods. After a 9-month follow-up, the differences among treatment results were even greater. Members of TOPS chapters in which behavior modification was introduced by professionals lost significantly more weight (P = 0.05) than those taught the same program by the TOPS chapter leaders. In this study, then, self-help was less effective than treatment directed by a professional.

Self-monitoring. The systematic self-presentation of rewards has become an increasingly popular clinical technique. Bandura (1969) emphasized three core elements in self-reward operations: (1) self-monitoring, the systematic observation of one's behavior, (2) self-evaluation, the comparison of one's performance with a standard of achievement, and (3) self-reinforcement, presenting oneself with a tangible reward if one's performance matches or exceeds the chosen standard.

Mahoney (1974) studied self-reward and self-monitoring techniques in weight-control programs. Forty-nine obese adults were assigned randomly to one of four groups: (1) self-reward for weight loss, (2) self-reward for habit improvement, (3) self-monitoring, and (4) delayed treatment (the control group). Individuals in the first three groups were given information on basic stimulus-control techniques for losing weight, and they monitored their own eating habits during a base period of 2 weeks. Thereafter, self-monitoring subjects continued their recording and were given standardized goals for weight loss and habit change at individual weekly weigh-ins. In addition to the monitoring procedure, self-rewarding subjects made deposits of their own money and awarded themselves portions of their deposits when they attained their goal (either weight loss or habit improvement). Control subjects received no treatment during the first 8 weeks, but thereafter they participated in a program which combined the procedures of the two self-rewarding groups.

Analysis of Mahoney's data revealed short-term and variable weight losses during the 2-week base period of self-monitoring. Even when definite goals were set for the subjects, these reductions did not prove to be either enduring or significant. However, when subjects were allowed to reward themselves in addition to monitoring their eating habits, they lost substantially more weight. Those who lost the most belonged to the group who rewarded themselves for habit change rather than weight loss. A significant relationship was found between successful weight reduction and the degree to which eating habits improved.

Bellack (1976) compared self-monitoring of food intake with self-reinforcement of eating behavior in thirty-eight obese subjects in a weight-reduction program. Two levels of therapist contact were used to control for possible confounding by external reinforcement, making four groups in all. Subjects in both of the self-rewarding groups lost significantly more weight than their self-monitoring counterparts; in fact, they lost at a rate of more than 1 pound per week. Differences related to the level of therapist contact were not significant.

Generalizations

The following generalizations can be made regarding the eleven studies that have been discussed.

The number of subjects was small, ranging from six to seventy-three and averaging nineteen per study. Subjects in four of the studies were university students. Two studies included subjects of low socioeconomic status; all other subjects were middle class, many of them private patients. The subjects were primarily female (92 percent) and ranged in age from 16 to 61. No children were studied.

The treatment periods varied greatly, ranging from 6 to 16 weeks and averaging 10.8 weeks. The most frequent treatment period (the mode) was 12 weeks. (Jordan and Levitz [1973] compared the results of several studies on the basis of 12-week treatment periods.) The mean weight loss during treatment was 0.46 kilograms (1.02 pounds) per week. For the six 12-week studies, weight loss ranged from 1.91 to 9.55 kilograms (4.2 to 21.0 pounds), with a mean of 5.41 kilograms (11.9 pounds), and the mean weight loss per week was 0.45 kilograms (0.99 pound). Follow-up periods also varied greatly, ranging from 4 to 52 weeks and averaging 20.8 weeks. The mean weight loss during follow-up was 0.16 kilogram (0.36 pound) per week. The ratio of therapists to subjects was high, ranging from 1:1 in Stuart's 1967 report to 1:18 in Levitz and Stunkard's self-help group study (1974). Bellack (1976) used no therapist in one group. The average ratio of therapists to subjects was 1:7.

These generalizations indicate a need for standardized treatment and follow-up periods in order that results may be more effectively compared and evaluated. Although the average weight loss of subjects in active behavior therapy is encouraging, the average weight loss during follow-up is quite disappointing. The high ratio of therapists to subjects raises the question of practicability and indicates a need for further evaluation of self-help groups.

What's Missing in Behavior Modification?

Weisenberg and Fray (1974) raised the question, What's missing in behavior modification? They cited the fact that, except for a study by Penick et al., the reported investigations of behavioral treatment of obesity were conducted with college students, patients of private physicians, or other middle-class subjects. In the study by Penick et al. (1971), the only study to include lower-class subjects, both the best and the worst results were obtained.

Weisenberg and Fray (1974) tried the behavior modification approach with an ethnically and racially mixed group to see if it would be as effective with and applicable to the routine population of an urban outpatient clinic as it had been with the middle-class group. Overall, behavior modification was either less effective or not significantly different from standard methods of group therapy. Weisenberg and Fray suggested that for lower socioeconomic groups, one-to-one treatment might be more effective than group treatment and that simplified forms should be developed which would require only a minimum of writing or reading skill.

Conclusion

The treatment of obesity has been the subject of an overwhelming number of books and articles over many decades. The common feature of all the treatments and techniques that have been proposed is their failure to effect weight loss in all obese persons, although each new technique has had some major success with some individuals.

Ferster, Nurnberger, and Levitt (1962) suggested that health professionals should not be concerned with whether one or another program can effect weight loss. Many individual and group therapy programs do lead to temporary loss of weight; however, what one should be concerned about, according to them, is the "development of self-control in eating which will endure and become an available part of the individual's future repertoire." Most conventional programs have not focused on the food intake patterns or food behaviors available to the subject before or after losing weight, nor have they presented techniques for developing control of food behavior and food intake patterns. To date, behavior modification has produced the best results. This relatively new technique aims at identifying, assessing, and changing the food behavior of obese persons. Behavior therapy was first formally applied to weight control by Ferster, Nurnberger, and Levitt in 1962, and since the mid-1960s there has been a modest increase in the use of this technique—an increase that has been accelerating during the 1970s. With more research and continued refinement, techniques for modifying behavior can have a more significant impact upon the food intake patterns of obese persons.

REFERENCES

Axler, B. H., and Schwarz, A. 1972. Selling students. *School Foodservice Journal* 26 (3):45.
Babcock, C. G. 1961. Attitudes and the use of food. *Journal of the American Dietetic Association* 38:546.
Bandura, A. 1969. *Principles of behavior modification.* New York: Holt, Rinehart and Winston.
Bellack, A. S. 1976. A comparison of self-reinforcement and self-monitoring in a weight reduction program. *Behavior Therapy* 7:68.

Bleibtreau, H. K. 1973. An anthropologist views the nutrition profession. *Journal of Nutrition Education* 5:11.

Bradfield, R. B.; Paulos, J.; and Grossman, L. 1971. Energy expenditure and heart rate of obese high school girls. *American Journal of Clinical Nutrition* 24:1482.

Bray, G. A. 1974. Fogarty conference on obesity. *American Journal of Clinical Nutrition* 27:423.

Bruch, H. 1971. Family transactions in eating disorders. *Comprehensive Psychiatry* 12:238.

Bruch, H. 1973a. *Eating disorders: Obesity, anorexia nervosa and the person within.* New York: Basic Books.

Bruch, H. 1973b. Psychological aspects of obesity. *Medical Insight* 5 (7):23.

Bullen, B. A.; Monello, L. F.; Cohen, H.; and Mayer, J. 1963. Attitudes toward physical activity, food and family in obese and non-obese adolescent girls. *American Journal of Clinical Nutrition* 12:1.

Bullen, B. A.; Reed, R. B.; and Mayer, J. 1964. Physical activity of obese and non-obese adolescent girls measured by motion picture sampling. *American Journal of Clinical Nutrition* 14:211.

Canning, H., and Mayer, J. 1966. Obesity—Its possible effect on college acceptance. *New England Journal of Medicine* 275:1172.

Carlisle, J. C. 1975. Food intake practices of high school students in Shelby County, Alabama. Ph.D. thesis, University of Tennessee (Knoxville).

Duddleston, A. K., and Bennion, M. 1970. Effect of diet and/or exercise on obese college women. *Journal of the American Dietetic Association* 56:126.

Dwyer, J. T.; Feldman, J. J.; and Mayer, J. 1967. Adolescent dieters: Who are they? *American Journal of Clinical Nutrition* 20:1045.

Dwyer, J., and Mayer, J. 1968-69. Psychological effects of variations in physical appearance during adolescence. *Adolescence* 3:353.

Eppright, E. S. 1947. Factors influencing food acceptance. *Journal of the American Dietetic Association* 23:579.

Faterson, H. F., and Witkin, H. A. 1970. Longitudinal study of development of the body concept. *Developmental Psychology* 2:429.

Ferguson, J. M. 1975. *Learning to eat: Behavior modification for weight control.* Palo Alto, Calif.: Bull.

Ferster, C. B.; Nurnberger, J. I.; and Levitt, E. B. 1962. The control of eating. *Journal of Mathetics* 1:87.

Fewster, W. F.; Bostian, L. R.; and Powers, R. D. 1973. Measuring the connotative meanings of foods. *Home Economics Research Journal* 2:44.

Garn, S. M. 1972. The measurement of obesity. *Ecology of Food and Nutrition* 1:333.

Garn, S. M., and Clark, D. C. 1974. Economics and fatness. *Ecology of Food and Nutrition* 3:19.

Garn, S. M., and Clark, D. C. 1975. Nutrition, growth, development and maturation: Findings from the Ten-State Nutrition Survey of 1968-70. *Pediatrics* 56:306.

Garn, S. M.; Clark, D. C.; and Guire, K. E. 1975. Growth, body composition, and development of obese and lean children. In *Childhood obesity*, ed. M. Winick, pp. 23-46. New York: Wiley.

Garn, S. M.; Clark, D. C.; and Ullman, B. M. 1975. Does obesity have a genetic basis in man? *Ecology of Food and Nutrition* 4:57.

Gates, J. C.; Huenemann, R. D.; and Brand, R. J. 1975. Food choices of obese and non-obese persons. *Journal of the American Dietetic Association* 67:339.

Gaul, D. J.; Craighead, W. E.; and Mahoney, M. J. 1975. Relationship between eating rates and obesity. *Journal of Consulting and Clinical Psychology* 43:123.

Gifft, H. H.; Washbon, M. B.; and Harrison, G. G. 1972. *Nutrition, behavior, and change.* Englewood Cliffs, N.J.: Prentice-Hall.

Goldblatt, P. B.; Moore, M. E.; and Stunkard, A. 1965. Social factors in obesity. *Journal of the American Medical Association* 192:1039.

Goldman, R.; Jaffa, M.; and Schachter, S. 1968. Yom Kippur, Air France, dormitory food and the eating behavior of obese and normal persons. *Journal of Personality and Social Psychology* 10:117.

Grinker, J. A. 1975. Symposium: Chemical senses and nutrition: 3. Taste factors and obesity. *Food Technology* 29 (8):76.

Grinker, J. A.; Hirsch, J.; and Smith, D. V. 1972. Taste sensitivity and susceptibility to external influence in obese and normal weight subjects. *Journal of Personality and Social Psychology* 22:320.

Grinker, J. A.; Price, J. M.; and Greenwood, M. R. C. 1976. Studies of taste in childhood obesity. In *Hunger: Basic mechanisms and clinical implications*, ed. D. Novin, W. Wyrwicke, and G. A. Bray, pp. 444-457. New York: Raven Press.

Hagen, R. L. 1974. Group therapy versus bibliotherapy in weight reduction. *Behavior Therapy* 5:222.

Hammar, S. L.; Campbell, M. M.; Campbell, V. A.; Moores, N. L.; Sareen, C.; Gareis, F. J.; and Lucas, B. 1972. An interdisciplinary study of adolescent obesity. *Journal of Pediatrics* 80:373.

Hampton, M. C.; Huenemann, R. L.; Shapiro, L. R.; Mitchell, B. W.; and Behnke, A. R. 1966. A longitudinal study of gross body composition and body conformation and their association with food and activity in a teen-age population: 2. Anthropometric evaluation of body build. *American Journal of Clinical Nutrition* 19:422.

Harmatz, M. G., and Lapuc, P. 1968. Behavior modification of overeating in a psychiatric population. *Journal of Consulting and Clinical Psychology* 32:583.

Harris, M. B. 1969. Self-directed program for weight control: A pilot study. *Journal of Abnormal Psychology* 74:263.

Hashim, S. A., and Van Itallie, T. B. 1965. Studies in normal and obese subjects with a monitored food dispensing device. *Annals of the New York Academy of Sciences* 131:654.

Heald, R. P. 1975. Juvenile obesity. In *Childhood obesity*, ed. M. Winick, pp. 87-88. New York: Wiley.

Hill, S. W., and McCutcheon, N. B. 1975. Eating responses of obese and non-obese humans during dinner meals. *Psychosomatic Medicine* 37:395.

Hirsch, J., and Knittle, J. L. 1970. Cellularity of obese and non-obese human adipose tissue. *Proceedings of the Federation of American Societies for Experimental Biology* 29:1516.

Huenemann, R. L.; Hampton, M. C.; Behnke, A. R.; Shapiro, L. R.; and Mitchell, B. W. 1974. *Teenage nutrition and physique*. Springfield, Ill.: Charles C. Thomas.

Huenemann, R. L.; Hampton, M. C.; Shapiro, L. R.; and Behnke, A. R. 1966. Adolescent food practices associated with obesity. *Proceedings of the Federation of American Societies for Experimental Biology* 25:4.

Huenemann, R. L.; Shapiro, L. R.; Hampton, M. C.; and Mitchell, B. W. 1966. A longitudinal study of gross body composition and body conformation and their association with food and activity in a teenage population: 1. Views of teenage subjects on body conformation, food and activity. *American Journal of Clinical Nutrition* 18:325.

Huenemann, R. L.; Shapiro, L. R.; Hampton, M. C.; and Mitchell, B. W. 1967. Teenagers' activities and attitudes toward activity. *Journal of the American Dietetic Association* 51:433.

Huenemann, R. L.; Shapiro, L. R.; Hampton, M. C.; and Mitchell, B. W. 1968. Food and eating practices of teenagers. *Journal of the American Dietetic Association* 53:17.

Johnson, M. L.; Burke, B. S.; and Mayer, J. 1956. Relative importance of inactivity and overeating in the energy balance of obese high school girls. *American Journal of Clinical Nutrition* 4:37.

Johnson, R. E.; Mastropaolo, J. A.; and Wharton, M. A. 1972. Exercise, dietary intake and body composition. *Journal of the American Dietetic Association* 61:399.

Jones, H. E. 1972. The fat child. *Practitioner* 208:212.

Jordan, H. A., and Levitz, L. S. 1973. Behavior modification in a self-help group. *Journal of the American Dietetic Association* 62:27.

Kozlowski, L. T., and Schachter, S. 1975. Effects of cue prominence and palatability on the drinking behavior of obese and normal humans. *Journal of Personality and Social Psychology* 32:1055.

Krech, D.; Crutchfield, R.; and Ballachey, E. 1962. *Individual in society*, pp. 279-281. New York: McGraw-Hill.

Lerner, R. M., and Gellert, E. 1969. Body build identification, preference and aversion in children. *Developmental Psychology* 1:456.

Levitz, L. S. 1973. Behavior therapy in treating obesity. *Journal of the American Dietetic Association* 62:22.

Levitz, L. S., and Stunkard, A. J. 1974. A therapeutic coalition for obesity: Behavior modification and patient self-help. *American Journal of Psychiatry* 131:423.

McConnell, S. 1974. Selected food preferences and some connotative meanings of foods by high school students in Hancock County, Tennessee. M.S. thesis, University of Tennessee (Knoxville).

McKenna, R. J. 1972. Some effects of anxiety level and food cues on the eating behavior of obese and normal subjects: A comparison of the Schachterian and psychosomatic conceptions. *Journal of Personality and Social Psychology* 22:311.

Mahoney, M. J. 1974. Self-reward and self-monitoring techniques for weight control. *Behavior Therapy* 5:48.

Mayer, J. 1975. Obesity during childhood. In *Childhood obesity*, ed. M. Winick, pp. 73-88. New York: Wiley.

Mobbs, J. 1970. Childhood obesity. *International Journal of Nursing Studies* 7:3.

Monello, L. F., and Mayer, J. 1963. Obese adolescent girls: An unrecognized minority group. *American Journal of Clinical Nutrition* 13:35.

Moore, H. B. 1957. The meaning of food. *American Journal of Clinical Nutrition* 5:77.

Moore, M. F.; Stunkard, A.; and Stole, L. 1962. Obesity, social class and mental illness. *Journal of the American Medical Association* 181:962.

Nathan, S. 1973. Body image in chronically obese children as reflected in figure drawings. *Journal of Personality Assessment* 37:456.

Nathan, S., and Pisula, D. 1970. Psychological observations of obese adolescents during starvation treatment. *Journal of the American Academy of Child Psychiatry* 9:722.

Nisbett, R. E. 1968a. Determinants of food intake in obesity. *Science* 159:1254.

Nisbett, R. E. 1968b. Taste, deprivation, and weight determinants of eating behavior. *Journal of Personality and Social Psychology* 10:107.

Nisbett, R. E., and Gurwitz, S. B. 1970. Obesity, food deprivation and supermarket shopping behavior. *Journal of Personality and Social Psychology* 12:289.

Nordsiek, F. W. 1972. The sweet tooth. *American Scientist* 60:41.

Osgood, C. E.; Suci, G. J.; and Tannenbaum, P. H. 1957. *The measurement of meaning.* Urbana, Ill.: University of Illinois Press.

Pangborn, R. M., and Simone, M. 1958. Body size and sweetness preference. *Journal of the American Dietetic Association* 34:924.

Penick, S. B.; Filion, R.; Fox, S.; and Stunkard, A. 1971. Behavior modification in the treatment of obesity. *Psychosomatic Medicine* 33:49.

Pomerleau, O.; Bass, F.; and Crown, V. 1975. Role of behavior modification in preventive medicine. *New England Journal of Medicine* 292:1277.

Price, J. M., and Grinker, J. 1973. Effects of degree of obesity, food deprivation and palatability on eating behavior of humans. *Journal of Comparative and Physiological Psychology* 85:265.

Pumpian-Mindlin, E. 1954. The meanings of food. *Journal of the American Dietetic Association* 30:576.

Sallade, J. 1973. A comparison of the psychological adjustment of obese versus non-obese children. *Journal of Psychosomatic Research* 17:89.

Schachter, S. 1968. Obesity and eating. *Science* 161:753.

Schachter, S. 1971a. *Emotion, obesity and crime.* New York: Academic Press.

Schachter, S. 1971b. Some extraordinary facts about obese humans and rats. *American Psychologist* 26:129.

Schachter, S.; Goldman, R.; and Gordon, A. 1968. Effects of fear, food deprivation and obesity on eating. *Journal of Personality and Social Psychology* 10:91.

Schachter, S., and Gross, L. P. 1968. Manipulated time and eating behavior. *Journal of Personality and Social Psychology* 10:98.

Schafer, R., and Yetley, E. A. 1975. Social psychology of food faddism. *Journal of the American Dietetic Association* 66:129.

Seltzer, C. C., and Mayer, J. 1970. An effective weight control program in a public school system. *American Journal of Public Health* 60:679.

Stanley, E. J.; Glaser, H. H.; Levin, D. G.; Adams, P. A.; and Coley, I. L. 1970. Overcoming obesity in adolescents: A description of a promising endeavor to improve management. *Clinical Pediatrics* 9:29.

Steelman, V. P. 1974. *The cultural context of food: A study of food habits and their social signifi-cance in selected areas of Louisiana.* Bulletin 681. Baton Rouge: Louisiana State University Agricultural Experiment Station.

Stefanik, P. A.; Heald, F. P.; and Mayer, J. 1959. Caloric intake in relation to energy output of obese and non-obese adolescent boys. *American Journal of Clinical Nutrition* 7:55.

Stuart, R. B. 1967. Behavioral control of overeating. *Behaviour Research and Therapy* 5:357.

Stuart, R. B. 1971. A three-dimensional program for the treatment of obesity. *Behaviour Research and Therapy* 9:177.

Stuart, R. B., and Davis, B. 1972. *Slim chance in a fat world: Behavioral control of obesity.* Champaign, Ill.: Research Press.

Stunkard, A. J. 1958. The results of treatment for obesity. *New York State Journal of Medicine* 58:79.

Stunkard, A. J. 1972. New therapies for the eating disorders: Behavior modification of obesity and anorexia nervosa. *Archives of General Psychiatry* 26:391.

Stunkard, A. J. 1976. *The pain of obesity.* Palo Alto, Calif.: Bull.

Stunkard, A. J., and Burt, V. 1967. Obesity and the body image: II. Age at onset of disturbances in the body image. *American Journal of Psychiatry* 123:11.

Stunkard, A. J.; d'Aquile, E.; Fox, S.; and Filion, R. D. L. 1972. Influence of social class on obesity and thinness in children. *Journal of the American Medical Association* 221:579.

Stunkard, A. J., and McLaren-Hume, M. 1959. The results of treatment for obesity. *Archives of Internal Medicine* 103:79.

Stunkard, A. J., and Mendelson, M. 1967. Obesity and the body image: I. Characteristics of distur-bances in the body image of some obese persons. *American Journal of Psychiatry* 123:1296.

Todhunter, E. N. 1972. Food is more than nutrients. *Food and Nutrition News* 43 (6-7):1.

Van Itallie, T. B., and Campbell, R. G. 1972. Multidisciplinary approach to the problems of obesity. *Journal of the American Dietetic Association* 61:385.

Wagner, M., and Hewitt, M. I. 1975. Oral satiety in the obese and non-obese. *Journal of the American Dietetic Association* 67:344.

Weinseir, R. 1976. Nutritional considerations in the treatment of obesity. Presented at the Child Nutrition Workshop, 30 November 1976, Birmingham, Ala.

Weisenberg, M., and Fray, E. 1974. What's missing in the treatment of obesity of behavior modifica-tion? *Journal of the American Dietetic Association* 65:410.

Winick, M. 1974. Childhood obesity. *Nutrition Today* 9 (3):6.

Winick, M., ed. 1975. *Childhood obesity.* New York: Wiley.

Wollersheim, J. P. 1970. Effectiveness of group therapy based upon learning principles in the treat-ment of overweight women. *Journal of Abnormal Psychology* 76:462.

Wooley, C. W.; Wooley, S. C.; and Dunham, R. B. 1972. Can calories be perceived and do they affect hunger in obese and non-obese humans? *Journal of Comparative and Physiological Psychology* 80:250.

Wooley, S. C. 1972. Physiologic versus cognitive factors in short-term food regulation in the obese and non-obese. *Psychosomatic Medicine* 34:62.

CHAPTER 10

Food Behavior Research

The effects of nutrient intake on the growth patterns and health of individuals have been established, but there has been little systematic focusing of attention on the food behavior of the individual. Studies restricted in time and place have been conducted to describe individual food behavior or to suggest how food behavior might be altered to alleviate nutritional problems at different stages of the life cycle or within different subcultures in the United States; however, the cumulative effects of food behavior on a person's health are not completely understood. The effects of food patterning, the actual development of an individual's food behavior, are currently under discussion by nutritionists, dietitians, and other health professionals. Truisms such as "food habits are established during infancy and are difficult to change" are espoused, and yet there is little evidence to support them.

Community food and nutrition professionals working in the United States and in international programs are admonished first to learn about the culture of the people they intend to serve and then to design and implement nutrition programs. They are instructed to find out about the religious beliefs, political organization, agricultural production, health resources, socioeconomic stratifications, housing, school programs, transportation, educational level, occupations, social welfare programs, geography, environment, energy resources, food habits, food attitudes, food beliefs, and food preferences of the people. In summary, they are told to assess the community. Yet, the tools for learning about food behavior have not been carefully developed and tested, and the methodology for obtaining the data and information needed by food and nutrition professionals who want to modify food behavior or reinforce good food behavior is not well defined.

Although it is simplistic to say that good or poor nutrition depends on nutrient intake, too many professionals forget that good or poor nutrition is often the result of the food choices people make. Community food and nutrition professionals need to be acutely aware that individual food behavior reflects a person's relationship to food throughout his or her life and that it is constantly being modified. Knowledge of how people feel about food can be used in developing new food products and in promoting food behavior that contributes to optimum nutritional status.

Studying an individual's food behavior means, essentially, studying the four parameters that describe or limit a person's relationship to food: availability, safety, acceptability, and nutritive quality. Nutrition educators need to know what factors affect each of these parameters and how they are interrelated. Research in this area would contribute a great deal to the understanding of food behavior. At present, many field-workers are especially interested in the food behavior and special food and nutrition needs of American ethnic groups. The agricultural focus of United States assistance to developing countries has sparked a new interest in food behavior and in the influence of food behavior on food supply and food consumption in foreign countries.

Since community nutrition workers are expected to learn about food behavior in a systematic way, a brief discussion of the state of food behavior research, past and present, is appropriate.

BACKGROUND: THE COMMITTEE ON FOOD HABITS

A look at some highlights of past research on food behavior in the United States should help to clarify the present state of research on food habits.

In 1940 the National Research Council established two committees, the Committee on Food and Nutrition (concerned with the biological and physiological aspects of nutrition) and the Committee on Food Habits (concerned with the psychological and cultural patterns of nutrition). Since little information about food habits was available, the task of the Committee on Food Habits was considered a pioneering one. The committee collected existing knowledge on food likes and dislikes and on the processes of formulating and changing food habits. Its 1943 report, *The Problem of Changing Food Habits* (National Research Council 1943), heralded the new science of food behavior. The committee also promoted limited research projects for demonstrating changes in food habits. Perhaps the best known of those projects is the one that was conducted by Kurt Lewin (1943), describing the gatekeeper and the channel theory of food. (The channel theory explains how and why food comes to the table; the gatekeeper is the person who controls the channels to the table.)

American participation in World War II, food rationing, and the distribution of food under lend-lease agreements all occurred during the committee's first 3 years of existence. The availability of foods, or perhaps the lack of availability of certain foods, in the United States had both short- and long-term effects on the development of American foodways. It is not surprising that efforts were devoted to studying the impact of working odd shifts on the food habits of war workers, or the acceptability of emergency rations, or the wartime role of nutrition professionals.

The need for a standard methodology to study food behavior was pointed out at the beginning of this chapter. The Committee on Food Habits recognized this need in 1945. Now, as then, the question is, How can professional nutritionists help people to develop food behavior that is both stable and flexible, that promotes health, and that allows them to adjust to whatever food conditions exist? In the 1970s community nutrition workers are faced with clients whose lives and food behavior may be affected by unemployment, rising food prices, contamination of food, and the global food supply. Food technologists, nutritionists, and policymakers have debated the same questions for over 30 years: Should we alter the constituents of food or try to change people's behavior? Should we fortify or nutrify food or should we teach consumers about nutrition?

Baseline data describing food behavior are needed for use in that debate. The *Manual for the Study of Food Habits,* prepared by the Committee on Food Habits in 1945, included specifications for obtaining data on food patterns, social organization and food, the ideology of food, the induction of new generations into food patterns, the material culture and technology of food, food pathology, and stability and changes in culture. The committee defined the unit of study as "a *given human being* (whose whole behavior has been modified by his social experience) *consuming a given item of food* (the constitution of which has often been modified by human means) *at a given place* (where the availability and quality of the food will have been determined partly by local geographical conditions and partly by man-made improvements . . .) *at a given period in history* (with the climatic and social conditions characteristic of that period)."

The committee functioned little after the war ended. In 1964 Margaret Mead, renowned anthropologist and a member of the original committee, noted that food habit research in the 1960s differed little from that conducted in the 1940s, and she remarked that there had been few advances in either theory or research methods. The code that she proposed for describing dietary patterns, along with some further discussion, is reprinted here (Mead 1964, pp. 22-23).

Needed: A Multidimensional Code for Describing a Dietary Pattern

Early in our work on food habits it became evident that there was a need for a code that would make possible a formal description of a people's dietary pattern. Such a code would allow for the description of food in all its different aspects:

1. *in physiological sensory terms,* including such factors as taste, smell, texture, temperature control, resistance to chewing, etc.
2. *in terms of its chemistry*
3. *in nutritional terms,* including methods for calculating the significant ratios of nutrients to one another in a diet
4. *in cultural terms*
   a. *agricultural,* including the nutritionally relevant details of soil conditions, planting, growing, and harvesting, the use of fertilizers, and methods of storing, processing, and preparing foods for use
   b. *economic,* including the economic arrangements surrounding food distribution and provision, its relation to the transportation system (particularly important in countries where a basic item in the diet is produced only in one region; also in countries with poor interregional communication, where abundance of food in one region may be no indicator of the presence or absence of supplies in another), etc.
   c. *socio-cultural,* including those aspects of social organization which significantly affect nutrition, such as differential access to food by sex, age, special state (e.g., puberty, pregnancy, lactation, mourning, illness), caste or class, region, occupation, etc.
   d. *educational,* including methods of teaching and learning the dietary pattern, the extent to which food enters into disciplinary practices, the extent to which weight, growth, and aging are involved with prestige patterns, social approval and disapproval, etc.
   e. *related to food handling,* including styles of serving (all the cultural factors that enter into meal style), use of color, types of fixed combinations, eating utensils, disposal of leftovers, garbage disposal, and the disposal of human feces
   f. *related to dietary patterning,* including the geographic and other origins of specific patterns and the seasonal character of each version.

A formal code of this kind should be constructed in such a way that comparable units can be used both to provide stimuli and to record responses, and it should be so organized that the responses can be suitably referred to individual differences, specific kinds of experience, emotional disturbance, disease, etc.

Until we do construct a formal code for the recording and description of a dietary pattern, the science of food habits will remain essentially what it is today—a fragmented set of associations casually related to the relevant disciplines. The fragmentation existing at present is well illustrated by the summary statement made by Gottlieb and Rossi. . . .

> While some attention has been given to the physical components and the psychophysical attributes of foods, additional attention needs to be given to. the social-psychological aspects. For example, we know that foods vary in their desirability (an aspect which the food preference ratings measure so well). It may well be that there are other dimensions of considerable importance: For example, foods may vary in their "centrality"—the extent to which they are considered essential to a diet; in their perceived nutritional value; and in their prestige.

The proliferation of scales and the accumulation of masses of detail, as in the studies made by W. O. Jones, or by P. J. Quin, or by the Cornell University group who worked in Thailand, serve only to underline the difficulties that are encountered, the imbalances that occur, and the narrowness of view that may result when those who are working on one problem lack a frame of reference through which their research can be related to the field as a whole.

In spite of its desirability, the construction of a code seemed to be a utopian idea as recently as fifteen years ago. But today, with improved methods of carrying out chemical, physiological, and biological assays and of studying the senses, and with the development of computer techniques that make possible the simultaneous handling of many variables and reduce the tediousness of the necessary processes of computation, the construction of an adequate code becomes feasible.

The problem today is a different one. It is essentially the problem of choosing a model which will ensure the building of an open system—one which will remain responsive to new knowledge in every relevant field.

> The fact that a code already existed would encourage scientists working in the field to draw on the organized knowledge made available through this means and to enrich and refine its resources by the addition of knowledge as it developed through new research.

It has been more than a decade since Mead called for a multidimensional code for describing dietary patterns, a code that would include physiological and sensory terms, chemical terms, nutritional terms, and cultural terms. Although that code has not been established, advances in theory and methodology have been made. It is not in the proliferation of articles entitled "Eating Habits of ——" or "The Food Habits of ——" that developments in methodology occur, but in systematic efforts to develop appropriate research tools.

Grivetti and Pangborn (1973) reviewed the approaches and methods used in food behavior research. They categorized them as (1) environmental, (2) regional, (3) ecological, and (4) functional. They believed that no one approach is better—the nature of the problem should determine the approach to be used.

RECENT RESEARCH

Since the late 1960s there has been renewed interest in food behavior research. Ecological and multidisciplinary methodologies have been evolving and in recent years the focus of research has shifted from description of individual food behavior to description and analysis of family food-related behavior. The research has incorporated multidimensional elements, using the theoretical, scientific, and practical expertise of anthropologists, economists, nutritionists, psychologists, physiologists, and sociologists.

Jerome (1967) employed observations, informal interviews, life histories, frequency tests, 7-day family food consumption records, participant observations, and documents and newspapers to study food habits and acculturation. Jerome's work built on the previous work of Cussler and de Give (1952), which identified means to study the psychosocial elements complexing and interacting in food habit research. "This intensive study of food habits of a population group represents an effort to establish the *whys* of dietary practice as well as the *whats* in household food consumption."

Sanjur (1968) applied the technique of participant observation to "evaluate the general dimensions of the ecology of malnutrition and further identify the nature and magnitude of infant nutrition problems in a rural community of Latin America." Her work drew on Cravioto Dehicardie, and Birch's (1966) work on the biosocial factors affecting malnutrition. Open-ended questionnaires and interviews provided the general data necessary to explore health, education, social, community, food, and general background variables. Scalogram analysis, cross tabulation, and the "gamma" test of association were used to obtain descriptive patterning of the converging factors observed and recorded. The results furthered the understanding of the link between social and health correlates and increasing dietary complexity.

Although Jerome and Sanjur both were participant observers collecting data related to food behavior, their orientations and means of analysis differed greatly. Jerome's work is an ethnological study incorporating quantitative data to further define the realm of food behavior of the population she describes. Sanjur used participant observation to define a set of variables and statistically establish the degrees of association between the set and nutrition problems related to infancy. Sanjur (Sanjur and Scoma 1971) later rephrased Mead's multidimensional code and described dietary patterns in terms of food consumption, food preference items, food ideology, and culture.

Kolasa (1974) used participant observation in addition to a random sample survey to substantiate her field study interviewing of a smaller purposive sample. The survey questionnaire and interviewing techniques were employed to isolate factors involved in the cultural transmission of foodways and changes in foodways. These methods developed out of extensive preliminary observations, surveys, and informal and formal interviews to identify similarities and differences in the food-related behavior of mothers and their adult daughters residing in east Tennessee. The random sample survey provided a more general reference upon which statistical comparisons could be based to indicate possible bias introduced by the interviews of the purposive sample or to broaden the generalizations that could be made from the study.

Survey testing is often used to clarify a formulated set of hypotheses, and case analyses provide the means to develop the set of hypotheses. Case analysis is a qualitative research method that uses observation, participant observation, interviews, life histories, diaries, documents, and other sources of information to gather data that go beyond descriptions and present explanations.

Lackey (1974) used case analysis to study family food purchasing, hoping that she could define new areas for hypothesis testing. Her analyses yielded detailed accounts useful in understanding the complexities of human behavior. This approach allows for intensive consideration of the cultural, sociological, economic, psychological, and environmental aspects of smaller purposive populations that may lead to a more general increased awareness of attitudes, beliefs, and values. Lackey used interviews, observations, and record-keeping instruments to collect data on demographic, behavioral, and attitudinal elements. The analysis of the qualitative and quantitative data provides a unique picture of the participants in sample groups and supports the implication that this approach is a useful tool for future program development, delivery, and evaluation.

As an outgrowth of participant observation experiences, data collection, and surveys, conceptual framworks have been formulated.

A conceptual framework describing the nutritional status of a group was presented by Sims, Paolucci, and Morris (1973). They thought an ecological approach would be useful for studying food behavior, since food behavior can be viewed as a "result of the transactional patterns between resources which may enter the family from the distal environment, and the family's use of such resources which may vary as a result of that family's decision-making and valuing processes."

Caliendo et al. (1977) used a modified Sims "unidirectional" ecological conceptual framework to expand the understanding of factors involved in the dietary and nutritional status of the preschool child. Interviews, questionnaires, 24-hour recalls, and simplified biochemical and anthropometric measures provided the data which were analyzed by Pearson product-moment correlation, multiple and stepwise regression, and path analysis. These means were used to explore the statistical relationship between the dependent variables and independent variables assessed from the nonprobability purposive sample studied. The dependent variables were related to nutritional status and the selected independent variables included those of demography and family resources, maternal psychosocial and attitudinal qualities, and selected variables peculiar to each child.

Yetley (1974) used a causal model to analyze food behavior. She did multiple regression analyses on all possible relationships among variables in the model and applied path analysis and other causal model techniques to the data, which yielded descriptive information and an empirically modified causal model.

The methodologies and techniques used in research on food habits were, at first, suited mainly to studies on individuals—specific studies with limited application. But they have been developed and expanded for more general studies whose results have broader applicability. For example, Bass and students at the University of Tennessee have been developing instruments for assessing the food behavior of high school students. They are using the semantic differential scale for assessing the connotative meaning of food, as well as instruments that measure students' food preferences and their knowledge of and misconceptions about food and nutrition, an instrument for identifying food terminology, and the 24-hour recall in combination with the question What do you usually eat? This type of information is needed for each community in our country, but acquiring it is time-consuming and expensive.

Lund and Burk (1969) published a conceptual framework for analyzing children's consumer behavior related to food. They conducted a pilot study, based on the conceptual framework, that was designed to test hypotheses about the nature of children's food consumption behavior. The publication describes many of their instruments and gives a detailed explanation of the statistics used in establishing the conceptual framework.

Now that the food behavior of individuals is better understood, it has become important to understand group processes as well. It is especially important to understand the relationships between two people, such as mother and child, or husband and wife. Gradually, the emphasis of research is shifting to the food behavior of the family unit.

The examples of recent research in food behavior that have been presented here show that the methodologies for studying food behavior have not yet been standardized.

Granted that any methodology will have to be adjusted for the particular situation, it should nevertheless be possible to develop some standard instruments or groups of instruments. The need for a holistic approach is recognized, but getting financial support for multidisciplinary research is difficult.

OBJECTIVES OF RESEARCH

Nutritional assessment, nutritional surveillance, and food behavior research often are confused and the terms used interchangeably. They are not the same and do not measure the same variables. *Nutritional assessment* is the appraisal of available information to provide a description of the existing nutritional situation. *Nutritional surveillance* is the monitoring of specific parameters indicative of nutritional status. *Food behavior research* has already been discussed. Each is a bona fide area of research—they may overlap in emphasis, but they measure different parameters; however, a multidisciplinary approach is essential for a full understanding of people's nutritional needs and the various aspects of their need for food. *Nutritional status* is determined by (1) comparing dietary studies of nutrient intake with accepted standards, (2) clinically evaluating physical signs of nutritional health and/or disease, and (3) measuring (biochemically) the nutrients within the body.

Nutritional assessment and nutritional status will not be discussed in detail here. Christakis (1973) outlined the anthropometric, biochemical, clinical, and dietary methodologies. The World Health Organization published a *Manual for Nutritional Surveillance* (FAO/UNICEF/WHO Expert Committee 1976). McLaren (1976) edited a text for community workers to assist them in assessing nutritional status. Jelliffe (1966) prepared the classic manual describing methods of assessing the nutritional status of a community. And Burgess and Burgess (1975) prepared a guide to field methods for conducting nutritional assessment.

It is important to recognize the reason for doing a nutritional assessment. An assessment may be done in order to learn what the nutritional problems and related health problems of people actually are, or it may be done to document the existence of problems already recognized. The documentation may be used as a baseline to which other data can be compared, and it may be used to draw attention to nutritional problems and show that intervention programs are needed.

Physical signs of malnutrition, such as delayed growth, slowed development (compared to that of persons in similar groups), pallid skin, and faults in the mucous membranes of the mouth and eyes, are symptoms of nutritional deficiencies. Persons with severe deficiencies may show symptoms such as edema or changes in the consistency or color of their hair. The World Health Organization Expert Committee on Medical Assessment of Nutritional Status proposed a classification of physical signs (Jelliffe 1966). (Sometimes the signs do not indicate a diseased state, but rather poor hygiene or excessive exposure to the elements.)

1. *Group one* signs are considered valuable in nutritional assessment. These are signs of malnutrition that are apt to be caused by deficiency of one or more nutrients.
2. *Group two* signs need further investigation. They may be related to health and environment or to poverty.
3. *Group three* signs are physical signs that are not related to nutrition.

This classification is extremely useful in mass screening. The measurements indicated in table 12 are useful in making classifications of physical signs.

TABLE 12. MEASUREMENTS FOR CLASSIFYING PHYSICAL SIGNS OF MALNUTRITION

	Neonates and Infants	Preschool	School Age	Adults and Aging
Weight[a]	X	X	X	X
Tricepts skin fold[b]	X	X	X	X
Head circumference	X	X		
Chest circumference	X	X		
Length recumbent[c]	X	X	X	X
Arm circumference	X	X	X	X
Standard height				

Data should be judged in relation to the characteristics of the population and the standardized norms for that population.

[a]Weight on a beam balance is preferred.

[b]Lange and Harpender calipers can be used for measuring skin fold thickness. This requires training and standardization of techniques.

[c]Height should be measured without shoes.

An integral part of determining nutritional status is the laboratory assessment. Laboratory tests can give a precise indication of a person's nutritional state. For example, biochemical analysis of blood and urine or analysis of physiological functions shows a great deal about an individual's physiological and nutritional state. Laboratory tests are used to determine deficiencies of:

1. The blood-forming nutrients iron, folacin, vitamin B_6, and vitamin B_{12}.
2. The water soluble vitamins thiamine, riboflavin, niacin, and vitamin C.
3. The fat soluble vitamins A, D, E, and K.
4. Serum albumin.
5. The minerals iron and iodine.
6. Blood lipids.

The purpose of these tests is to detect marginal nutritional deficiencies in individuals, to supplement a nutritional assessment of a community, and to isolate nutritional problems.

Nutritional assessment relates the quality of life to nutritional status. Demographic information, socioeconomic stratification, health and morbidity statistics, school transportation, occupation, and geographic environment are measured in relation to nutrient intake. (Much of the same information is needed for a description of food behavior.) To find out how these factors contribute to the food behavior of the individual, more information is needed on such topics as the meaning of food, food preferences and food choices, and family composition. Studies of food behavior provide information for the development of educational materials and programs, whereas nutritional assessment points out a population's need for specific nutrients.

For community food and nutrition professionals, the objectives of research into food behavior are:

1. To obtain knowledge of food behavior in the community, that is, knowledge of food habits, preferences, intake, and patterns and practices (including selection, procurement, manipulation, storage, consumption, terminology and meaning, and use in the community.
2. To identify the technological, economic, political, philosophical, and ideological forces influencing food behavior.
3. To discover the interrelationships among all of these factors.

The results of research must then be organized into practical plans for dealing with the specific nutritional problems of individuals and communities. At present little is known about the development of food preferences, food habits, and food attitudes, and less about their interrelationships with the developmental stages (both physical and psychological) of the individual. More information about their interrelationship with the environment is also needed. Clearly there is much work yet to be done.

ETHICS IN RESEARCH

In recent years, there has been much concern about ethics and research. Black and Champion (1976) pointed out four types of interpersonal relationships that are involved in research into the social and behavioral aspects of human beings.

1. The relationship of the researchers with those sponsoring the research. Most government agencies, such as the Department of Health, Education and Welfare, have their own printed form that assures protection of the human rights of the research subjects. This form must be included with the request for funds. It indicates that a project involving research on human subjects has been approved by the institution.

2. The relationship of the researchers with those permitting or supporting access to the source of data, whether documents or human beings. First, the cooperation of these people must be secured and certain conditions agreed upon (for example, the degree of anonymity the sponsor desires and the procedure for collecting and handling data to ensure this). Second, the amount of information that the sponsor needs about the specific project must be determined. And third, the form in which the results of the study will be made available must be agreed upon.

3. The relationships with other investigators in the project. Conflicts can be avoided by clarifying the specific responsibilities of each researcher. Statistics or food beliefs or food attitudes might be the responsibility of a particular person with expertise in that area. Even so, the principal investigator has to manage interpersonal problems.

4. The relationship with the subjects. Consent forms are a necessary part of most research. Care must be taken so that the subjects are not harmed in any way by their participation in the research.

Persons in the field of applied anthropology have tended to define three categories of responsibility (Foster 1969). First, researchers are responsible to science. That means they must avoid any action or recommendation that would impede the advancement of scientific knowledge. Second, they must respect the dignity and consider the general well-being of their fellow human beings. They must take the greatest care to protect those who provide the data. Third, they are responsible to their clients or to the sponsors of the research. They must use the best scientific knowledge and skill available to them, but they must not make promises or raise expectations that cannot be fulfilled or that conflict with their responsibilities to science and to other people.

Much discussion on ethics and the control of research has taken place in the past few years in response to specific instances both in behavioral research and in physical and biochemical research with humans. Researchers need to be aware of ethical problems and how they affect the climate for a particular type of research. The right to privacy is very basic to the American way of life. The subjects or participants in a study have the right to (1) have their anonymity preserved, (2) refuse to answer any question and/or to quit at any time, and (3) receive a report of the results of the study.

Needless to say, the approach one makes both to those controlling access to the data and to the subjects themselves, as well as the manner in which collected data are handled and the uses to which they are put, are of utmost importance to research. For example, in the negotiation of a research project on older people's eating habits in a low-income urban area, the gerontologist who gave final approval would not allow income data to be collected because she felt it would unduly disturb her clients. In another instance, a psychologist would not allow a person's age to be asked unless the researcher could indicate a real value for that data. The psychologist insisted that declaration of age would cause psychological distress for some people.

RESEARCH METHODS

There are many methods of obtaining information about a community's food behavior. The particular method used depends upon the information sought.

Much information can be gathered from secondary sources. Local newspapers, bulletin boards in public places, and radio and television stations provide information on food terminology, the use of food as a focus for social functions, the availability of food items, customs involving foods, types of information the people are exposed to, and so on. These sources do not require cooperation from other people and therefore present fewer problems than the collection of data from primary sources. The local librarian is usually eager to suggest sources of information.

The yellow pages of the local telephone book contain many basic facts about a community. Often there is a chamber of commerce to promote the community's commercial interests. Information from this source can give insight into what local leaders believe will persuade others to view their community in a positive way. This reveals to the researcher the relative importance of specific aspects of the community in the eyes of its business and political leaders.

Census tape for the community will give statistics on age, sex, occupation and income, place of residence, and marital status. These census reports are public documents and available to anyone.

Other sources of valuable information that has been collected for use in planning and policymaking in the community include the following.

1. County and city courthouses. City and county maps showing the locations of homes and the lines of population density can often be obtained at courthouses.
2. Professionals within the community, health workers at all levels, and others involved in food and nutrition education, such as extension agents, public health nurses, and social workers. It is desirable to develop and maintain a helping and sharing type of relationship with these people. It is equally important that one recognize the prejudices and personality differences of other professionals and make decisions based on facts rather than on other people's perceptions of events.
3. School administrators. Information on school populations over the years may indicate changes within the community, for example, in the mobility of families with children, the percentage of children who come from poverty-level homes, the comparative achievement level of the school, and the aspirations of the students.
4. Local associations. Realtors and restaurant associations may have information on the mobility patterns of the community.
5. Visible evidence. Large industrial complexes, government housing for military personnel, and universities are clues to who the people are.

Observation

Observation is a valuable means of learning about the foodways of a community. Of course, observations are made in relation to the observer's own frame of reference, and that can be a problem. Another problem is that it is almost impossible to observe without influencing what is being observed. Nevertheless, observation can provide a lot of information about how a community operates and what the people consider important. Observations should be done systematically and often they can be quantified.

Participant observation was discussed by Kolasa and Bass (1974). Becoming an active participant while one observes has its disadvantages. It is difficult to observe and to be involved in an activity at the same time. However, with some practice, one can become adept at this and make participant observations of food selection, procurement, storage, distribution, manipulation, consumption, and waste disposal. Food terminology and the use and meaning of food in the community can also be learned in this way. Problems inherent in participant observation are (1) adding a new element (oneself) to the situation and thus changing the behavior, (2) interpreting observations according to a personal frame of reference, and (3) losing one's objectivity.

All observations should be recorded as soon as possible in a data record book, often referred to as a *field notebook*. This can be an effective way of collecting data for a program development or for research. Sometimes the data in a field notebook are used only to generate hypotheses. But for those involved in research on food behavior, the notebook, in addition to being a valuable research tool, provides insight into the food behavior of a community that no other method can.

Participant observation requires making contacts within the community and *interacting with others*. In doing this, it is important that community food and nutrition professionals recognize and appreciate people's privacy and individualism and also their frequent willingness to help others. The first approach to members of a community may be a deciding factor in the future effectiveness of a researcher or an educator.

Interviews

Interviews may be informal and relatively unstructured, or they may be formal and highly structured. An informal interview might be used to acquire basic information on the location of services in a community. A formal, highly structured interview would be appropriate for research purposes, for example, gathering information to elucidate food behavior. An interview should proceed systematically and the information should be recorded as quickly as possible, since many people do not like to have what they say recorded.

Many interviews are structured and an interview *schedule* or questionnaire is used to ensure that the interviewer gets the information desired. Probing questions to elicit more information may be used in some instances, while in others, the data would be biased by probing questions. In an informal interview, the answer to one question may lead to another question which will further clarify the first answer or elicit more information. A field notebook should be used to record the interviewer's perception of the events surrounding an interview. Black and Champion (1976) discussed the types of interviews and their relative merits.

Key Informants. Someone in a community who is recognized as knowledgeable about the food practices of most of the people in the community is chosen to be interviewed. Information concerning all aspects of the community's foodways can be obtained from this person. Two or three other key informants should also be interviewed and all of the responses compared.

Questionnaires. Questionnaires may be handed out to a group, mailed out, placed in a prominent place to be picked up, or used as interview schedules. A questionnaire should be developed and tested under conditions similar to those in which it will be used. Discussions of how to develop clear questions and valid questionnaires can be found in Jacobs (1974), Backstrom and Hursh (1963), Black and Champion (1976), and VanDalen (1973). The degree to which a questionnaire should be tested depends upon how the results will be used.

A questionnaire must ask the right question, and ask it in such a way that the investigator will find out what he or she needs to know (Jacobs 1974). When constructing a questionnaire an investigator should consider the following.

1. Who needs the information?
2. What decision will be made based on the information?
3. What facts will affect the decision?
4. Who is being questioned?
5. What are the consequences, to the research project and to the respondent, of a "wrong" answer (e.g., an answer indicating that a subject participating in a program is violating the program's regulations)?

Three types of questions can be used in questionnaires—open-ended, two-way, and multiple-choice. Several factors must be considered in deciding which type of question to use.

1. How much you know about the range of possible answers.
2. How much time your respondents have, or are willing, to give you.
3. The number of subjects needed to get satisfactory reliability, and the data analysis techniques that will be required.

An apparent advantage of the open-ended question is that it is easy to ask. However, the disadvantages outnumber the advantages in that (1) it will take more time to obtain written responses to the questions, (2) the respondent may give an incomplete answer or no answer at all after seeing how much work is involved in filling out the questionnaire, (3) analysis of open-ended questions is very difficult and time-consuming and must be done by someone who understands the questions' content, and (4) open-ended questions may easily be misinterpreted by the respondent since there is no fixed set of answers to serve as a guide.

The two-way question is quickly and easily answered because the respondent has only to choose one of two alternatives. This type of question is easy to develop and can be rapidly analyzed. But, as with the open-ended question, the disadvantages are often greater than the advantages: (1) two alternatives might not be enough to answer some questions, (2) some respondents tend to choose the first or last answer they see, and (3) the two alternatives may overlap instead of being mutually exclusive.

Multiple-choice questions have many advantages. They can be scored easily, and the data analysis is relatively inexpensive since no special knowledge of the content is required. Respondents can answer multiple-choice questions much more quickly than open-ended questions and thus are more likely to complete the questionnaire. All respondents are put on an equal basis; they have the same set of alternatives to choose from. One problem with the multiple-choice question is that the question maker is required to know all of the significant possible alternatives when formulating the question.

A poorly made questionnaire can cause unnecessary problems for the respondents. Every instance of ambiguity, poor wording, inconvenient spacing, awkward format, or whatever should be pointed out while the questionnaire is being developed and tested. The respondents' and interviewers' reactions to the subject matter and to the length of the questionnaire must also be taken into account in drafting the final form. A questionnaire needs to be tested and retested under circumstances like those it will ultimately be used in.

Statistics

Statistics is a vital tool which has an important place in research on community food and nutrition. Computer services, statistical services, and the latest techniques available should be used to control error in the transfer of data and to ensure that the analysis is appropriate to the level of the data. Mark sense cards and computer tape can be adapted for use if one works with computer center personnel, informing them of the type of data to be gathered, tabulated, and statistically analyzed. It is important to discuss and arrange these matters while a project is still in the planning stages. Interviewers can be trained to record responses directly on mark sense cards or score sheets so that the key punch operation can be omitted or very much simplified, and questionnaires can be coded in a way that allows key punching to be done directly from the questionnaire.

Statistics is only one of many tools and skills; it has its place and its proper use. Incorrect use of statistics can mask findings or lead to erroneous conclusions.

SUMMARY OF THE RESEARCH PROCESS

1. Make an assumption (based on observations) about food behavior.
2. Refine the hypothesis by participant observation and study of the relevant literature. Develop a conceptual framework of possible relationships, based on observation and literature search.
3. Investigate funding sources.
4. Define the sample population and discuss appropriate sampling techniques with a statistician.
5. Determine the possibility of carrying out the research (the willingness of those in authority to cooperate). Make any necessary adjustments in the population and the sampling technique.
6. Develop appropriate instruments (validation and reliability are essential) to meet research objectives and to evaluate the research project.
7. Formulate a statistical design that includes methods of statistical analysis and mechanical processes of data collection.
8. Obtain appropriate authorization or consent and human rights clearance.
9. Secure appropriate funding.
10. Pretest instruments. Validation, reliability, and field testing under conditions similar to those of the research project are important processes in the development of instruments.
11. Train personnel in data collection methods, including fiscal controls and field site management.
12. Oversee the collection of data.
13. Analyze the data.
14. Evaluate the research project.

REFERENCES

General

Backstrom, C. H., and Hursh, G. D. 1963. *Survey research.* Handbooks for Research in Political Behavior Series. Evanston, Ill.: Northwestern University Press.
Black, J., and Champion, D. 1976. *Methods and issues in social research.* New York: Wiley.

Burgess, H. J. L., and Burgess, A. 1975. A field worker's guide to a nutritional status survey. *American Journal of Clinical Nutrition* 28:1299.

Caliendo, M. A.; Sanjur, D.; Wright, J.; and Cummings, G. 1977. Nutritional status of preschool children—An ecological analysis. *Journal of the American Dietetic Association* 71:20.

Christakis, G. 1973. *Nutritional assessments in health programs.* Washington, D.C.: American Public Health Association.

Clarke, M., and Wakefield, L. 1975. Food choices of institutionalized vs. independent-living elderly. *Journal of the American Dietetic Association* 66:600.

Committee on Food Habits. 1945. *Manual for the study of food habits.* National Research Council, Bulletin 111. Washington, D.C.: National Academy of Sciences.

Cosper, B., and Wakefield, L. 1975. Food choices of women: Personal, attitudinal and motivational factors. *Journal of the American Dietetic Association* 66:152.

Cravioto, J.; Dehicardie, E. R.; and Birch, H. G. 1966. Nutrition, growth, and neurointegrative development: An experiment and ecologic study. *Pediatrics* 38:319.

Cussler, M., and de Give, M. 1952. *Twixt the cup and the lip.* New York: Twayne.

FAO/UNICEF/WHO Expert Committee. 1976. *Methodology of nutritional surveillance.* World Health Organization Technological Report no. 593. Geneva: World Health Organization.

Foster, G. 1969. *Applied anthropology.* Boston: Little, Brown.

Grivetti, L., and Pangborn, R. 1973. Food research: A review of approaches and methods. *Journal of Nutrition Education* 5:205.

Jacobs, T. O. 1974. *Developing questionnaire items.* Alexandria, Va.: Human Resources Research Organization.

Jelliffe, D. B. 1966. *The assessment of the nutritional status of the community.* World Health Organization Monograph Series no. 53. Geneva: World Health Organization.

Jerome, N. 1967. Food habits and acculturation: Dietary practices and nutrition of families headed by southern-born Negroes residing in a northern metropolis. Ph.D. thesis, University of Wisconsin (Madison).

Kolasa, K. 1974. Foodways of selected mothers and their adult daughters in upper east Tennessee. Ph.D. thesis, University of Tennessee (Knoxville).

Kolasa, K., and Bass, M. A. 1974. Participant observation in nutrition education program development. *Journal of Nutrition Education* 6:89.

Lackey, C. J. 1974. Family food buying: A consumer education program. Ph.D. thesis, University of Tennessee (Knoxville).

Lewin, K. 1943. Focus behind food habits and methods of change. In *The problem of changing food habits.* National Research Council, Bulletin no. 108. Washington, D.C.: National Academy of Sciences.

Lund M., and Burk, M. C. 1969. *A multidisciplinary analysis of children's food consumption behavior.* Bulletin 265. St. Paul: University of Minnesota Agricultural Experiment Station.

McLaren, D. S., ed. 1976. *Nutrition in the community.* New York: Wiley.

Mead, M. 1964. *Food habit research: Problems of the 1960's.* National Research Council, publication 1225. Washington, D.C.: National Academy of Sciences.

National Research Council. 1943. *The problem of changing food habits.* Bulletin no. 108. Washington, D.C.: National Academy of Sciences.

Sanjur, D. 1968. A socio-cultural approach to the study of infant feeding practices and weaning habits in a Mexican village. Ph.D. thesis, Cornell University (Ithaca).

Sanjur, D., and Scoma, A. D. 1971. Food habits of low-income children in northern New York. *Journal of Nutrition Education* 3:85.

Sims, L. 1973. A theoretical model for the study of nutritional status: An ecosystem approach. Ph.D. thesis, Michigan State University (East Lansing).

Sims, L. S.; Paolucci, B.; and Morris, P. M. 1972. A theoretical model for the study of nutritional status: An ecosystem approach. *Ecology of Food and Nutrition* 1:197.

Szczensniak, A. S., and Kahn, E. L. 1975. Consumer awareness and attitudes to food texture. *Journal of Texture Studies* 2:280.

VanDalen, D. B. 1973. *Understanding educational research: An introduction.* New York: McGraw-Hill.

Yetley, E. 1974. A causal model analysis of food behavior. Ph.D. thesis, Iowa State University (Ames).

Ethics in Research

Anonymous. 1968. Ethical standards of psychologists. *American Psychologist* 23:357.

Anonymous. 1971. Needed: An ethical code for behavioral scientists. *American Journal of Economics and Sociology* 30:45.

Black, J., and Champion, D. 1976. *Methods and issues in social research.* New York: Wiley.

Boruch, R. F. 1971a. Assuring confidentiality of responses in social research: A note on strategies. *American Sociologist* 6:308.

Boruch, R. F. 1971b. Maintaining confidentiality of data in educational research: A systematic analysis. *American Psychologist* 26:413.

Conrad, H. S. 1967. Clearance of questionnaires with respect to invasion of privacy, public sensitiveness, ethical standards, etc. *American Psychologist* 22:356.

Research Methods

Alexander, J., and Norman, C. 1966. Attitude as a scientific concept. *Social Forces* 45:278.

Anderson, A. R. 1970. Personalizing mailed questionnaires correspondence. *Public Opinion Quarterly* 37:273.

Arthur, A. Z. 1966. Response bias in the semantic differential. *British Journal of Social and Clinical Psychology* 5:103.

Back, K. W., and Brookover, L. 1966. Time sampling as a field technique. *Human Organization* 25:64.

Backstrom, C. H., and Hursh, G. D. 1963. *Survey research.* Handbooks for Research in Political Behavior Series. Evanston, Ill.: Northwestern University Press.

Becker, J., and Geer, B. 1960. Participant observation: The analysis of qualitative field data. In *Human organization research,* ed. R. Adamo and J. Preim. Homewood, Ill.: Dorsey Press.

Bernsman, J., and Vidich, A. 1960. Social theory in field research. *American Journal of Sociology* 65:577.

Black, J., and Champion, D. 1976. *Methods and issues in social research.* New York: Wiley.

Brown, M. L. 1965. Use of the postcard query in mail surveys. *Public Opinion Quarterly* 29:635.

Bruyn, S. 1966. *The human perspective in sociology: The methodology of participant observation.* Englewood Cliffs, N.J.: Prentice-Hall.

Bruyn, S. 1967. The new empiricists: The participant observer and the phenomenologist. *Sociology and Social Research* 51:317.

Burgess, H. J. L., and Burgess, A. 1975. A field worker's guide to a nutritional status survey. *American Journal of Clinical Nutrition* 28:1299.

Burk, M. C., and Pao, E. M. 1976. *Methodology for large-scale surveys of household and individual diets.* Washington, D.C.: Government Printing Office.

Dexter, L. 1970. *Elite and specialized interviewing.* Evanston, Ill.: Northwestern University Press.

Ehrlich, H. J. 1969. Attitudes, behavior and the intervening variables. *American Sociologist* 4:29.

Glass, J. F., and Frankiel, H. H. 1968. The influence of subjects on the research: A problem in observing social interaction. *Pacific Sociological Review* 11:75.

Gordon, R. 1969. *Interviewing: Strategy, techniques, and tactics.* Homewood, Ill.: Dorsey Press.

Hayes, D. P. 1965. Item order and Guttman scales. *American Journal of Sociology* 70:51.

Heise, D. R. 1966. Social status attitudes and word connotations. *Sociological Inquiry* 36:227.

Heise, D. R. 1969. Some methodological issues in semantic differential research. *Psychological Bulletin* 72:406.

Heise, D. R. 1970. The semantic differential and attitude research. In *Attitude measurement,* ed. G. Summers. Chicago: Rand-McNally.

Jacobs, T. O. 1974. *Developing questionnaire items.* Alexandria, Va.: Human Resources Research Organization.

Kolaja, J. 1956. A contribution to the theory of participant observation. *Social Forces* 35:159.

Kolasa, K., and Bass, M. A. 1974. Participant observation in nutrition education program development. *Journal of Nutrition Education* 6:89.

Komorita, S. S., and Bass, A. R. 1967. Attitude differential and evaluative scales of the semantic differential. *Journal of Personality and Social Psychology* 6:241.

McCormick, T. 1945. Simple percentage analysis of attitude questionnaires. *American Journal of Sociology* 50:390.

McDonagh, E. D., and Rosenblum, A. L. 1965. A comparison of mailed questionnaires and subsequent structured interviews. *Public Opinion Quarterly* 29:131.

Mead, M. 1968. Research with human beings: A model derived from anthropological field practice. *Daedalus* 98:361.

Pelto, P. 1970. *Anthropological research.* New York: Harper and Row.

Reiss, I. L. 1965. Hayes item order, and Guttman scales. *American Journal of Sociology* 70:629.

Schooler, C. 1969. A note of extreme caution on the use of Guttman scales. *American Journal of Sociology* 74:296.

Seiler, L. H., and Hough, R. L. 1970. Empirical comparisons of the Thurston and Likert techniques. In *Attitude measurement,* ed. G. Summers. Chicago: Rand-McNally.

Sherif, M.; Sherif, C.; and Neperdall. 1965. *Attitude and attitude change.* Philadelphia: W. B. Saunders.

VanDalen, D. B. 1973. *Understanding educational research: An introduction.* New York: McGraw-Hill.

Whiting, J. and Whiting, B. 1970. Methods for observing and recording behavior. In *A handbook of method in cultural anthropology,* ed. B. Maroll and R. Cohen. Garden City, N.Y.: National History Press.

Williams, T. 1967. *Field methods in the study of culture.* New York: Holt, Rinehart and Winston.

Zelditch, M., Jr. 1962. Some methodological problems of field studies. *American Journal of Sociology* 67:566.

CHAPTER 11

The Community Food and Nutrition Professional

What is the scope of practice of community food and nutrition professionals? What are the skills required of these people and what exactly do they do? If one compiled a list of the myriad activities that food and nutrition professionals or community nutritionists perform, it would be easy to understand why there is no concise definition of community nutrition. One might say that a community food and nutrition professional is a person trained in the science of foods and nutrition who applies that science to the lives of people. Or, it might be equally correct to say that a community food and nutrition professional is one who assesses the nutritional needs of the community and then mobilizes resources to meet or reduce those needs. Both definitions are quite general; therefore, the role of the community nutritionist will be discussed in more detail in this chapter.

WHAT'S IN A TITLE?

Public health nutritionist, community nutritionist, food and nutrition worker, food and nutrition educator, nutritionist, extension home economist, nutritional anthropologist, and community dietitian are all titles assumed by professionals and sometimes by paraprofessionals. These workers assess community nutritional problems and act to alleviate them. At this writing, no legal definitions for these terms exist, nor are these professions generally described in state public health statutes. As all community nutritionists well know, anyone can pose in public as a nutritionist. Food faddists, hucksters of quick-weight-loss plans, and health food producers and promoters often call themselves nutritionists. It is not unusual to find the public in a state of confusion, attempting to determine the accuracy of information and claims about nutrition when differing views and purported facts are all presented by "nutritionists."

A LOOK AT THE TRADITIONAL ROLES

One way to describe the professionals who assess nutritional problems and provide nutritional services and education is by their academic training and by the tasks they have performed as providers of nutritional services. A review of the traditional classifications of workers involved in nutrition will establish the baseline for a description of the community food and nutrition professional. The *Dictionary of Occupational Titles*, compiled by the United States Department of Labor (1965), includes definitions of many occupations available in the United States. The dietitian's work is described as follows (p. 202).

> Plans and directs food service programs in hospitals, schools, restaurants and other public or private institutions. Plans menus and diets providing required food and nutrients to feed individuals and groups. Directs workers engaged in preparation and serving of meals. Purchases or requisitions food, equipment and supplies. Maintains and analyzes food cost control records to determine improved methods for purchasing and utilization of food, equipment and supplies. Inspects work areas and store facilities to insure observance of sanitary standards. When employed in schools, hospitals or similar organizations, instructs individuals and groups in application of principles of food. May prepare educational materials on nutritional values of food and methods of preparation.

The *Dictionary* also includes descriptions of administrative, chief, research, teaching, and therapeutic dietitians. The listing for nutritionist varies significantly from that for dietitian.

> [A nutritionist] organizes, plans and conducts programs concerning nutrition to assist in promotion of health and control of disease. Instructs auxiliary medical personnel and allied professional workers on food values and utilization of foods by human body. Advises health and other agencies on nutritional phases of their food programs. Conducts in-service courses pertaining to nutrition in clinics and similar institutions. Interprets and evaluates food and nutrient information designed for public acceptance and use. Studies and analyzes scientific discoveries in nutrition for adaption and application to various food problems. May be employed by public health agency and be designated as Nutritionist, Public Health.

And the listing for "Nutritionist, Public Health," repeats this definition of nutritionist.

Although many dietitians now may find the definition of dietitian very narrow and limiting, it is similar to the definition accepted by the Executive Board of the American Dietetic Association in 1940. (The American Dietetic Association is the professional organization that sets qualifications and is responsible for the registration of dietitians in the United States.) According to this definition, a dietitian is "one who has had college training in the science of nutrition and management and is proficient in the art of feeding individuals or groups." The traditional nutritionist, too, has had college training in nutrition but is expected to interpret the principles of nutrition to individuals and groups.

The traditional role and educational qualifications of the public health nutritionist have been discussed in the literature (Anonymous 1962; Huenemann and Peck 1971; Huenemann 1973). Generally, the public health nutritionist is described as a nutritionist employed by a state or county health department, who has earned a Master of Public Health degree by completing appropriate public health, nutrition, and food courses, as well as fieldwork for a health agency. The American Public Health Association, founded to promote personal and environmental health, invites the membership of professionals representing all disciplines and specialities in public health, including nutrition.

Traditionally, the dietitian with a Bachelor of Science degree in dietetics and an internship experience has focused on the nutritional care of individuals in an institution such as a hospital, nursing home, school, or camp. Such care might have included counseling clients of the outpatient clinic and of private physicians and referring clients to appropriate social service agencies, with little or no follow-up of the client expected.

The dietitian was concerned with immediate, often therapeutic, health care. For example, a dietitian employed at a weight-reduction camp for children might have ensured that the children ate low-calorie, balanced meals but would have provided little or no follow-up care for the children after their return home. The hospital dietitian might have provided an appropriate diet for a diebetic patient (upon a physician's order) and perhaps even offered diabetic counseling and education but, again, would have made limited provision, or none at all, for the patient's continuing care after discharge. This role is changing today, and there are many dietitians providing follow-up care and working in community settings.

A professional who has traditionally met some of the community's nutritional needs is the county extension home economics agent. Since the early 1900s, extension agents, possibly trained in dietetics or public health nutrition but more often in home economics, have presented information on nutrition and food to their local communities. Perhaps extension home economists are usually pictured as showing farm women methods of preparing and preserving the home food supply to better meet their families' nutritional needs. But some home economics agents, employed in localities with no dietitian or public health nutritionist, often did work not traditionally assigned to home economists. Where public health and dietetic personnel are scarce, this practice continues today. For example, home economics agents may be asked to check the nutritional adequacy of menus for community programs like senior citizens' nutrition programs.

CHANGING ROLES

The food supply in the United States has increased and become more varied, health care delivery systems—preventive and curative—continue to evolve, and the standard of living for most Americans has risen; yet malnutrition, of various descriptions and degrees, exists. To cope with this and with problems of surplus food production, federal food commodity programs and then food stamp programs were instituted, along with supplemental food programs, to meet the needs of malnourished Americans. School-age children have benefited from school milk and school lunch programs, and, more recently, school breakfast programs (free, reduced price, and full price) and summer feeding programs have been initiated. Head Start and day-care programs and the Title VII senior nutrition program, with their food-service components, have forced changes in the traditional roles of the nutritionist and the dietitian. The programs mentioned here and others, will be discussed in detail in chapter 13.

In recent years, the role of the dietitian has been defined in many ways. Todhunter (1970) said a dietitian was "one who is professionally qualified by education and experience to provide nutritional care, and apply the science and art of nutrition in helping people of all ages, sick or well, individually or in groups, to meet their nutritional needs."

The American Dietetic Association has recognized the expanding role of the dietitian. In 1974, a committee of that association prepared a report defining titles and responsibilities for the profession of dietetics. The committee defined administrative, clinical, community, consultant, research, and teaching dietitians and dietetic assistants and technicians, and the definition of the generic term *dietitian* was expanded.

[A dietitian is] a specialist educated for a profession responsible for the nutritional care of individuals and groups. This care includes the application of the science and art of human nutrition in helping people select and obtain food for the primary purpose of nourishing their bodies in health or disease throughout the life cycle. This participation may be in single or combined functions; in foodservice systems management; in extending knowledge of food and nutrition principles; in teaching these principles for application according to particular situations; or in dietary counseling.

The dietitian specializing in public health nutrition is involved in planning programs to protect the public from misinformation, providing normal and therapeutic diet counseling to individuals and groups, supervising paraprofessional workers, advocating legislation, and supervising the operation of a federally supported community nutrition program.

THE PARAPROFESSIONAL NUTRITION WORKER

The creation of certain food and nutrition programs—such as the Expanded Food and Nutrition Education Program, the Cooperative Extension Service, and the Special Supplemental Food Program for Women, Infants and Children—and of nutrition delivery systems such as that described by Yanochik (1973) has introduced another kind of nutrition worker to the community. These workers are generally paraprofessionals trained by dietitians, public health nutritionists, or extension home economists to deliver nutritional services and nutrition education to the public and, in some cases, to complete routine assessments of nutritional status. These providers of nutrition counseling are called auxiliary nutrition workers, community nutrition workers, nutrition aides, nutrition program assistants, dietetic assistants, or dietetic technicians, depending upon the program.

The entrance of the paraprofessional nutrition worker into the field of community nutrition has meant increased manpower and delivery of services to the public at a reduced cost. It has, however, sometimes caused misunderstandings about who the community nutritionist is. For example, a public health nutritionist was charged with the task of providing direct, individual nutrition education to participants in the Women, Infants, and Children Program. For a time she was puzzled because several clients refused nutrition education services, saying they had their own personal nutritionist from the state university. She was astounded by the possibility that any of the university nutrition staff would be acting as "private nutritionist" to low-income consumers. After some time it became clear that the women refusing nutrition education from the public health nutritionist were enrolled in the Expanded Food and Nutrition Education Program, affiliated with the land-grant university, and were being visited by the assistant or aide for that program and not by a university nutritionist.

OTHER NUTRITION WORKERS

In addition to the growing cadre of auxiliary workers in nutrition, other professional groups, also represented by professional organizations, are interested in assessing nutritional needs or delivering nutritional services or studying food behavior. Of particular interest are the nutrition educators who have established the Society for Nutrition Education and the Institute for Nutrition Today and the nutritional anthropologists who belong to the Committee on Nutritional Anthropology of the American Anthropological Association.

The Society for Nutrition Education continues to grow. Among its members are persons trained in dietetics, public health nutrition, medicine, nursing, health education, home economics, and food technology. Many of these professionals would consider themselves community nutritionists. Community nutritionists focus on educating people to maintain food behavior conducive to optimal nutritional status and to modify food behavior detrimental to health.

The Institute for Nutrition Today is an outgrowth of *Nutrition Today,* a journal originally sponsored by the citrus industry of Florida. The institute members include physicians, food and nutrition professionals, and anyone else who is interested in nutrition.

The more recently formed nutritional anthropology group has an eye to describing food behaviors that are either conducive to or detrimental to good nutritional status. The Committee on Nutritional Anthropology, formed in 1974, has among its members nutritionists, cultural and medical anthropologists, physical anthropologists, dietitians, nutritional anthropologists, public health nutritionists, and physicians. Much of their work involves assessing the nutritional needs of the community. The group was formed to encourage professionals to study food behavior, food habits, and the culture of food and its implications for nutritional status.

WORKING TOGETHER

Egan (1964) noted the changing roles of dietitians and public health nutritionists and believed the most useful nutrition programs would result from all working together. She described, too, three groups of workers providing nutritional services to the community: (1) nutrition specialists (those with training and experience in nutrition), (2) professional workers with training in nutrition (those who received training in nutrition along with preparation in medicine, nursing, social work, education, or home economics), and (3) auxiliary nutrition workers (those with short-term and applied training in nutrition and foods). Perhaps these classifications are still appropriate today.

WHAT'S THE DIFFERENCE?

Does it make a difference if someone is called a community nutritionist and others are called public health nutritionist, community dietitian, extension home economist, nutritionist, or nutrition educator? A distinction between professional and paraprofessional community nutrition workers must be maintained. For nutrition programs to be successful, the distinctive roles, responsibilities, and qualifications of the professional and paraprofessional must be understood. For example, paraprofessionals have been effective in presenting basic nutrition information to selected audiences; however, they do not have the expertise to interpret therapeutic diets.

The titles of community dietitian, public health nutrition educator, nutritional anthropologist, nutritionist, and extension home economist all signify some degree of differing specialization. Some would argue that the distinctions are important and should be maintained, while others would say that if the job gets done—if the nutritional needs of the community are assessed and met—it really doesn't make any difference who does the job. As mentioned earlier, the scope of practice of community nutrition workers has not been defined. Many committees throughout the country are attempting to complete the task.

If community food and nutrition professionals are to be effective educators and planners, they must understand people's food behavior and the factors that influence it. It is assumed that they have a knowledge both of food and nutrition and of methods for assessing nutritional status. Also important are skill in counseling, interpersonal communications, and planning and evaluation. The community food and nutrition professional is responsible for helping clients to assess their problems and to plan and initiate action. It is the obligation of food and nutrition educators to present scientific facts in such a manner that clients can integrate them into their lives. Clients can, of course, choose whether they will accept or reject the nutritionist's recommendations.

If a client rejects the recommendation, it may be that the assessments and educational methods of the professionals are at fault. The attitudes and goals of both client and professional must be considered in this assessment. Understanding the relationship of foodways and food behavior to the total culture of the individual and the group is essential if food and nutrition educators are to develop effective food and nutrition programs.

REFERENCES

American Dietetic Association. 1975. *Professional standards review procedure manual.* Chicago: American Dietetic Association.

American Dietetic Association, Committee on Professional Standards Review. 1974. Community dietitian or nutritionist: Draft of PSR standards. Mimeographed. Chicago: American Dietetic Association.

American Dietetic Association, Committee on Community Nutrition and Diet Therapy. 1969. Guidelines for developing dietary counseling services in the community. *Journal of the American Dietetic Association* 55:343.

Anonymous, 1962. Educational qualifications of nutritionists in health agencies. *American Journal of Public Health* 52:116.

Barney, H. S., and Egan, M. C. 1968. Home economists as members of health teams. *Journal of Home Economics* 60 (6):427.

Bosley, B. 1975. Nutritionists and dietitians in the seventies: Trends in education. *World Review of Nutrition and Dietetics* 20:49.

Burgess, H. J. L. and Burgess, A. 1975. A field worker's guide to nutritional status survey. *American Journal of Clinical Nutrition* 28:1299.

Christakis, G., ed. 1973. Nutritional assessment in health programs. *American Journal of Public Health* 63 (November supplement).

Egan, M. 1964. Working together in community nutrition. *Journal of the American Dietetic Association* 45:355.

Egan, M. 1975. *The skilled helper.* Monterey, Calif.: Brooks-Cole.

Frankle, R. T., and Christakis, G. 1973. Community nutrition teams: Cooperation between a large urban medical complex and community agencies brings nutritional and medical care to the community. *Hospitals* 47 (24):56.

Frankle, R. T.; McGregor, B.; Wylie, J.; and McCann, M. B. 1973. Nutrition and lifestyle: I. The Door, a center of alternatives—The nutritionist in a free clinic for adolescents. *Journal of the American Dietetic Associaton* 63:269.

Hammar, S. L. 1966. The role of the nutritionist in an adolescent clinic. *Children.* 13 (6):217.

Heseltine, M. M. 1959. Dietitians and nutritionists in community health programs. *Journal of the American Dietetic Association* 35:793.

Holmes, D. 1972. Nutrition and health-screening services for the elderly. *Journal of the American Dietetic Association* 60:301.

Huenemann, R. L. 1973. Public-health nutritionists in state and local programs. In *U.S. nutrition policies in the seventies,* ed. J. Mayer. San Francisco: W. H. Freeman:

Huenemann, R. L., and Murai, M. 1972. Philosophy and status of an educational program for public health nutritionist-dietitians. *Journal of the American Dietetic Association* 61:669.

Huenemann, R. L., and Peck, E. B. 1971. Who is a public health nutritionist? *Journal of the American Dietetic Association* 58:327.

Nichaman, M. Z., and Collins, G. E. 1974. Nutrition programs in state health agencies. *Nutrition Review* 32:65.

Peck, E. B. 1974. The public health nutritionist-dietitian: An historical perspective. *Journal of the American Dietetic Association* 64:642.

Piper, G. M. 1964. Planning new community nutrition services. *Journal of the American Dietetic Association* 44:461.

Robert-Sargeant, S., and Essex-Cater, A. 1973. The role of the nutritionist in the community health service. *Community Health* 5:137.

Shimoda, N. 1973. Observations of a nutritionist in a free clinic. *Journal of the American Dietetic Association* 63:273.

Todhunter, N. E. 1970. *A guide to nutrition terminology for indexing and retrieval.* U.S. Department of Health, Education and Welfare, Public Health Service, National Institute of Health Publications. Washington, D.C.: Government Printing Office.

Tremolieres, J. 1973. Nutrition in public health. *World Review of Nutrition and Dietetics* 18:275.

U.S. Department of Health, Education and Welfare, Office of Human Development, Office of Child Development. 1975. *Handbook for Local Head Start nutrition specialists.* Washington, D.C.: U.S. Department of Health, Education and Welfare.

U.S. Department of Labor. 1965. *Dictionary of occupational titles: Definition of titles.* Washington, D.C.: Government Printing Office.

Washburn, A. B. 1974. Nutrition counseling for drug addicts in rehabilitation. *Journal of Nutrition Education* 6:13.

Weber, M. 1973. A look at a working nutrition program in Appalachia. *Public Health Currents* 13 (4):1. (Ross Laboratories, Columbus, Ohio)

Yanochik, A. 1973. Community nutrition workers—Their effectiveness in a nutrition delivery system. *Public Health Currents* 13 (5):1. (Ross Laboratories, Columbus, Ohio)

CHAPTER 12

Food and Nutrition Education in the Community

Community food and nutrition education can usually be categorized as nonformal rather than formal. Nonformal education is defined as "all learning processes taking place outside of school" or, in a more restricted sense, "out of school learning which is consciously undertaken or planned" (Rainey 1976). While there are opportunities for formal food and nutrition education in many communities, this chapter will focus on nonformal community nutrition education.

PLANNING FOOD AND NUTRITION EDUCATION

Planning a food and nutrition education program means finding the most appropriate and effective ways to proceed with community food and nutrition education. It involves many different but interrelated steps and implies much more than simply developing nutrition education programs on specific topics in reaction to community problems and needs. Close consideration must be given to the processes that will follow the planning stage—implementation, evaluation, and revision; for unless all of these phases are integrated, the program's effectiveness will be diminished. Planning includes the decision-making stage that determines whether a nutrition education program is developed holistically or is merely a fragmented effort.

The planning of a nutrition education program can be broken down into several distinct, yet interrelated, phases: assessment of community food and nutriton education needs, assessment of the community, identification of other food and nutrition programs and cooperating agencies, and program design. Those phases are presented here in a logical sequence leading to final program development. Community nutritionists will realize, however, that many of the phases occur simultaneously and that different educational situations may require a different sequence or emphasis than is given here.

This chapter was written by Dr. Carolyn Lackey specially for this book.

Assessment of Community Food and Nutrition Education Needs

Assessing a community's food and nutrition education needs means evaluating the community in terms of the prevalence of malnutrition, the availability of food and nutrition services, and the food and nutrition problems that are not being addressed by an existing agency or program. The community nutritionist will identify problems that can be approached exclusively through food and nutrition education and also problems requiring such action as referral to medical, social, job rehabilitation, and other community services provided by qualified agencies. Some problems that the community nutritionist can deal with through education are lack of skills for preparing and preserving food, ignorance of what constitutes a well-balanced diet for persons of various ages and physical conditions, incorrect methods of feeding infants, inadequate diets of individuals who qualify for but do not participate in food assistance programs, inadequate nutrition resulting from food faddism and nutritional quackery, and culture and language barriers that hinder participation in existing nutrition programs.

To plan a program effectively, the community nutritionist must first appraise the community's food and nutrition problems and translate them into educational objectives. The appraisal will be a time-consuming, systematic, and detailed process if no assessment of nutritional needs has been conducted. However, community nutritionists may have access to data that have been collected by agencies or individuals, for example, the Expanded Food and Nutrition Education Program, universities, community nutrition councils, or special nutrition and health screening programs. Data from these sources may provide valuable information on the typical dietary patterns of the community, the number of persons already involved in food and nutrition education and what they are being taught, nutritional problems that have already been identified by special research projects or by other food and nutrition professionals in the community, and the types and prevalence of nutrition-related health problems as determined by health screening and medical records. In either case, the community nutritionist needs to amass and study data carefully before beginning to plan a program.

What information should be included in an assessment of community food and nutrition education needs and how can it be obtained? The following assessment tools can help identify and quantify a community's most prevalent food and nutrition problems: observation and participant observation; interviews with other food and nutrition professionals and health professionals; dietary recalls, records, or histories; screening for biochemical and clinical signs of malnutrition; and anthropometric measurements that relate to present and past nutritional status. The design and use of dietary, clinical, biochemical, and anthropometric measurements have been discussed at length by Christakis (1973) and Jelliffe (1966). The following discussion will concentrate on the use of data from community agencies, from observation, and from questionnaires and interviews.

The community nutritionist will first want to find any available information that is directly or indirectly related to problems of food and nutrition. Such data can be obtained from the files of food and nutrition agencies and public health offices, from the records of health care facilities and courthouses, and from agricultural forecasts, school health-service reports, and other agencies within the community.

In addition to gathering data that have already been collected and sometimes even summarized, the community nutritionist may rely heavily upon the technique of observation and participant observation. Observation includes looking at a community's housing conditions, sources of food supply, typical life-style, and general social, political, cultural, and economic atmosphere. This technique requires close attention to the visible and verbal signs that characterize the people's mode of living and their attitudes toward general issues. Observation is often the easiest way to identify program target audiences where a combination of poverty, joblessness, low educational level, or other factors may contribute to food and nutrition problems. Once population groups have been identified, the community nutritionist needs to acquire more data on the specific types of problems that people have and to find out whether other programs or agencies are already addressing those problems.

More in-depth data can be collected through participant observation. The nutritionist engages in day-to-day activities with the people and in this way becomes able to understand and explain the conditions that have been identified through observation. Acculturation of this sort should enable the community nutritionist to plan more effective educational programs, programs that are adapted to the life-styles and living conditions of those in the community.

Personal interviews and contacts with other community professionals are also valuable assessment tools. The community nutritionist should interview local physicians and other medical professionals, including public health, hospital, and school nurses; school lunch personnel; Cooperative Extension home economists; and dentists and other professionals working with food and nutrition or health services. Their past work in the community, and their knowledge of the insight into community programs provide the community nutritionist with a variety of opinions on existing conditions and on work that has been done or is being planned to help alleviate the food and nutrition problems.

Questionnaires should be designed to elicit a person's expressed needs for food and nutrition information. They may have fixed responses from which the respondent chooses an answer, or they may be open-ended, with no set of responses to choose from. Questionnaires must be carefully constructed and developed so that the time and energy expended in gathering data by this method are not wasted. Community nutritionists can use questionnaires to determine whether an educational need they perceive as important to the community is indeed one the community would respond to if a program were offered. The response to a questionnaire may indicate a lack of interest in some aspect of nutrition that the nutritionist considers very important. In such an instance, the nutritionist may decide to employ an awareness campaign to alert the community or influential community organizations to an important educational need that has not been recognized by the community.

Assessment through questionnaires can also identify persons who need to be referred to community agencies that deal with problems which are outside the scope of food and nutrition but which affect a person's ability to deal with food and nutrition problems. For example, some people with low incomes may have inadequate diets not because they are poor or lack knowledge of food and nutrition, but because failing eyesight makes it hard for them to get to and from stores, to select food from shelves, or to prepare food in the kitchen. Problems like this can often be solved by referring the person to an agency that can supply medical treatment at reduced cost or to a center that provides help for people with impaired sight.

After determining that, in general, there are food and nutrition problems, the community nutritionist must identify the specific problems and classify them into categories that can be addressed through appropriate food and nutrition education programs. While the assessment is being carried out, the community nutritionist will be determining program priorities and developing educational strategies.

The needs assessment should be a continuing process that remains an integral part of program planning. Any community, no matter how small or isolated, is constantly changing; social, political, economic, and educational forces are not static. The community nutritionist must be sensitive to community change and reflect this in program planning. As assessment continues, the focus of educational programs will shift. Needs assessment can also be used to evaluate the effectiveness of current programs and to give the community nutritionist an indication that programs effective in the past need to be reactivated and/or revised in response to community change.

Community nutritionists need not be passive individuals whose educational programs are the outcome of community needs assessment only. As professionals trained in food and nutrition, they will often observe needs that would not be identified by any assessment technique currently in use.

Identifying food and nutrition problems is not the only function of the assessment phase. Other essential information needs to be gathered from people in the community if educational programs are to be relevant and successful. That includes information on people's attitudes and beliefs regarding the foods available to them and the relationship between food and health. The techniques of observation, personal interviews, and questionnaires can be used to obtain that information. Without it, even the best-designed educational program may be ineffective. The social, economic, psychological, cultural, and other meanings of food discussed elsewhere in this book are some of the most important factors in the final program design.

Assessment of the Community

In addition to identifying the food and nutrition problems of the community, the community nutritionist must look at the community as a whole, that is, at its social, political, educational (both formal and nonformal), and religious orientations. Distinct cultural and ethnic groups, influential organizations and individuals, and the community power structure must all be identified.

Generalizations based on demographic data—including population distribution according to age; sex per capita income and community income distribution; education; occupation; family size; and racial and ethnic groups—give the nutritionist an overall view of the community's population. The same type of information is needed about individuals participating in food and nutrition education programs, so that the programs can be tailored to the group's characteristics. (Of course, individual variations within a group must always be taken into account.) It is also useful to know about local mass media, transportation facilities, sources of food supply, sanitation conditions, and geography and climate.

Like assessment of community food and nutrition education needs, assessment of the community as a whole will aid the community nutritionist in planning relevant educational programs. As pointed out in previous chapters, food behavior is not an isolated behavior but is affected by a person's environment, including social and cultural surroundings.

Identification of Other Food and Nutrition Programs and Cooperating Agencies

Unless a community is extremely isolated, there will usually be agencies or programs that deal in some way with food and nutrition. The community nutritionist should make contact with those groups and find out what programs and services related to food and nutrition are already being offered. Then the community nutritionist can (1) help other agencies plan effective food and nutrition education programs, (2) develop a referral system, (3) establish program priorities among the existing agencies, (4) organize cooperative programs in cases where audiences and objectives overlap among agencies, and (5) help unify and strengthen the food and nutrition services available to the community by combining the efforts of several agencies.

For example, the Cooperative Extension Service and the state public health services have worked together to develop educational bulletins and programs on infant feeding. Even this one instance of coordination has resulted in savings of time and effort and money. Or coordination might take the form of contractual agreements between agencies, either for the development of educational materials and programs or for the conduct of food and nutrition research related to any of the four steps of food and nutrition education (i.e., planning, implementation, evaluation, and revision).

After reviewing the work of other agencies that are directly or indirectly involved in food and nutrition education, community nutritionists should be better equipped to set their own program priorities, based on needs assessment and knowledge of existing programs. What may have looked like an impossible situation according to the needs assessment can now be pictured as a more clearly delineated working situation.

Unfortunately, cooperation, coordination, and close contact with other food and nutrition programs and related agencies may not be an easy task. Agencies may have previously established objectives that preclude cooperation in joint educational efforts, and their bureaucratic structures may hinder coordination of programs. Personality conflicts between community nutritionists and other food and nutrition professionals can also be a problem. However, all professionals concerned with the nutritional status of individuals should work together to eliminate barriers that hinder cooperation and coordination of efforts. That is the most logical way to use limited funds and community resources to the best advantage.

Program Design

At this point, the community nutritionist has assessed the food and nutrition problems and needs of the community and determined which ones can be handled through educational programs. Other agencies dealing with food and nutrition assistance and education have been identified and their work assessed. In addition, the community nutritionist should by now have a clear picture of the community situation in which food and nutrition education will be offered. It is time to set program priorities and to design educational experiences.

Since not all food and nutrition problems and needs can be handled effectively at once, the community nutritionist, alone or in cooperation with other agencies, must decide which problems, needs, and audiences should be addressed first. There are no guidelines showing which population groups or nutritional needs ought to have top priority; the community nutritionist must rely on his or her trained judgment to decide the matter. Once priorities have been determined, program planning takes shape in the form of program objectives, program scope, educational format, and facilities and equipment for delivering the program and evaluating its effectiveness.

Program Objectives. The nutrition education objectives of agencies providing food and nutrition services ought to be of two basic types: (1) objectives directed by federal, state, or local legislation or agency function and (2) behavioral objectives for participants in nutrition education programs. Both types should be considered in the planning process.

Examples of actual objectives might be to provide nutrition programs for children enrolled in a school for the deaf; to provide mandatory nutrition education for specially funded programs (such as the Women, Infants and Children Program) that stipulate a nutrition education component; to develop a specified number of public service radio announcements for each month; to publish pamphlets on food and nutrition topics; to draw attention to the agency through news media coverage; and to enroll new members in the agency's structured programs. It is easy to tell when objectives like these have been accomplished. They are all valid objectives for an agency; however, they are incomplete because they do not stipulate any change in the behavior of the target audience. The underlying purpose of each could be documentation of the agency's activity in order to garner support for continued funding.

In the past, programs and agencies received funding on the basis of the number of people reached through feeding programs, the number of people attending food and nutrition education programs, or the number of pamphlets distributed. But now they are not only held accountable for the time spent in program development and education, they are also required to document changes in the nutritional status and food behavior of the people reached by their programs. Therefore, in addition to stating objectives in terms of audiences to be reached and methods of program delivery, much attention must be given to changing the food behavior of the target audiences.

A well-designed nutrition education program needs clear and detailed objectives that designate the target audience, the delivery method, and measurable changes in behavior or nutritional status that will be beneficial to the community. The problems and needs of the community, as determined by assessment of the community and its food and nutrition education needs, should guide the community nutritionist in developing behavioral objectives for the target audiences. Other texts can be consulted for suggestions on how to write objectives (Cyrs 1973) and plan programs around them. The important things to keep in mind are that objectives should be written to include measurable changes in the nutritional status and food behavior of the target audiences and that community and needs assessment must precede formulation of the program objectives.

Program Scope. A community nutrition education program may be the result of careful planning based on needs assessment, or it may be a response to a crisis. In the first instance the nutritionist is working in accordance with a detailed, long-range plan; in the second, the program is a reaction to a situation that does not permit the development of long-range objectives or of plans for a systematic accumulation of nutritional knowledge by the program participants. The community nutritionist responding to a crisis does not build long-range programs to anticipate future crises but is concerned instead with creating a short-term educational program of narrow scope that meets immediate needs. The nutritionist involved in a systematic, long-range program has assessed the problems and needs of the community and has a program plan that reflects nutrition education priorities. This approach is designed to provide the community with programs that lead to lifelong acquisition of nutrition knowledge by the participants.

A combination of the two approaches allows the most flexibility in programming and is the most responsive to community problems and needs. It can be achieved by responding to crises in the context of a systematic, objective-based, long-range program. The community nutritionist thus has a well-defined set of objectives but is free to react when the need arises, to situations not covered in the established plan.

For example, assume that a community nutritionist assessed a community's need for education in infant nutrition and found that many young parents knew little about the subject. The nutritionist then developed a well-planned educational program with the following objectives: (1) to increase knowledge of infant nutrition, (2) to change behavior in cases where infant feeding practices were incorrect, and (3) to improve the infants' nutritional status. The program was under way and the nutritionist had already discussed breast-feeding when researchers reported that human milk may become contaminated if lactating mothers eat meat from animals that have eaten contaminated feed. In response to this crisis, the nutritionist, instead of proceeding according to the program plan, immediately returned to the subject of breast-feeding and pointed out how the new research findings affected what had been said about it in the earlier discussion. Once the crisis had been dealt with, the nutritionist returned to the program plan.

Educational Format. When the program objectives have been established and the scope of the program determined, the next step is to work out an appropriate educational format. This process includes (1) deciding what information will help the audience meet the stated behavioral objectives, (2) selecting methods of delivery, (3) determining which available resource materials can be adapted to serve the program objectives, (4) estimating the amount of time that both the nutrition educator and the audience can devote to the program, and (5) developing a strategy to motivate the intended audience to participate in the program. Each of these processes will be discussed in some detail.

Subject Matter. Once behavioral objectives have been set for a specific program, the subject matter must be tailored to the objectives. The character of the prospective audience will partially determine the program content. The community nutrition educator determines not only the information needed by the audience but also the level at which to present it. Earlier assessment of the community and of individuals will aid in determining the audience's current level of knowledge and their capacity to understand and assimilate information at various educational levels.

Delivery Method. After the community nutritionist has determined what information will be presented and at what educational level, the method of delivery should be selected. In choosing a method of delivery, one must consider the accessibility of various systems such as radio and television, the number of people one wishes to reach, the educational level of the people and their motivation to either attend meetings or read pamphlets, the amount of time that can be spent, and the physical and monetary resources available for conducting the program. Systems available for delivery may include mass media such as radio, television, newspapers, and other printed materials. The accessibility of these media to both the community nutritionist and the intended audience will help determine whether they can be effective for program delivery. For example, if printed materials are distributed to a large proportion of the community but most of the intended audience cannot read them, then this medium is not very effective.

Other delivery systems include group meetings or one-to-one contact. These methods allow for greater interaction between the nutritionist and the program participants but may prove to be too time-consuming. Also, many who need the program may be persons who will not attend group meetings. Often the people most in need of assistance from the community nutritionist are insecure in unfamiliar surroundings or have time, transportation, and child-care constraints that prevent their attendance at meetings. Motivation to learn about nutrition has to be high for an individual to attend a nutrition education program in today's society, where so many other options for leisure time are available.

One-to-one contact is a delivery system that has been used successfully in the Expanded Food and Nutrition Education Program. In one-to-one contact the community nutritionist works with people on an individual basis through home visits or individual counseling in the nutritionist's office or other designated place. Although this delivery system may be too time-consuming for programs in which many people require assistance, it can be a good way to deal with individuals whose foods and nutrition needs are too specific to be covered in a more general public program. Trained auxiliary workers can assist the nutritionist with this method of delivery.

Telephone and mail may be effective means of exchanging information with some persons. Again, while time-consuming, they permit the community nutritionist to handle the very specific problems of a small segment of the population whose needs are not met by large-scale community food and nutrition education programs. For example, a food and nutrition information center manned by trained graduate students or paraprofessionals or volunteers, with extensive files and resource people, can serve as a telephone question-answer base. Persons with specific problems or questions related to food and nutrition can receive information immediately, simply by calling the information center.

From this limited discussion of program delivery systems, it should be clear that the method must be chosen with full awareness of the educational level and motivation of the intended audience. A recognized need for nutrition education does not guarantee a captive audience for the community nutritionist. Selecting the medium that will most effectively reach the intended audience is a very important part of program design. Sometimes trial and error is the only way to find the right medium, but often other community professionals who also develop educational programs can guide the community nutritionist in selecting effective delivery systems.

Available Resources. After the delivery system has been decided upon, an appropriate mode of presentation must be chosen, for example, lecture, film, discussion, demonstration, pamphlet, or slide/tape series. The resources of time, money, personal talent, and materials available to the community nutritionist will influence the choice.

The community nutritionist does not always need to develop original food and nutrition education materials. Often films, filmstrips, lesson plans, and pamphlets are available from the Cooperative Extension Service and from industries, professional organizations, and nonprofit agencies whose work involves food and nutrition. The most efficient community nutritionist is one who can select from such materials and adapt them, if necessary, to specific program objectives. However, developing and testing new ways to present food and nutrition education not only adds a different and exciting dimension to the community nutritionist's job, it also adds to the resources available to other community nutritionists. The wheel need not be reinvented for each food and nutrition education program, but materials and delivery methods must be carefully evaluated with regard to the assessed characteristics of the intended audience.

In addition to the educational materials that are available from various sources, there may be persons in the community who can contribute to the community nutritionist's educational efforts. These individuals may include not only other food and nutrition professionals who are already engaged in educational programs, but also people with specific expertise who are not generally asked to function as educators. The community nutritionist may find that one of the important aspects of the job is discovering such people and making use of their knowledge. Once they have been identified and have expressed a willingness to share their skills and knowledge, they become a volunteer force of potential educators which the nutritionist must coordinate and use to the community's advantage. For example, the manager of a local restaurant may never have had formal training in quantity food service but may nonetheless be well qualified to help with a program to train operators of newly formed day-care centers, especially if the community nutritionist does not have a strong background in quantity food service.

Another aid to the community nutritionist are paraprofessionals whom the nutritionist trains to deliver programs, identify target audiences, perform follow-up evaluations, and identify or develop educational materials and activities. They may be paid staff or volunteers interested in food and nutrition education. Usually they are members of the community, and their familiarity with the community and its long-standing food and nutrition problems and needs is valuable. They can give the community nutritionist a grass-roots appraisal of situations and often are able to suggest effective ways to approach problems. Having someone with whom to test ideas before the program design is finished and implementation begun can result in more creative approaches to education that are better adapted to the intended audiences.

Time. Another aspect of program design is the length of time the audience is willing to devote to food and nutrition education. The transportation available and the distance to be traveled, child-care needs, work schedules, and other personal situations will affect attendance at group meetings. In addition to the length of time the audience is willing to devote to attending programs, the time of day or year the program is given may affect attendance. Many of these considerations apply not only to a group meeting at a specific date, time, and place, but also to the other delivery systems that have been discussed. It is important that the time demanded by the delivery system be evaluated during the planning process. The community nutritionist should also attempt to learn as much as possible about the audience in advance in order to plan around factors that might reduce participation.

Even when people are willing to make adjustments in their daily routines to attend programs, there is a limit to how long one can expect to hold their attention. It depends partly on their interest in the subject but also on the fact that they are learning something new. A person's ability to concentrate and to recall information at a later date is affected by the amount of information presented. Too often nutrition educators try to teach in one or two programs all that they have learned about a subject during years of study. Some audiences respond better to programs or materials that focus on a single concept. This is true not only for lecture, demonstration, and participation methods of delivery but for printed materials as well. It is worth restating that the community nutritionist can gain insight and guidance from others in the community who are engaged in similar educational efforts.

Motivation. The community nutritionist has worked diligently planning and designing an effective educational program. However, people will not be attracted to a program simply because it has been efficiently planned or even because they themselves have requested it. They must be motivated. And the community nutritionist must find a way to motivate them. Why should a young mother, even though she would like to know more about infant feeding, hire a baby-sitter so that she can attend a program? Why should a 45-year-old woman who has been preserving food as her mother did 25 years ago attend a program on how to preserve food? Why should a young father leave his television football game to go to a Parent-Teacher Association meeting on proposed revisions to the school lunch program? Why? Especially since food and nutrition education has had the reputation of being dull and unexciting to much of the public. The community nutritionist has a formidable task ahead: to motivate people to attend programs, or listen to a specific radio program, or watch a certain television program, or read pamphlets. Yet the task is not impossible if one can capitalize on the public's current interest in food and nutrition, physical fitness, and the world food supply.

There is no quick and easy way to motivate people. Involving persons from the intended audience in the phases of program planning may help them become motivated to learn and participate. For example, they might serve on community committees or specific task forces or simply form a group of individuals who have expressed their common desire for information about food and nutrition. When people are involved in its planning phases they are better able to see a program's relevance for themselves and others, and their word-of-mouth promotion of the nutrition education program can be a great asset.

Once the community nutritionist has established a reputation for developing useful and interesting programs that reflect the community's input, motivational strategy becomes less important; however, it must not be neglected. As communities change, so do the factors that motivate people to continue learning. The community nutritionist must be sensitive to changes and meet them with creatively designed programs and innovative motivational techniques.

Facilities and Equipment for Program Delivery. While designing the educational programs, the community nutritionist must always be aware of the physical and monetary resources available within the community or easily accessible elsewhere. Regarding physical resources, the following questions must be attended to while the program is still in the planning stage.

If the educational program is in the form of a group meeting, does the community nutritionist have access to a meeting place? Is it free or will rent be charged? Must it be reserved far in advance? Will audiovisual equipment be used in the program, and, if so, is it available at the meeting place? If the delivery system is printed matter, does the community nutritionist have a budget for this or must the funds be supplied by other community organizations that must first be convinced of its merit? Does an allocation exist for mailing printed materials to individuals? Are there public places where printed matter or short programs can be delivered to people?

The community nutritionist should include the physical arrangements as part of the program design. For example, programs for the elderly should be held in places with few or no stairs to climb, easily accessible by walking or public transportation, with good lighting and acoustics. The community nutritionist's plan may have to be altered if physical facilities and resources are inadequate or unavailable. For example, suppose the community nutritionist has heard that a computer dietary analysis was very successful in another community and so wishes to use the computer dietary analysis as part of an awareness approach to nutrition. An investigation of what it would require to conduct such a program reveals that the nearest portable computer terminal is 150 miles away and a special telephone hookup is required for access to the main computer. The time and money required to conduct such a program must be evaluated in terms of the program's potential success and the number of people who would be reached. Moreover, the nutritionist must decide whether this particular program is in accord with long-range objectives, time allocations, and total budget.

Many nutrition educators have learned that even the simplest oversight, such as the lack of a three-pronged plug adapter or an extension cord, can foil even the best program if it was planned around an audiovisual presentation. Care must be taken to obtain all the equipment needed. The community nutritionist should not assume that physical requirements can be handled after a program has been designed; they are an integral part of program design at all stages.

Budgetary requirements for program development may be an even greater obstacle to producing the "ideal" educational program. Budgets for foods and nutrition education usually are not in keeping with the importance of the subject. Additional sources of money might be contractual agreements with other agencies or tax-deductable donations from organizations outside the food and nutrition field. The pooling of budgetary allowances by cooperating agencies can increase the amount of educational materials or programs that can be developed or distributed. For instance, one community nutritionist without travel funds heard that a church community development committee was sponsoring a seminar in a distant section of her state and that the population to be served by the seminar had requested information on food preservation. The nutritionist approached the organizers of the seminar and agreed to participate in the seminar and also to give a program on food preservation if they would provide transportation. The organizers of the seminar recognized the role of food preservation in community self-help and accepted the community nutritionist's plan.

IMPLEMENTING FOOD AND NUTRITION EDUCATION

Implementation of food and nutrition education is very simple to detail. As a community nutritionist you have planned to the best of your ability an educational situation designed to fulfill a program objective. Now, *do it.*

Many of the aspects discussed under program planning were included so that no further planning would be necessary at this point. No matter what delivery system was chosen — radio, public meetings, or pamphlets — the community nutritionist is now ready to accomplish the objective of making food and nutrition education available to the intended audience. However, lest the community nutritionist think she or he is "home free" now, it must be remembered that flexibility is a key concept here, also. Implementing a food and nutrition education program may required last-minute changes in delivery system or method, subject matter, or objectives.

Assume that an agency involved in food and nutrition has asked the community nutritionist to give a program on infant feeding to a group of mothers with children under the age of 1 year. The community nutritionist knows who the intended audience is, where and when the program is to be given, the audiovisual facilities that are available, and the audience's sociocultural and economic characteristics as described by the requesting agency. The community nutritionist arrives at the appointed time and greets the audience, a small informal group. A quick look shows that approximately two-thirds of the women are past the child bearing age. They were to have been young mothers with young children but they don't seem to fit that description. Something seems amiss. The community nutritionist asks how many women in the audience have children under 1 year of age and discovers one such woman and a woman who is expecting a baby in 2 months. The representative from the agency notices the speaker's surprise and quickly explains that the attendance she had anticipated at the program seemed small the previous day so she had contacted the director of migrant day-care centers in the area, who then required the food-service personnel of the day-care center to attend the program. Now, should the community nutritionist continue with the well-organized program on mothers' feeding their own infants or change the topic to quantity food service for infants whose mothers leave them in day-care centers? Obviously, some change in the program is needed so that the entire audience can benefit from it. The community nutritionist is in control of the situation now and can adapt the program to the audience's expectations and needs, although prior notification of the audience mix would have been helpful.

EVALUATING FOOD AND NUTRITION EDUCATION

The community nutritionist must evaluate food and nutrition education in terms of the program objectives that were developed in the planning stage. Some objectives, such as those concerning the number of educational programs to be offered, the number of people to be reached by the programs, and the written materials to be distributed, are easy to evaluate numerically. But, as stated earlier, evaluation of food and nutrition education must be more than numerical. Programs should be accountable for accomplishing behavioral objectives that stipulate changes in the participants' behavior and/or improvement in their nutritional status. Changes in food and nutrition knowledge can be determined to see whether cognitive learning has occurred; however, cognitive learning cannot be assumed to lead directly to behavioral change. These are two distinctly different aspects for evaluation.

All program evaluations need not be made in terms of agency or behavioral objectives. While less easily documented for program accountability, on-the-spot evaluations through verbal responses and group interaction can give the community nutritionist valuable immediate feedback.

Evaluation methods should be designed at the same time as the program format so that in the evaluation phase data are collected on information or behavioral change that is stressed in the program. Although making evaluations adds time to the program, it is essential if the community nutritionist is striving to improve educational programs so that they provide the greatest possible learning opportunity for the audience and encourage necessary behavioral change. If a community nutritionist uses the same educational strategy and subject matter for any length of time, it should be evaluated periodically. The community is not static, and program evaluations can help the community nutritionist note changes in the community that should be reflected in programming.

REVISING FOOD AND NUTRITION EDUCATION

Educational needs assessment and program evaluation will help the community nutritionist find the areas of program planning that need revision. First, the program's effectiveness must be determined by evaluation. Then, the particular aspects of the situation that contributed to the program's success or ineffectiveness must be pinpointed. This entails close evaluation of all aspects of program development and implementation. It may be that only slight revisions in one area will correct the situation that limited the program's success. On the other hand, many aspects of the food and nutrition education process may have been overlooked or misinterpreted during program planning and thus greater revision will be necessary. Many educational programs will require some revision the first time they are presented, and other revisions will be needed as the community itself changes.

SUMMARY

Program development must not be carried out in isolation from the community environment. The community nutritionist has to be aware of all the factors that are involved in a complete appraisal of the social, cultural, economic, physical, and attitudinal aspects of the community and that must be taken into account in developing a nutrition education program. While assessing a community's food and nutrition needs, the community nutritionist should study the foodways of the citizens. The nutritionist must also identify existing programs that affect the nutritional status of the population. This includes knowing who the other professionals are and how the programs relate to each other — what their objectives are, how they are administered, and what portion of the community they serve. It is important that the community nutritionist know what resources are available, not only material, professional, and monetary resources, but also volunteers, including local citizens and food and nutrition students from colleges.

Limiting educational objectives and developing long-range program plans is crucial if the community nutritionist is to serve the community's most pressing needs as efficiently as possible. Access to basic data on food behavior is essential. The nutritionist needs such data to determine target audiences and program topics. Knowing whether food behavior is core, secondary, or peripheral helps the community nutritionist to select target areas where behavior is more easily modified. The assessment phase of program planning provides the community nutritionist with the information necessary to begin program design. Designing a program includes developing an appropriate approach to food and nutrition education and working out a plan for implementing the program. Identifying and evaluating a variety of approaches and reviewing the literature are helpful procedures at this time.

Involving community citizens in some of the decision-making processes of program planning helps them recognize their own and their community's nutritional problems and encourages them to seek the necessary resources (knowledge, food, health care, monetary assistance, etc.) to alleviate the problems. Community involvement in program implementation and evaluation also contributes to a program's relevance and effectiveness.

The community nutritionist's role as educator is not complete until the program has been evaluated and, if necessary, revised. Once this has been accomplished, the nutritionist can make recommendations regarding continuation of the program and then move on to other problem areas.

REFERENCES

Christakis, G. B. 1973. *Nutritional assessment in health programs.* Washington, D.C.: American Public Health Association.

Cyrs, T. E. 1973. *You, behavioral objectives and nutrition education.* Chicago: National Dairy Council.

Jelliffe, D. B. 1966. *The assessment of the nutritional status of the community.* WHO Monograph no. 53. Geneva: World Health Organization.

Rainey, M. C. 1976. Non-formal education: Definitions and distinctions. *Interaction 'ECO'* 6:1. (Michigan State University)

CHAPTER 13

Programs and Agencies Providing Nutritional Services and Education

Now that the myriad activities that a community food and nutrition professional might participate in have been described, a discussion of some specific programs and agencies that provide food and nutrition services is appropriate. Some programs, such as Head Start, have well-defined roles for the community food and nutrition professional. However, jobs for professionals trained in community food and nutrition are limited only by the imagination, drive, and salesmanship of those professionals.

There are both nationwide and local programs that typically employ community food and nutrition professionals. Capsule descriptions of these programs and the role of food and nutrition professionals in them will be given in this chapter. Only a skeleton view will be provided, since a program's existence may depend on legislation, state or local interest or jurisdiction, local need, availability of matching or supporting funds, availability of trained and interested personnel, or a host of other factors. Furthermore, regulations for programs continually change and implementation may vary with locality. Examples of publicly and privately funded national and local programs will be presented, beginning with the major food program supported by the federal government, a program that receives either praise or criticism from all sectors of the community — the Food Stamp Program.

THE FOOD STAMP PROGRAM

Neither the Food Stamp Act of 1964 nor the Food Stamp Act of 1977 specified a nutrition education component beyond handouts on meal planning and the effective use of food stamps. But since community nutritionists must be aware of all food programs assistance operating within the community, a discussion of the Food Stamp Program is included here.

The Food Stamp Program was implemented nationwide in 1964, following a pilot project program, as a replacement for commodity food distribution programs. It has become the major food program conducted by the federal government, growing at a rate of 9 percent per year. It is a transfer payment program administered by the Food and Nutrition Service of the Department of Agriculture in cooperation with state and county welfare agencies. The purpose of the program is to enable low-income housholds to buy the right kind of food, or to buy more food of greater variety, to improve their diets. This is done by increasing the purchasing power of a household's food dollars. According to the 1964 Act 5 with a given amount of money participants could purchase stamps and a bonus. When shopping in an authorized store, they could purchase more food than their dollars would otherwise allow. The Food Stamp Act of 1977 has eliminated the purchase requirement, and food stamp benefits will be given to eligible households at no charge. Specific regulations and allotments of the program will not be given here since they change often. At the time of this writing, the rules for the Food Stamp Act of 1977 have not been announced, but some general information about the requirements and benefits of the program as it existed in 1976 should provide an idea of the program's scope. Current regulations and allotments can be obtained by consulting the *Federal Register* or the Food and Nutrition Service.

Eligibility

Households were eligible for food stamps if they were receiving public assistance, were unemployed and registered with their state employment office, or were employed and receiving a low income. (The 1977 rules will contain a work registration requirement.) A household receiving Aid to Dependent Children assistance or social security pensions through the welfare system automatically qualified but still had to submit an application. For others, eligibility was based on the household's net income and resources and the number of persons in the household. Items such as medical bills and high housing costs were deducted from gross income before eligibility was calculated. For most participants, certification for food stamp benefits was for a 3-month period, but households with stable incomes could be certified for as long as 6 months while those with fluctuating incomes, like migrant workers, were often certified for only 1 month at a time. (The rules of the Food Stamp Act of 1977 will change much of this.)

The eligibility of segments of the population such as the "voluntary poor" has been debated from time to time. Many opponents of the Food Stamp Program believe that students, strikers, and other voluntary poor should not receive assistance.

Purchase of Stamps

Households certified for the program were issued identification cards allowing them to buy a specified allotment of stamps on a monthly basis. The allotment was adjusted twice yearly to reflect changes in the cost of food as documented by Bureau of Labor statistics. The *purchase price* or the amount each household had to pay for the stamps, was determined by the household's income. While those with extremely low incomes received stamps free, others paid up to 30 percent of their net income for stamps.

The purchase requirement was a very controversial facet of the Food Stamp Program. Some people advocated eliminating it completely and others thought that the figure of 30 percent of net income should be raised or lowered. The Food Stamp Act of 1977 has done away with the purchase requirement, and food stamp benefits will be free, probably after January 1979.

The tasks of processing applications, determining eligibility, and certifying participants, as well as providing outreach, have been carried out by welfare agencies. The selling of food stamp coupons has been conducted by banks, post offices, and other authorized outlets. In some areas, it is possible to get food stamps through the mail.

The Thrifty Food Plan

The allotment of food stamps is calculated to provide household members with enough stamps to purchase food according to the Department of Agriculture's Thrifty Food Plan. This food plan was developed by the Agricultural Research Service and released in September 1975. It provides for adequate quantities of most nutrients but only marginal quantities of others. The Thrifty Food Plan was designed for participants as a guide to wise selection of food products for human consumption and of seeds or plants used to product food. (Nonfood items, such as paper goods, pet food, soap, beer, and cigarettes, cannot be purchased with food stamps.) Some professional community food and nutrition workers, as well as other advocates of the program, have suggested that the Thrifty Food Plan provides a nutritious diet only to people who have excellent skills in food purchasing, budgeting, preparing, and storing. These advocates have testified in state and national legislative hearing on hunger and malnutrition in the United States that many participants in the Food Stamp Program do not possess the necessary food-related skills and do not have sufficient knowledge of food and nutrition to provide an adequately nutritious diet for all members of the household using the Thrifty Food Plan. Complete descriptions of the Thrifty Food Plan, recipes, and other information are available from the Food Stamp Division, Food and Nutrition Service, United States Department of Agriculture, Washington, D.C. 20250.

Role of the Community Food and Nutrition Professional

Perhaps no other food assistance program receives more political attention and public criticism than the Food Stamp Program. Community food and nutrition professionals should be familiar with how the program operates both nationally and locally, so that they can comment on proposed regulations, testify at hearings, and make constructive suggestions to legislators. For example, if one believes that nutrition education should be a mandated and funded component of the Food Stamp Program, one can become an advocate for nutrition education legislation. Community food and nutrition workers can also assist recipients in planning food purchases and nutritious meals and teach them the skills required to prepare and store food.

THE COOPERATIVE EXTENSION SERVICE

Administered jointly by the federal, state, and county governments, the Cooperative Extension Service has been helping people in the United States improve their home life, their farms, their communities since Congress authorized it in 1914. Funding for informal and alternate sources of education and information to the community is provided by the Department of Agriculture, state and local governments, and land-grant colleges and universities. The funding is often supplemented by grants from the public and private sectors of the community. Although specific programs may not be national in scope, the Cooperative Extension Service functions in every county of all fifty states and in Puerto Rico, the Virgin Islands, and the District of Columbia. Many foreign countries also have extension services patterned after that of the United States.

In providing public services and education, the Cooperative Extension Service acts as a bridge between the scientific community and the public. For example, specialists in agriculture and family living present research findings in everyday language and help apply them to specific problems within a community. In addition to employing specialists and fieldworkers to conduct its programs, the Cooperative Extension Service also enlists the aid of volunteers. The leadership capabilities of adults and youth are encouraged and developed in this way.

The Cooperative Extension Service is undergoing reorganization at the federal level, but at present there are four main program areas: home economics, expanded food and nutrition education, youth (including the 4-H Program), and agriculture. While the community food and nutrition professional may work in any one or all four of these areas, the role of food and nutrition is more clearly defined in the first three program areas, and therefore they will be discussed further here.

Home Economics Education or Family Living Education

Home economics became a recognized component of the Cooperative Extension Service in 1918, 4 years after the Smith-Lever Act authorized the Service. Programs on nutrition, management of resources, consumer education, child development and family relationships, housing and home environment, health, community leadership development, and public policy education form the basis of the education and information dissemination conducted by the Family Living Education section of the Cooperative Extension Service.

Many people carry an image of the home economics agent as the professional who advised the farmer's wife on the care and feeding of her family and who organized home demonstration clubs. Such a characterization no longer describes the home economics agent of today, who uses radio, television, newspapers, newsletters, and correspondence courses to bring timely information to all members of the community, rural and urban alike. Programs are designed specifically to reach target audiences, and the methods employed are specific for each group. Programs on a wide variety of topics may be planned primarily for mothers, teenagers, senior citizens, singles, minorities, the handicapped, the unemployed, or others. Clubs or groups organized according to the members' interests learn through discussions and practice experiences. Many forms of education, including workshops, siminars, tours, exhibits, demonstrations, and meetings, are used to inform the consumer. Extension Service personnel may present programs on meal patterns designed to fit family income and life-style, weight control, food preservation to conserve nutrients, use of nutrition labels in food selection, and meal planning.

In 1974 a national task force identified areas of concern for Home Economics Extension that included human nutrition, consumer problems, children and families, housing, health, and community development. Specific nutritional concerns included nutrient adequacy, especially for families with limited resources and individuals at high nutritional risk, health problems related to nutrition, food consumption pattern, food technology as it relates to nutrition, use of the U.S. Recommended Daily Allowances (U.S. RDA) and the Recommended Dietary Allowances (RDA), and nutrition labeling. The task force recommended that existing programs focusing on these issues be emphasized and that new programs be developed.

Although the recommendations from the task force are distributed nationally, most programs are developed at the state or county level. Extension Service specialists at land-grant institutions assist county staff in developing programs. Locally, needed programs may be initiated by Extension Service field staff assigned to the county. Several states have direct information access centers: consumers calling a central location receive answers to questions or information on a variety of topics, including food and nutrition. Community food and nutrition specialists answer questions about food and nutrition directly, prepare situation statements, prepare and record telephone tapes on current food and nutrition issues, and present lectures to interested groups. During the mid-1970s, Cooperative Extension Service personnel observed the renewed interest in home gardening and assisted gardeners by providing information about gardening, food preservation, and food safety.

The public service and educational programs of the Cooperative Extension Service are available to everyone, regardless of income, education, race, or sex, and most of them are provided without charge.

The Expanded Food and Nutrition Education Program (EFNEP)

The Expanded Food and Nutrition Education Program (EFNEP) is designed to teach nutrition to low-income families on a person-to-person basis. It was authorized by section 32 of the 1969 agricultural bill. Funds to support the EFNEP are provided in large measure from the taxes levied against agricultural commodities brought into the United States. Although the EFNEP is a Cooperative Extension Service program, limited funding has restricted its implementation to only a small proportion of all counties in the nation. For the most part, the program serves low-income urban families belonging to minority ethnic groups.

The educators in this program are low-income paraprofessionals who may have backgrounds similar to the participants'. They are recruited from the target population and trained in food and nutrition skills by the home economics extension agent. After their initial training they receive continual in-service training in nutrition, food preparation, family relations, child rearing, money management, shopping, general housekeeping, and sanitation.

Since families eligible for the EFNEP have low incomes and generally poor food and nutrition skills, they are referred to the program by social service agencies, health departments, public schools, and, occasionally, the courts. Some families hear about the EFNEP by word of mouth and seek it out by themselves, and others are recruited by aides going door-to-door in low-income districts.

The EFNEP offers no economic benefits such as money or free food, although nutrition aides do direct eligible families to programs that offer direct food benefits. Rather, the nutrition aide provides information and may visit a new family in their home once a week. When they appear to be managing resources better, the aide may visit them less often, with the goal of "graduating" them. The aim of the program is not to foster dependence upon the aide, but to teach meal preparers the skills that allow them to function independently and meet their family's nutritional needs.

Most of the education carried out through the EFNEP is on a one-to-one basis in the family's home. Homemakers most in need of food and nutrition education may not learn well in group situations or may find it difficult to attend classes or meetings. The aide teaches through practical experiences such as helping the homemaker cook a meal or accompanying her grocery shopping. In general, the aides present the nutrition education program to the homemaker; however, it may be directed to an adult male, a grandmother residing in the home, or teenage boys or girls. Several studies documenting the effectiveness of this program have been conducted. In general, the greatest improvement in dietary patterns and life-style is seen in the aides themselves. With families, the greatest improvement is seen after 12 to 18 months in the program. Many improvements in the life of the family have not been documented scientifically but are recorded in testimonials.

The EFNEP Youth Program. Extension home economists, 4-H agents, and program assistants work with EFNEP nutrition aides to get disadvantages youth involved and interested in nutrition. The program, coordinated with state 4-H plans, provides programs such as "Mulligan Stew," nutrition puppets, and nutrition projects in and after school. Aides often follow up the school contact with home visits. Summer camps are also a part of many programs. One goal of the EFNEP Youth Program is to move young people into 4-H programs.

Role of the Community Food and Nutrition Professional. Professional food and nutrition workers do not, in general, work directly with the families participating in the EFNEP. Rather, their role is to train nutrition aides in basic nutrition and in methods of teaching poorly educated low-income families about food and nutrition. They must help the aides both to understand nutrition science and to translate that knowledge into activities and lessons for low-income rural and urban homemakers of various ethnic and racial backgrounds.

The professional may present special meetings for homemakers in the program or visit and counsel homemakers with special nutritional or dietary problems. The professional also may design, or assist the aides in producing, audio or visual instructional materials.

Youth Program, Including the 4-H Program

The Youth Program is designed to help young people gain competence in specific subjects while developing personal character and leadership. Most 4-H activities are centered in local clubs of youth 7 to 17 years old that are supervised by an adult volunteer leader trained by a county agent. The club members select projects written by federal or state professionals that focus on a specific subject such as home repairs, care of farm or domestic animals, clothing construction, or food and nutrition. The entire club may choose one project, devoting six to ten meetings to its completion. Individual projects may be completed at home, under the supervision of the club leader.

Projects in food and nutrition usually include both basic nutrition and practical cooking experience. Additional work that can be completed at home is often included to extend the practical aspect of learning. Typical food and nutrition projects might focus on eating breakfast, yeast bread preparation, or understanding international foods.

THE SPECIAL SUPPLEMENTAL FOOD PROGRAM FOR WOMEN, INFANTS AND CHILDREN (WIC)

The recognition that certain groups of Americans are nutritionally at risk at various times during their lives has supported the development of food and nutrition programs with well-defined audiences and goals. The Special Supplemental Food Program for Women, Infants and Children (WIC) is a nationwide program designed to provide supplemental food as a health service to low-income, high-risk pregnant and lactating women and to infants and children under the age of 5 years. It is expected that the supplemental food will contribute to a more favorable outcome of pregnancy and to improved health status for all participants.

The WIC Program was mandated by the Child Nutrition Act of 1966 and is funded through the United States Department of Agriculture. The funds to support the program are channeled through state health departments or other comparable state agencies which in turn award grants to local agencies such as county health departments. The local agencies then administer the WIC Program. While the actual descriptions of local WIC programs vary widely, all local programs are required to follow the federal guidelines for eligibility and benefits. WIC legislation is under consideration in 1978, and many of the provisions may be changed. The following paragraphs describe the program as it existed prior to September 1978.

To qualify for WIC supplemental foods a pregnant or lactating woman, a woman up to 6 months after giving birth to a child, or a child under 5 years old must also be eligible to receive free or reduced-price medical care and be medically or nutritionally at risk. The idea of risk is central to the WIC Program's philosophy: the foods provided are considered a form of medical treatment rather than an income benefit. Therefore, receiving food through the WIC Program does not affect a recipient's benefits under other social service programs such as the Food Stamp Program.

A participant can be classed as "at risk" for many specific reasons, including anemia, complications at birth, unacceptable weight gain in pregnancy, slow growth rate, food allergies, congenital defects, chronic infant or childhood diseases, or an inadequate diet as measured by a 24-hour food recall. Clients must be referred to the WIC Program by a physician, a nurse, a dietitian, or some other health professional.

The original legislation mandating the WIC Program did not mandate nutrition education as a component of the program. More recent legislation has made nutrition education a mandatory part of all WIC programs. Nutrition education is to be available to all participants and to all parents and guardians of children participating in the program.

Since the WIC Program provides specific foods, initial nutrition education efforts have focused on the value and use of those foods. The foods provided for pregnant and lactating women and for children 1 to 5 years old are the same and include whole milk, canned or forzen citrus juice, iron-fortified cereal, and eggs. Infants receive iron-fortified formula, infant juice, and dry infant cereal. At 6 months of age the infant package can be changed to include half iron-fortified formula and half whole milk. The Food and Nutrition Service is responsible for the food-packaging requirement and can be contacted for those regulations.

Public Law 93-150, which amended section 17 of the Child Nutrition Act authorizing the WIC Program, expired 30 June 1975. Interim proposals and regulations existed until legislation was enacted making $680 million available for the WIC Program for 27 months, ending in September 1978. Since the new legislation requires nutrition education, agencies in each state responsible for administering the WIC Program may develop goals and objectives for nutrition education. In general, long-term goals for the nutrition education of WIC participants might include (1) making them aware that a wide variety of food is necessary for good health and that the food they eat influences their health and (2) teaching them ways to use fruits, vegetables, and WIC foods to their best advantage. Nutrition education could be presented to groups of participants by a professional or paraprofessional, and individual nutrition counseling might be provided for participants needing special advice.

Role of the Community Food and Nutrition Professional

The role of the community food and nutrition worker depends in part on the availability of other professionals to help deliver nutrition education. In the past, case loads have been large and professional food and nutrition staff too small to provide more than stopgap nutrition education. If the community food and nutrition professional is solely responsible for the nutrition education component of the program, one-to-one counseling will be limited and group food demonstrations and lectures will be routine. The professional might also be responsible for developing local nutrition education goals, objectives, and evaluation schemes as well as handouts, booklets, shopping hints, recipes, and displays. Another function of the community food and nutrition professional is to help certify WIC participants by taking dietary recalls from clients and making anthropometric measurements.

In some cases the professional may train paraprofessional aides to provide general nutrition education to participants and their families, thus leaving the professional more time for intensive nutrition counseling with clients. If paraprofessionals are employed, the professional has the ongoing job of training, supervising, and evaluating them.

PRESCRIPTION COMMODITY FOOD PROGRAMS – FOCUS:HOPE

For several years the number of commodity food distribution programs has been declining. In 1976 there were fewer than twenty such programs in the United States. The largest is the Food Prescription Program, administered by Focus:Hope in Detroit, Michigan. It is a commodity food program designed to meet the needs of a population nutritionally at risk. Focus:Hope, an organization formed by community leaders following the 1967 Detroit riots, has attempted to better black-white relationships in that city. In 1970 it assumed responsibility for providing Department of Agriculture commodity foods to women during pregnancy and for 1 year after childbirth and to children until their sixth birthday if they are nutritionally at risk because of inadequate nutrition and income.

In many respects the Food Prescription Program is similar to the WIC Program. A physician, nurse, nutritionist, dietitian, or other health professional must certify that the woman or child is nutritionally at risk. Anyone participating in maternal and child health programs, public assistance programs, or the Food Stamp Program or receiving substantially free medical care at a health clinic automatically meets the income limitation. Other potential participants can declare that they are unable to afford private medical care. Only in cases of questionable representation is an evaluation of income and resources required. Participants must be recertified every 6 months. Women or children who receive food supplements through the WIC Program are not eligible for Focus:Hope food supplements. In a recent survey of participants of the Focus:Hope program, it was found that commodities acquired through the program were being eaten by all members of the family, not just those eligible for the program (Kass 1977).

The foods provided by the Department of Agriculture for this program have been selected to offset the health hazards of chronic hunger. Unlike some commodity food programs, Focus:Hope has a guaranteed supply of specific commodities, including canned meats, vegetables and fruit juices, instant nonfat dry milk, cereal, egg mix, evaporated milk, corn syrup, instant mashed potatoes, and peanut butter. Participants come to the warehouse, where they proceed as if in a grocery store, selecting from the shelves the food items in quantities they are alotted. Transportation by volunteers is provided as a support service.

The staff and advocates for Focus:Hope believe that the Food Stamp Program does not extend a household's food-buying power enough to provide a high-quality diet for mothers, infants, and young children. The Food Prescription Program functions like the WIC Program to provide food as a medical supplement rather than an income supplement, but it provides a wider variety of foods than the WIC Program and children can receive supplements for a longer period of time.

Funding for the program operation has come from the Office of Economic Opportunity. Several staff members are paid, but the program is largely dependent on volunteer staff. Volunteer workers distribute recipes which use foods available through Focus:Hope, and they also demonstrate the use of foods. This constitutes the only nutrition education provided directly to participants, though they can also receive nutrition education at the health centers where they are certified for the program or by participating in the EFNEP.

Role of the Community Food and Nutrition Professional

Although most community food and nutrition professionals are involved in nutrition counseling or other forms of nutrition education, it is not unreasonable to expect that some would become advocates for or administrators of commodity food distribution programs. If a commodity food program meets the needs of some segments of the community, the professional might work to maintain or expand the program's services by contacting appropriate government officials, testifying at public hearings, or arranging for positive media coverage. In a more traditional mode, the community food and nutritional professional may develop low-cost recipes incorporating commodity foods, experiment with simple preparation methods that would make some commodities more palatable and therefore more acceptable, provide nutrition education, as feasible, in a grocery-store atmosphere, and encourage nutrition education at the city and county clinics where the program participants get their health care.

NUTRITION REHABILITATION OR MOTHERCRAFT CENTERS

Although the focus of this book is the food behavior of Americans and community nutritional problems and programs in the United States, it is useful, in a discussion of mothers and children, to look at the nutrition rehabilitation centers or mothercraft centers found in communities throughout the developing and undeveloped world. At these centers malnourished children receive nutritional care and their mothers are given nutrition education. The idea of educating the mother to feed her children better at the same time that she is taking an active part in the rehabilitation of her malnourished child was proposed in the mid-1950s. Education, not rehabilitation, is the central goal of these centers, for only a change in the mother's child-rearing practices can bring long-term improvement in her child's nutritional status.

Since education is the most important facet of the work done at the centers, it is imperative that only methods available to the mother be used in rehabilitating her children. Thus, only locally available and inexpensive equipment, utensils, and food are used. The mother learns how to cure the child with food and how to use proper food to prevent the reoccurrence of malnutrition in the family. Nutrition rehabilitation centers will have little success if no economically and culturally feasible alternatives for feeding children exist. Therefore, these centers are a viable means of treating malnutrition only when the malnutrition results not from a lack of food supplies but rather from inadequate or incorrect child-feeding practices.

While rehabilitation centers vary in their method of operation (some are attached to a health center or hospital and others are not), a typical center might admit twenty-four to forty 1- to 4-year-old children at a time. It would be open 6 days a week, with the children arriving before breakfast and leaving after the evening meal. About six mothers would attend on a given day to assist the coordinator of the center with food preparation and child care and to receive nutrition education. The center coordinator would usually be a paraprofessional woman having a cultural background similar to that of the population being served and a high-school-level education with additional training in nutrition. She might have served an apprenticeship under an experienced paraprofessional at another center before taking charge of a center herself. Professional medical and nutritional staff would make periodic visits for supervision.

Role of the Community Food and Nutrition Professional

For the most part, paraprofessionals who receive training from the professional community food and nutrition worker prove to be effective rehabilitation center workers. The task of the professional is to determine whether there are malnourished children and if the food supply is sufficient, to establish a rehabilitation center. The professional might measure the food and nutrition knowledge of mothers to determine whether a rehabilitation center would be useful. If the need for a center is documented the professional might then design, implement, and evaluate the program. The task of finding the community resources to support the center, as well as training and supervising the paraprofessional, may fall to the community food and nutrition professional.

HEAD START PROGRAM

The care and feeding of children is an important function of any society. While acute malnutrition is rarely diagnosed in the United States, the care and feeding of American children is of concern to food and nutrition professionals, legislators, and the public at large, as witnessed by a variety of programs including Head Start and its food component, school breakfasts and lunches, and summer feeding programs.

The principal objective of the Head Start Program is to allow children of low-income families the opportunity to develop a greater degree of social competence. The children's nutritional needs, as well as other factors that allow them to interact effectively in society and with the environment, are recognized in the Head Start goals. The Office of Child Development funds the Head Start Program and issues performance standards to which all local Head Start programs must conform. Standards have been issued for education, health, dental health, nutrition, social services, and parent involvement. For the health performance standards, growth assessment (including head circumference measurements of children under 2 years old, height, weight, and age) must be completed. A hemoglobin or hematocrit determination for screening for anemia is also required.

As a part of the nutrition performance standards, parents are to be interviewed early in the year about family eating habits and any special dietary needs and feeding problems of the child. In general, the nutritional status of the family, the child, and the community is to be assessed. The rest of the nutrition performance objectives are specific to nutrition education and the provision of food to supplement what the child eats at home.

Children in part-day programs are allowed to receive food that will provide one-third of the Recommended Dietary Allowances. Children enrolled in full-day programs receive food providing one-half to two-thirds of Recommended Dietary Allowances. Guidelines and standards for the kinds of foods, the meal patterns, and the quantities of foods are given.

Standards that take into account the eating environment (length of eating periods, ventilation, lighting, utensils, furnishings) are promoted. Attention is also given to the social function of food. Staff are encouraged to include a variety of foods in the meals to meet cultural and ethnic needs, and they try to involve the children in preparing and serving meals and cleaning up afterwards. They are told not to use food as a punishment or a reward and not to force the children to eat every food that is served.

The Head Start Program is to include a plan for the nutrition education of staff, parents, and children. Food and meal periods are to be planned and used as an integral part of the educational program, which will focus on the selection and preparation of foods that meet the family's nutritional requirements and are within their budget. In addition, the program is to assist families that qualify for other food programs (for example, the Food Stamp Program, the WIC Program, and reduced-price school meals) to obtain their benefits.

Role of the Community Food and Nutrition Professional

Food and nutrition professionals who spend a suggested minimum of 8 hours per month per Head Start center are charged with many duties. These include the development, implementation, and supervision of a feeding program and the assessment of the community's and the children's needs, followed by the development, implementation, and supervision of nutrition education and counseling.

SCHOOL LUNCH AND BREAKFAST AND SUMMER FEEDING PROGRAMS

As children spend more time outside of the home at a younger age, the provision of nutritious meals in a variety of day-care centers is of concern to nutrition professionals and child development experts. In 1976 Public Law 94-105 expanded child-care food programs so that children cared for in tax-exampt facilities or in facilities sponsored by a tax-exempt organization could receive food supported in part by funds from the Department of Agriculture. Community food and nutrition professionals need to be aware of the changes that occur in programs available for feeding the pre-school child. Reimbursement for feeding children can be obtained by licensed day-care centers, nursery schools, and day-care homes.

Milk and lunch programs have been provided for school-age children for many years, and recently school breakfasts and summer feeding programs have been implemented. A discussion of these programs as they operated in 1977 follows. The Child Nutrition Act of 1978 may make some changes in the programs.

The National School Lunch Program

The earliest reported organized school lunch program was a free lunch program for poor children in New York vocational schools operated by the Children's Aid Society. Since that time many communities have sponsored lunch programs. During the 1930s, the federal government initiated a program assistance to schools for their lunch programs in the form of agricultural produce that could not be sold elsewhere.

The National School Lunch Act of 1946 established food service in the schools. Stated objectives of the school lunch program included safeguarding the health of American children and encouraging the consumption of nutritious agricultural commodities. The act provided for Department of Agriculture commodity foods to be distributed to schools participating in the program. Federal legislation required that lunches supported by federal funds or commodities (called type A lunches) meet specific nutritional requirements. Type A lunches must contain 2 ounces of meat, poultry, fish, or cheese or one egg of 1/2 cup of cooked dry beans or peas or 1/4 cup of peanut butter or a combination of the foregoing; a 3/4-cup serving of two or more fruits, vegetables, or both; one slice of bread or the equivalent of a whole or enriched grain product; 1 teaspoon of butter or fortified margarine and 1/2 pint of milk.

The Child Nutrition Act of 1966 broadened the scope of the school feeding program. It required that free or reduced-price meals for poor children be made available in every school lunch program. Schools receive an additional payment from the Department of Agriculture for each free or reduced-price meal served. Supplying a nutritionally sound lunch that provides one-third of the child's Recommended Dietary Allowance has been a basic philosophy of the program. Although nutrition education has not been a mandatory component of the program. lunches can reinforce food and nutrition information. In November 1977 Public Law 95-166 authorized the secretary of agriculture to formulate and carry out a nutrition information and education program in the schools. The program will give children better opportunities to learn about food and nutrition and the relationship of nutrition to health, and it will give them a chance to use their knowledge to develop food and nutrition attitudes and practices that will be fundamental to their health and well-being throughout life. The program will tie the school cafeteria to the classroom. (At this writing only interim regulations have been announced.)

Criticism of school lunch programs has come from many quarters. Wastefulness, restriction of freedom of choice, inability to meet personal and ethnic food preferences, and mandatory provision of milk despite evidence that many children are lactase deficient or lactose intolerant are some of the faults that have been pointed out. In response to some of the criticism, Public Law 94-105 mandated that, by fall of 1976, secondary schools would have to allow children to choose no less than three but no more than five of the foods offered. With children free to select three, four, or five of the type A lunch foods rather than being served the entire type A lunch, nutrition education, especially concerning fruits and vegetables, seems imperative.

It is important to remember that school lunch is not served in all public schools in the United States. Assistance is available, but local school districts must choose to participate in the program. Specific information about the school lunch program can be obtained from the food and nutrition division or child nutrition unit of each state's department of education.

The National School Breakfast Program

In response to data indicating that only one in five children were eating an adequate breakfast before coming to school and that quality of breakfast and attention span might be linked, the Child Nutrition Act of 1966 authorized the National School Breakfast Program. Public Law 94-105, enacted in the fall of 1975, authorized the program as a permanent federal program and expanded it to all schools having children that need better nutrition. The program is operated by the Child Nutrition Division Service of the Department of Agriculture. Local districts wishing to participate must submit an application to the food-service division of their state's educational agency. Any participating school district will receive the funds necessary to operate the program.

The program provides children with free, reduced-price, or full-price hot or cold breakfasts. A breakfast must meet the following minimum requirements: 1/2 pint of fluid whole milk; 1/2 cup of fruit or 1/2 cup of full-strength fruit or vegetable juice; one slice of whole grain or enriched bread (or an equivalent serving of corn bread, biscuits, rolls, or muffins) or 3/4 cup of cereal, pancakes, or waffles; and protein-rich foods such as eggs, meat, poultry, fish, cheese, and peanut butter as often as possible.

School breakfast programs are not widespread. School officials have objected to breakfast programs for many reasons, including lack of desire to operate a new program, fear that the program will cost more than the reimbursement allowed, fear that expensive equipment will be needed, belief that breakfast belongs in the home with the family, bussing problems, and belief that schools are for educating children, not feeding them. Community food and nutrition professionals have been working to alleviate school officials' concerns about the program. The Child Nutrition Act of 1978 is expected to increase the availability of school breakfasts.

The Summer Food Program

The increasing employment of women and the continuing rise of food prices has created in some communities a need for child feeding programs outside of school. The Special Food Services Program for Children (known as the summer food program) was authorized by the National School Lunch Act of 1966 as amended in 1968 by

Public Law 90-302. For some time the summer food program for each state carried a ceiling for participation. Public Law 94-105 removed that ceiling and made funds for meals open-ended so that all eligible children could participate and the sponsor receive reimbursement.

All meals in the summer food program must be served free. Children eligible for the meals are the same children who qualify for free or reduced-price school lunches. Sponsors of the program provide food for the children when they are out of school, usually May through October, and are reimbursed for the meals served and for administrative costs. Because school districts have the facilities, they are encouraged, as are summer camps for the needy and other local groups, to sponsor summer feeding programs. In 1976 many groups abused the summer food program, and it is now monitored more closely in order to reduce fraud.

Role of the Community Food and Nutrition Professional

School breakfasts, lunches, and summer feeding programs not only provide meals for children but also influence the development of children's food behavior. Therefore, community food and nutrition professionals should have up-to-date information on the availability of these programs and on their qualification requirements. They should seek to improve the quality of food and education offered by the programs at both the state and the local level, and they should encourage and support such programs in their communities.

The professional whose work is directly related to these programs may become involved in preparing and submitting applications for the programs, implementing approved programs, and designing and carrying out nutrition education for the programs. In some communities, food and nutrition professionals have helped parents force reluctant school administrators to implement feeding programs and even to include nutrition education.

CENTERS FOR DRUG REHABILITATION OR EDUCATION

The programs of the Cooperative Extension Service and the schools have been the traditional means of supplying nutritional services and education to American children, adolescents, and young adults. However, there are other ways to reach those who need information about nutrition. Nutrition counseling in drug rehabilitation or education centers is one example of an alternative program.

Centers for drug rehabilitation or education are usually alternative mental and physical health centers. They often provide a wide range of free services to their clients, including crisis intervention, counseling for problem pregnancies and family and legal problems, and referral to other agencies and medical clinics. The clients of most drug education centers are adolescents and young adults. Funding comes from a variety of sources — local health departments, federal grants, and private funds. Many centers depended on donated funds and volunteer workers to begin with, and some continue to rely heavily on volunteers.

Nutrition education or counseling services have been provided at several centers as part of their medical clinics. The persons served by the centers are considered to have attitudes that would cause them to reject traditional sources of advice on health and nutrition. They might also be experimenting with unconventional food patterns and would therefore be an important target for nutrition counseling and education.

The nutritional goals of a drug rehabilitation or education center might be to assist clients with nutrition-related medical problems and to increase their awareness of their own nutritional needs. To meet these goals, the center would provide clients with a variety of opportunities for informal nutrition education. Group or one-to-one discussions of questions raised by clients in rap sessions might include such subjects as balancing vegetarian diets, good food sources of specific nutrients, or the relationship of nutrition to medical problems. Individual diet evaluations might be provided also. Nutrition education materials such as books, pamphlets, and handouts designed especially for alternative education would be accessible to clients in waiting rooms and lounges.

If clients are to make maximum use of the nutritional services available at these centers, they must be made aware of the services offered. Nurses, physicians, and counselors must be kept aware of the importance of nutrition and should be encouraged to refer patients to nutrition professionals.

Role of the Community Food and Nutrition Professional

Many drug education or rehabilitation centers still have no nutritional services for their clients but would be happy to add them if the energy and know-how of a food and nutrition professional were available. Professionals can assess the need for nutrition education in the alternative health care facilities in their communities, and if a need exists, they can design and implement programs, search for volunteers and funding, and develop educational materials that would appeal to the clients.

NUTRITION PROGRAMS FOR THE ELDERLY

Physicians and nutritionists, along with other health professionals, recognize that elderly citizens are a group nutritionally at risk. A government food program for senior citizens that includes a nutrition education component has been one answer to the problems of the elderly. Other assistance comes from community groups that deliver meals to the homebound.

Title VII Nutrition Program

A food and nutrition program for the elderly was mandated by the Older American Act of 1965. In March 1972 the National Nutrition Program for the Elderly was added as Title VII of that act. Title VII authorized funds to provide senior citizens with low-cost hot meals that would meet one-third of their Recommended Dietary Allowance. Since the philosophy of the program is to provide not only nutritious food but an opportunity for socialization as well, most meals are served in a group setting. Supportive services also were mandated. They include nutrition education, transportation, counseling, referrals to other agencies, and recreation and shopping assistance. Funding for these services is included in the provisions of Title VII, but the specific services for which the money is spent are determined at the state and local levels. Although the program is directed to low-income senior citizens, income means tests are not used to determine eligibility. Participants must be at least 60 years old or have a spouse over 60. The meals are free, but donations are accepted and in some cases encouraged.

Meals provided through the program must include a meat or meat substitute, milk, two servings of fruit and/or vegetables, bread and butter, and a dessert. In many programs money for coffee and tea is donated by participants. The meals are cooked at the serving site or catered and delivered by schools or commercial firms. Schools, churches, and senior citizen centers are the type of neighborhood centers where the meals are served.

The Older American Act also provided for the creation of state agencies to assist the elderly, and it is through those agencies that the programs are administered at the state level. Local groups apply for grants to administer the local programs. Community action programs, councils on aging, and human service agencies typically operate the local programs. Some local programs employ a community food and nutrition professional in a full-time, part-time, or consultant capacity to help make decisions about food service and to provide the mandatory nutrition education. Others use home economists from the Cooperative Extension Service, volunteer nutritionists or dietitians, or nutrition students to provide the nutrition education for the program.

Since the social component of the program may be as important as the food, outreach efforts are directed at elderly persons who are isolated and alienated. Yet, no matter what efforts are made, some who need the meals may be physically unable to come to the serving site. Regulations provide for a percentage of the meals to be delivered to people at home. The state agency on aging should be consulted for current regulations.

Home-delivered Meal Programs

Various community groups such as dietetic groups, hospitals, and church groups operate home-delivered meal programs. The programs are designed to meet the nutritional needs of elderly persons who experience physiological, social, and economic changes in their lives that may lead to undernutrition and who are generally homebound. Home-delivered meal programs provide nutritionally adequate, well-balanced, medically appropriate meals for those who cannot provide them for themselves. Such programs are an attempt to prevent further physical and psychological deterioration while allowing the person to continue living independently. Most home-delivered meal programs (other than those allowed under Title VII) are dependent on a variety of private and public monies and volunteer efforts.

Role of the Community Food and Nutrition Professional

As with all programs that require a community to make application, the professional may assess the need for senior nutrition programs, solicit support, and submit applications. The professional may then work to provide nutritious, safe, and acceptable meals for the program by planning menus and supervising food production and serving. If paraprofessionals are employed, the professional may be responsible for training and supervising the cooks, nutrition aides, and other workers. Devising and implementing a scheme to evaluate the effectiveness of both the food program and the nutrition education may be another job for the nutrition professional.

Nutrition education is a mandated component of the Title VII program but has been allocated little or no funding. Community food and nutrition professionals can encourage the appropriate agencies to give financial support to the nutrition education effort. Sometimes there is resistance from administrators who believe every available dollar should be spent for tangible goods such as food. The nutrition professional must be prepared with arguments to counter this attitude and must develop innovative methods for teaching appropriate food and nutrition information to the elderly.

PRIVATE OR NONPROFIT AGENCIES

The preceding discussion has focused on agencies and programs that are largely supported by public funding and that have regulations created through legislation. Communities are also served by many other food and nutrition programs and agencies that get little or no assistance from the government. Nonprofit organizations like the American Red Cross, the Visiting Nurses Association, the American Heart Association, the American Diabetes Association, and the Girl Scouts and Boy Scouts of

America may provide food and nutrition education and services. In some communities religious-affiliated groups such as the Salvation Army, the Saint Vincent de Paul Poor Society, and Bread for the World provide food relief and/or nutrition information. Industry, too, supports independent groups that provide food and nutrition information to the public. Some of these groups are the National Dairy Council, the Kansas Wheat Commission, the Cereal Institute, the Michigan Apple Commission, the Grocery Manufacturers of America, the National Lifestock and Meat Board, the Potato Board, the California Avocado Advisory Board, the American Lamb Council, and the Poultry and Egg National Board. The following discussion of the Visiting Nurses Association, Bread for the World, and the National Dairy Council presents examples of these groups.

The Visiting Nurses Association (VNA)

The VNA provides a variety of health services, primarily in the home, to mothers, children, young adults, and the elderly. Services such as nursing; nutrition counseling; homemaking guidance; and physical, occupational, and speech therapy are performed by health professionals in the homes of the sick and disabled. The association is accredited by the National League for Nursing and the American Public Health Association and approved by the National Council for Homemaker-Home Health Aid Service.

In many areas the staff, with the nutritionist's guidance, instruct and aid patients with both normal and modified diets. Specialized assistance is given by the nutrition consultant, who also keeps staff members informed of new developments and research in the nutrition field. In some localities, the VNA offers maternal and child health services, at clinics as well as in the home, to mothers and infants with serious health problems. Expectant and new mothers can receive instruction and aid in self-care and child care from various health professionals, including nutritionists. The VNA also supports Mom and Tot centers, community-oriented multiservice centers that may include day care, maternity clinics, planned parenthood clinics, pediatric clinics, screening clinics, club activities, and general assistance with health and social needs. One goal of VNA professionals is to help the elderly maintain their personal independence for as long as possible. The VNA provides professional and volunteer staff to help senior citizens obtain the health and social services necessary for remaining independent.

Anyone living in the VNA service area who needs health services at home and receives medical care from a physician associated with the VNA is eligible. Physicians, hospitals, patients themselves, families and friends of patients, or community agencies may request services for the patient. The patient can use Medicare, Medicaid, hospital insurance, and prepaid health plans to cover the cost of the services. Charges for services to patients without coverage can be reduced or cancelled, depending upon the family's financial position. The VNA is a nonprofit organization and therefore charges for its services are based upon the actual cost to the agency.

Bread for the World

The present concern for feeding the people of the world and protecting the environment has resulted in the formation of a variety of antihunger groups. In general, they seek to educate the American public about food and nutrition problems in the world. Some groups aid food relief efforts by collecting funds to send to areas where crops fail or natural disasters decimate the food supply.

The Bread for the World organization is a Christian citizen's movement against hunger and poverty. It is not a relief effort. Instead, Bread for the World urges citizens to tell legislators their views about United States policies and laws that affect hungry people in this country and elsewhere in the world. It encourages the formation of discussion groups that link concern for the poor and hungry with the Christian gospel. The issues discussed bear on hunger and poverty, assistance to poor countries, military spending, and international trade and investment. Bread for the World also publishes a monthly newsletter to inform members of current issues and to increase their impact on legislation by coordinating their efforts. Information on pending legislation and current issues and the names and addresses of key congressmen and congresswomen are provided. In addition to working to influence legislation, Bread for the World encourages its members to conserve the world's resources by eating lower on the food chain and decreasing their personal consumption of meat. A pamphlet containing a nutritionist's view on combining plant proteins to complement each other has been widely distributed in churches.

The National Dairy Council

The National Dairy Council is a nonprofit organization that promotes nutrition education based on the Basic Four. It was organized in 1925 by the dairy industry with the aim of promoting the achievement of optimal health. The Dairy Council acts as a resource center for reliable nutrition information. Dietitians, nutritionists, dental and medical professionals, teachers, and home economists all benefit from action-oriented workshops and lectures presented by community food and nutrition professionals employed by the National Dairy Council. Dairy Council professionals also present information for consumer and youth group leaders, senior citizens, and radio and television audiences. The Dairy Council makes available to educators and health professionals a variety of educational materials created by nutrition specialists. The booklets, posters, comparison cards, and other materials are available free or for a small charge.

REFERENCES

General

Guide to American Food Programs. 1977. San Francisco: California Rural Legal Assistance, Food Law Center. (115 Sansome Street, Suite 900, San Francisco, CA 94104)

The Food Stamp Program

Anonymous. 1967. Consumer food economics — A D.C. course on getting the most from food stamps. *Agricultural Marketing* 12 (6):4.

Consumer and Food Economics Institute. 1975. *The Thrifty Food Plan: Sample meals for a month.* Hyattsville, Md.: U.S. Department of Agriculture, Agricultural Research Service.

Federal Register 40 (231):55646, 1 December 1975. Rules and regulations — Thrifty Food Plan.

Federal Register 41 (40):8501, 27 February 1976. Proposed rules — Food Stamp Program.

Food and Nutrition Service. 1970. *Food stamps make the difference.* Washington, D.C.: U.S. Department of Agriculture.

Food and Nutrition Service. 1971. *Food stamps for you.* FNS-67, USDA. Washington, D.C.: Government Printng Office.

Food and Nutrition Service. 1975a. *The Food Stamp Program.* Washington, D.C.: U.S. Department of Agriculture.

Food and Nutrition Service. 1975b. *Shopping with food stamps.* USDA Program Aid no. 1109, PA-1123. Washington, D.C.: U.S. Department of Agriculture.

Food Research and Action Center. 1974. *FRAC's guide to the Food Stamp Program.* Washington, D.C.: Food Research and Action Center.

Goodwin, M., and Cowell, C. 1975. Nutritionists debate USDA Thrifty Food Plan. *Community Nutrition Institute Reports* 5 (46):3.

Hiemstra, J. S. 1972. Evaluation of USDA food programs. *Journal of the American Dietetic Association* 60:193.

Rada, E. L. 1974. Medicating the Food Stamp Program. *American Journal of Public Health* 64:477.

The Cooperative Extension Service

Coffer, E. 1972. Interdependence of research, teaching and extension in home economics. *Journal of Home Economics* 64 (1):32.

Extension Committee on Organization and Policy. 1974. *Focus II: Extension Home Economics*. (14000-3140108-74-R5000-3140159-74). Washington, D.C.: U.S. Department of Agriculture. Cooperative Extension Service.

Extension Service. 1971. *Extension Home Economics helps today's families build better lives*. PA-981, USDA. Washington, D.C.: U.S. Department of Agriculture.

Kelsey, L. D., and Hearne, C. C. 1963. *Cooperative Extension work*. Ithaca, N.Y.: Comstock Publishing Associates.

Lang, C. L. 1975. A historical review of the forces that contributed to the formation of the Cooperative Extension Service. Ed. D. thesis, Michigan State University (East Lansing).

Marion, B. W.; Simonds, L. A.; and Moore, D. E. 1969. *Food marketing in low-income area*. Columbus: Ohio State University, Cooperative Extension Service.

Paulsen, B. 1976. Results of a behavioral weight loss program with extension home economists as therapists. Presented at the 9th annual meeting of the Society for Nutrition Education, Kansas City, Mo.

Sanders, H. C., ed. 1966. *The Cooperative Extension Service*. Englewood Cliffs, N.J.: Prentice Hall.

Ugelow, E. I. 1965. Mobilizing the potential of home economics for low-income families. *Journal of Home Economics* 57:648.

Uhl, J. N., and Armstrong, J. 1971. Adult consumer education programs in the United States. *Journal of Home Economics* 63:591.

Ullrich, H. D., and Briggs, G. M. 1973. The general public. In *U.S. nutrition policies in the seventies*, ed. J. Mayer, pp. 175-187. San Francisco: W. H. Freeman.

U.S., Sixtieth Congress, first session, 1908. S-3392: Bill to Provide for the Advancement of Instruction in Agriculture, Manual Training and Home Economics, in the State Normal Schools of the United States.

Wang, V. L. 1971. Food information of homemakers and 4-H youth. *Journal of American Dietetic Association* 58:215.

The Expanded Food and Nutrition Education Program

Agricultural Economic Research Service. 1972. *Impact of the Expanded Nutrition Education Program on low-income families: An indepth analysis*. Agricultural Economics Report no. 220. Washington, D.C.: U.S. Department of Agriculture.

Agricultural Economic Research Service. 1973. *Families in the Expanded Food and Nutrition Education Program: Comparison of Food Stamp and Food Distribution Program participants and non-participants*. Agricultural Economics Report no. 246. Washington, D.C.: U.S. Department of Agriculture.

Anonymous. 1971. Nonprofessionals teach nutrition to low-income families in Maryland. *Appalachia* 4 (4):28.

Chase, H. P.; Larson, L. B.; Massoth, D. M.; Martin, D. L.; and Niernberg, M. 1973. Effectiveness of nutrition aides in a migrant population. *American Journal of Clinical Nutrition* 26:849.

Cook, F. 1969. Nutrition education via people to people. *Journal of Nutrition Education* 1 (2):9.

Eberhardt, L. W.; Jones, M.; Boyd, N. C.; and Harris, R. C. 1970. The Expanded Nutrition Program in Georgia. In *The food problem in Georgia*, ed. G. G. Dull, pp. 28-44. Report no. 2 of the Interdepartmental Institutional Committee on Nutrition, USDA-ARS. Athens, Ga.: Richard B. Russell Agricultural Research Center.

Frye, R. E. 1971. The Expanded Food and Nutrition Education Program. *Family Economics Review* 62-5 (March):30. (Agricultural Research Service)

Goldsmith, G. 1973. Professionals and paraprofessionals. In *U.S. nutrition policies in the seventies*, ed. J. Mayer, pp. 193-202. San Francisco: W. H. Freeman.

Green, L. W.; Li Wang, V.; and Ephross, P. H. 1974. A three-year, longitudinal study of the impact of nutrition aides on the knowledge, attitudes, and practices of rural poor homemakers. *American Journal of Public Health* 64:722.

Ikeda, J. 1975. Expressed nutrition information needs of low-income homemakers. *Journal of Nutrition Education* 7:104.

Jones, E. 1970. Program evaluation as an operational tool. *Journal of Nutrition Education* 2:19.

Miller, B. K. 1972. *Perceptions by aides, supervising aides and agents of the functions and training of an Extension aide in Michigan.* East Lansing: Michigan State University, Expanded Nutrition and Family Program.

Napier, T. L., and Wharton, C. 1974. *The Expanded Food and Nutrition Program: An experiment in behavior change.* Research Bulletin no. 1070. Columbus, Ohio: Agricultural Research and Development Center.

Prichard, K., and Hall, M. R. 1971. Attitudes of aides and clients in the Expanded Nutrition Program. *Journal of Home Economics* 63:545.

Schild, D. T. 1970. A converted bus takes EFNEP to the people. *Journal of Nutrition Education* 1 (3):22.

Wang, V. L., and Ephross, P. H. 1970a. EFNEP evaluated. *Journal of Nutrition Education* 2:148.

Wang, V. L., and Ephross, P. H. 1970b. *Poor but not forgotten.* Monograph 1. College Park: University of Maryland, Cooperative Extension Service.

The Special Supplemental Food Program for Women, Infants and Children

Bendick, M.; Campbell, T. H.; Bawden, D. L.; and Jones, M. 1976. *Toward efficiency and effectiveness in the WIC delivery system.* Washington, D. C.: The Urban Institute, 2100 M Street NW.

Editors. 1974. Position paper on child nutrition programs. *Journal of the American Dietetic Association* 64:520.

Federal Register 39 (250):44728, 27 December 1974. Regulations — Special Supplemental Food Program for Women, Infants and Children.

Food and Nutrition Service. 1975. New legislation for child nutrition and WIC programs. *Newsletter of the Food and Nutrition Service,* 26 November 1975, no. 44, p. 1. (U.S. Department of Agriculture).

Gamon, E., and Classen, L. 1975. The Special Supplemental Food Program for Women, Infants and Children (WIC). Presented at the 8th annual meeting of the Society for Nutrition Education, 19-22 August 1975, San Diego.

Kass, E. 1977. Supplemental commodity food use by Focus:Hope participants. M.S. thesis, Michigan State University (East Lansing).

Rush, D. 1974. The prenatal project: The first 20 months of operation. *Current Concepts in Nutrition* 2:95.

Swallow, K. A.; Mussenden, L. W.; Robinson, V. A.; and Crocetti, A. F. 1971. Tools for evaluation of diets of pregnant women. *Journal of Nutrition Education* 3:34.

Wilson, A. M. 1974. A.D.A. speaks on W.I.C. *Journal of the American Dietetic Association* 64:292.

Nutrition Rehabilitation Centers

Anonymous. 1975. Nutrition rehabilitation units. *British Medical Journal* 11:246.

Beghin, I. D. 1970. Nutritional rehabilitation centers in Latin America: A critical assessment. *American Journal of Clinical Nutrition* 23:1412.

Beghin, I. D. 1976. Centers for combating childhood malnutrition. In *Nutrition in the community*, ed. D. S. McLaren, pp. 169-184. New York: Wiley.

Grenville, C. M. 1976. *The Focus:Hope Food Prescription Program 1971-1976: A report to the community services administration.* Detroit: Focus:Hope.

Jelliffe, D. B. 1973. Observations on the teaching of nutrition at maternal and child health centers in some tropical communities. *Journal of Tropical Pediatrics* 20:232.

King, K. W. 1975. Mothercraft preventive centers. *American Journal of Clinical Nutrition* 28:435.

Office of Nutrition. Undated. *Nutrition education in child feeding programs in the developing countries.* Washington, D.C.: U.S. Department of State, Agency for International Development, Technical Assistance Bureau.

Suter, C. B. 1971. Nutrition education for mothers of Filipino preschool children. *Journal of Nutrition Education* 3:66.

The Head Start Program

U.S. Department of Health, Education and Welfare. 1975. *Handbook for local Head Start nutrition specialist.* Washington, D.C.: Office of Human Development and Office of Child Development.

Zimmerman, R. R., and Munro, N. 1972. Changing Head Start mother's food attitudes and practices. *Journal of Nutrition Education* 4:66.

School Lunch and Breakfast and Summer Feeding Programs

Anonymous. 1974a. Nutrition education in action in San Diego's school system. *Food Service Marketing* 36 (8):54.

Anonymous. 1974b. Washington, D.C.: A hot school lunch for every student. *Cooking for Profit* 43 (283):24.

Food Research and Action Committee. 1975a. *FRAC's guide to the National School Breakfast Program.* Washington, D.C.: Food Research and Action Committee.

Food Research and Action Committee. 1975b. *FRAC's guide to the National School Lunch and Breakfast programs.* Washington, D.C.: Food Research and Action Committee.

Food Research and Action Committee. 1977. *Out to lunch: A study of USDA's day-care and summer feeding program.* Washington, D.C.: Food Research and Action Committee.

Hiemstra, S. J. 1972. Evaluation of USDA food programs. *Journal of the American Dietetic Association* 60:193.

Lieberman, H. M.; Hunt, I.; Coulson, A. H.; Clerk, V. A.; Swendseid, M. E.; and Ho, L. 1976. Evaluation of a ghetto school breakfast program. *Journal of the American Dietetic Association* 68:132.

Mirenda, R., and Brooks, A. 1973. International food festival — A community action program. *American Journal of Public Health* 63:40.

Montoya, B. 1974. California's nutrition education project tests ways to reach kids. *Food and Nutrition* 4 (4):6. (U.S. Department of Agriculture)

National Agricultural Library. 1975. Food service programs for children: An annotated bibliography. Library List no. 99. Betsville, Md.: National Agricultural Library.

Parry, S. P., and Downen, M. L. 1961. *The federal school lunch and special milk program in Tennessee with implications for the dairy industry.* Bulletin 326. Knoxville: University of Tennessee Agricultural Experiment Station.

Schuchat, M. G. 1973. The school lunch and its cultural environment. *Journal of Nutrition Education* 5:116.

U.S. Public Law 94-105, 7 October 1975.

Drug Rehabilitation or Education

Brown, J. 1973. Diet and the new drugs: Eating habits of some drug users. *Ecology of Food and Nutrition* 2:21.

Brunswick, A. F. 1969. Health needs of the adolescent: How the adolescent sees them. *American Journal of Public Health* 59:1730.

Charalampous, K. D. 1971. Drug culture in the seventies. *American Journal of Public Health* 61:1225.

Erhard, D. 1971. Nutrition education for the Now generation. *Journal of Nutrition Education* 2:135.

Frankle, R. T.; McGregor, B.; Wylie, Jr.; and McCann, M. 1973. Nutrition and lifestyle: The Door, a center of alternatives — The nutritionist in a free clinic for adolescents. *Journal of the American Dietetic Association* 63:269.

Johnson, C. M. 1973. Nutrition and contemporary communal living. *Journal of the American Dietetic Association* 63:275.

Leevy, C. M.; Tamburro, C.; and Smith, F. 1970. Alcoholism, drug addiction and nutrition. *Medical Clinics of North America* 54 (6):1567.

Neumann, A. K.; Neumann, C. G.; and Ifekwunigew, A. 1973. Evaluation of small-scale nutrition programs. *American Journal of Clinical Nutrition* 26:446.

Schatz, B., and Ebrahimi, F. 1972. Free clinic patient characteristics. *American Journal of Public Health* 62:1354.

Shimode, N. 1973. Observations of a nutritionist in a free clinic. *Journal of the American Dietetic Association* 63:273.

Washburn, A. B. 1974. Nutrition counseling for drug addicts in rehabilitation. *Journal of Nutrition Education* 6:13.

Nutrition Programs for the Elderly

Anonymous. 1974. Elderly feeding in schools. *School Foodservice Journal* 28 (10):20.

Buchholtz, F. 1971. *A home-delivered meals program for the elderly*, pp. 1-140. U.S. Department of Health, Education and Welfare, Administration on Aging. Washington, D.C.: Government Printing Office.

Cronan, M. L., and Jewell, M. E. 1971. Feeding the elderly: The baby of school lunch. *School Foodservice Journal* 25 (8):76.

Hudson, G. 1971. *A Co-op approach to food for the elderly*. U.S. Department of Health, Education and Welfare, Social Rehabilitation Service, Administration on Aging. Washington, D.C.: Government Printing Office.

Knauer, V. 1971. Portable meals contribute to nutrition education efforts. *Journal of Nutrition Education* 3:59.

Kohrs, M. B. 1976. *Influence of the Congregate Meal Program in central Missouri on dietary practices and nutritional status of participants.* Jefferson City, Mo.: Lincoln University, Human Nutrition Research Program.

Pelcovits, J. 1973. Nutrition education in group meals programs for the aged. *Journal of Nutrition Education* 5:118.

Rankine, D. C., and Taylor, B. 1975. Are community nutrition programs meeting the needs of the elderly? *Journal of Home Economics* 67 (6):37.

Watkin, D. M. 1975. Nutrition programs for older Americans. *Nutrition and the M.D.* 1 (10):1127.

Wells, C. 1973. Nutrition programs under the Older American Act. *American Journal of Clinical Nutrition* 26 (10):1127.

Wylie, C. M. 1975. The delivery of health care to the elderly. *Public Health Currents* 15 (5):1.

Bread for the World

Pamphlets, newsletters, and *An Alternate Diet* can be obtained from Bread for the World, 235 East 49th Street, New York, NY 10017.

Student Exercises

CHAPTER 1 Foodways, Food Behavior, and Culture

EXERCISE 1

Objectives

1. To become familiar with the influence of the subsystems within our culture on the foodways of people in the United States
2. To find examples of the role of food in our culture.

Behavioral Objectives

After finishing this exercise you should be able to:
1. Cite examples of the influence of technology on foodways and food behavior.
2. Cite examples of the interrelationships of the subsystems within our culture and foodways.

Directions

1. Obtain recent issues of *Food Product Development, Institutions, Food Technology,* and *Food Services Management* and find examples in each of the influence of technology on the availability, safety, nutritive quality, and acceptability of food in the United States. Discuss each example in relation to the effect on foodways.
2. In the magazine articles, find acknowledgment of the influence of the political, philosophical, economic, technological, and social systems and the social institution on food. Discuss.
3. Find examples in the articles of food fulfilling specific functions within our culture.

EXERCISE 2

Objectives

1. To become familiar with differences in the use of language or terminology to describe food.
2. To recognize that terminology is neither right nor wrong so long as communication is clear.
3. To recognize that one's own terminology is a product of one's past and present environment.

Behavioral Objectives

After finishing this exercise you should be able to:
1. List terms used by different groups for the same food.
2. Determine what a product may be called by different groups within the same geographic area and by groups in other geographic areas.

Directions

Check each term that is used in your home. (Several terms for the same food may be used in your own home.) List any additional terms that you use. Terminology may vary according to situation, region of the United States, and ethnic group.

Snap beans	Baked beans
Green beans	Pinto beans
Pole beans	Kidney beans
String beans	Navy beans
Bunch beans	Soup beans
Bush beans	White southern beans
Shelly beans	Shuckie beans
Cornfield beans	
White corn	Sweet corn
Hickory cane corn	Field corn
White pearl corn	Fried corn
Yellow corn	Hickory king corn
Greens	Poke
Turnip greens	Dandelion
Tender greens	Lamb's quarter
Mustard greens	Spinach
Collards	Mixed greens

Sweet Potatoes

Boiled	Candied
Fried	Pie
Baked	Yams

White Potatoes

Creamed	Home fries
Boiled	Stewed
French fried	New
Hash brown	Steak fries
Baked	American fries
Irish	Whole
Mashed	

English peas	Green peas
Black-eyed peas	Lady peas
Crowder peas	Field peas
Purple hull peas	Butter peas
Pinkeye peas	Yellow eye

The single word *peas* is sometimes used by families instead of the words listed here. Does your family ever use the single word *peas?* If so, which of the types of peas listed here would you call *peas?*

Check the terms you use or know to describe a carbonated beverage.

Terms I Use	*Terms I Know*
Soda pop	Soda pop
Dope	Dope
Pop	Pop
Sody	Sody
Tonic	Tonic
Coke	Coke
Cola	Cola
Cold drink	Cold drink
Soft drink	Soft drink

What term do you use for the noon meal? What term do you use for the evening meal? Do you know most of the terms listed here? Why? If you do not know most of them, why not? You will note that some of the terms apply to the food itself and some to the method of preparation. The method of preparation is sometimes used in talking about a food to narrow the definition.

EXERCISE 3

Objectives

1. To become familiar with ethnic differences.
2. To become familiar with educational programs that exist for specific ethnic groups.

Behavioral Objectives

After finishing this exercise you should be able to:
1. Define what is meant by the terms *ethnic* and *ethnic differences.*
2. Give an example of a nutrition education program for a specific ethnic group.
3. Illustrate, by an example, the process of acculturation.
4. List factors that influence the development of an educational program.
5. List criteria that could be used to evaluate the effectiveness of an educational program.
6. List at least one program in your community that addresses the problem of ethnic acculturation.

Directions

1. From a recent issue of the *Journal of Nutrition Education* select one article concerned with an educational program for an ethnic group. Find examples of acculturation, and discuss factors that influenced the development of the program. What criteria were used for evaluating the effectiveness of this program?
2. What programs in your community address themselves to the problems of ethnic acculturation?

CHAPTER 2   Food Classifications and People

EXERCISE 1

Objectives
1. To become familiar with local classifications of food and compare them with those given in chapter 2.
2. To become familiar with the function of food in the local culture.

Behavioral Objectives
After finishing this exercise you should be able to:
1. Cite examples of local classifications of foods and compare them with the classifications listed in chapter 2.
2. List some of the functions of food in local culture.

Directions
1. In a Sunday edition of a local newspaper find examples of food classified according to the food classifications described in chapter 2.
2. Find examples of functions of food in the local culture. Discuss.

CHAPTER 3   The Individual and Food Behavior

EXERCISE 1

Objectives

1. To illustrate the use of the semantic differential scale as a tool for measuring the connotative meanings of foods.
2. To ascertain the meanings you yourself associate with foods.

Behavioral Objectives

After finishing this exercise you should be able to:
1. Use the semantic differential scale to determine the connotative meaning of a food.
2. Determine the meanings you yourself associate with various foods.

Directions

On each of the following lists check the box for each food that indicates the degree to which you associate that food with one of the two descriptive terms given. Think of other foods that could be added to these lists.

Do you associate the foods in this list with old persons or young persons?

		Extremely	Moderately	Slightly	Both	Slightly	Moderately	Extremely		Neither	Do Not Know Food
Hot dogs	Young								Old		
Cottage cheese	Young								Old		
Watermelon	Young								Old		
Gelatin salad	Young								Old		
Milk	Young								Old		
Hot tea	Young								Old		
Pizza	Young								Old		
Apple sauce	Young								Old		
Spinach	Young								Old		
Soda pop	Young								Old		
Orange juice	Young								Old		
Country fried steak	Young								Old		
Corn bread	Young								Old		
Mashed potatoes	Young								Old		
Bananas	Young								Old		
Carrot and raisin salad	Young								Old		
Johnnie cakes	Young								Old		
Coffee	Young								Old		
French fried potatoes	Young								Old		
Green beans	Young								Old		
Hamburger	Young								Old		
Roast beef	Young								Old		
Broccoli	Young								Old		
Deer meat	Young								Old		
Cabbage slaw	Young								Old		
Peanut butter cookies	Young								Old		
Fresh peaches	Young								Old		

Do you associate these terms with sick persons or well persons?

		Extremely	Moderately	Slightly	Both	Slightly	Moderately	Extremely		Neither	Do Not Know Food
Hot dogs	Sick								Well		
Cottage cheese	Sick								Well		
Watermelon	Sick								Well		
Gelatin salad	Sick								Well		
Milk	Sick								Well		
Hot tea	Sick								Well		
Pizza	Sick								Well		
Apple sauce	Sick								Well		
Spinach	Sick								Well		
Soda pop	Sick								Well		
Orange juice	Sick								Well		
Country fried steak	Sick								Well		
Corn bread	Sick								Well		
Mashed potatoes	Sick								Well		
Bananas	Sick								Well		
Carrot and raisin salad	Sick								Well		
Johnnie cakes	Sick								Well		
Coffee	Sick								Well		
French fried potatoes	Sick								Well		
Green beans	Sick								Well		
Hamburger	Sick								Well		
Roast beef	Sick								Well		
Broccoli	Sick								Well		
Deer meat	Sick								Well		
Cabbage slaw	Sick								Well		
Peanut butter cookies	Sick								Well		
Fresh peaches	Sick								Well		

Do you associate the foods in this list with males or females?

		Extremely	Moderately	Slightly	Both	Slightly	Moderately	Extremely		Neither	Do Not Know Food
Hot dogs	Male								Female		
Cottage cheese	Male								Female		
Watermelon	Male								Female		
Gelatin salad	Male								Female		
Milk	Male								Female		
Hot tea	Male								Female		
Pizza	Male								Female		
Apple sauce	Male								Female		
Spinach	Male								Female		
Soda pop	Male								Female		
Orange juice	Male								Female		
Country fried steak	Male								Female		
Corn bread	Male								Female		
Mashed potatoes	Male								Female		
Bananas	Male								Female		
Carrot and raisin salad	Male								Female		
Johnnie cakes	Male								Female		
Coffee	Male								Female		
French fried potatoes	Male								Female		
Green beans	Male								Female		
Hamburger	Male								Female		
Roast beef	Male								Female		
Broccoli	Male								Female		
Deer meat	Male								Female		
Cabbage slaw	Male								Female		
Peanut butter cookies	Male								Female		
Fresh peaches	Male								Female		

Do you think of the foods in this list as slimming or fattening?

		Extremely	Moderately	Slightly	Both	Slightly	Moderately	Extremely		Neither	Do Not Know Food
Hot dogs	Slimming								Fattening		
Cottage cheese	Slimming								Fattening		
Watermelon	Slimming								Fattening		
Jell-O	Slimming								Fattening		
Whole milk	Slimming								Fattening		
Hot tea	Slimming								Fattening		
Pizza	Slimming								Fattening		
Apple sauce	Slimming								Fattening		
Spinach	Slimming								Fattening		
Soda pop	Slimming								Fattening		
Orange juice	Slimming								Fattening		
Steak	Slimming								Fattening		
Corn bread	Slimming								Fattening		
Mashed potatoes	Slimming								Fattening		
Bananas	Slimming								Fattening		
Carrot and raisin salad	Slimming								Fattening		
Grits	Slimming								Fattening		
Coffee	Slimming								Fattening		
French fried potatoes	Slimming								Fattening		
Green beans	Slimming								Fattening		
Hamburger	Slimming								Fattening		
Roast beef	Slimming								Fattening		
Broccoli	Slimming								Fattening		
Cabbage slaw	Slimming								Fattening		
Chocolate chip cookies	Slimming								Fattening		
Fresh peaches	Slimming								Fattening		
Rolls	Slimming								Fattening		

EXERCISE 2

Objectives

1. To become familiar with the components of flavor.
2. To learn a technique of identifying the components of a food's flavor.
3. To ascertain the factors affecting the acceptability of a food to an individual.

Behavioral Objectives

After finishing this exercise you should be able to:
1. List the components of flavor.
2. List the components of flavor in a specific food sample.
3. List factors other than perception of flavor that contribute to a person's preference for a food.

Directions

Your instructor will place before you a glass dish containing the juice of mixed fruits or mixed vegetables at room temperature. Complete the following procedure.
1. Lean toward the juice and smell it.
    a. What is your first impression of the odor?
    b. What is your second impression of the odor?
2. Move your nose back and forth over the juice. Think.
    a. What is your total impression of the odor?
    b. From the combination of odor and appearance, make a list of words you can think of to describe the following.
        (1) Texture (e.g., *thick*)
        (2) Feelings (e.g., *earthy, strong*)
        (3) Components of the food (e.g., *tomato juice*)
3. Lift the container and place some of the juice in your mouth. Roll the juice back and forth in your mouth. Think. Then list your reactions to each of the following in order of observation.
    a. Components of food
    b. Texture
    c. Feelings
4. Give your overall reaction to the food by describing its flavor and answering the following questions.
    a. At what time of day and for what occasions would this food be suitable?
    b. What type of person you would expect to enjoy this food (extrovert, introvert, masculine, feminine, old, young, sick, well, fat, thin, etc.)?
    c. Do you relate this food to any person or incident in your life? If so, how does this influence your acceptance of the food?
    d. Should this food be served hot or cold?

EXERCISE 3

Objectives

1. To illustrate individual taste differences in response to physical stimuli.

Behavioral Objectives

After finishing this exercise you should be able to:
1. Determine if a person is a taster or nontaster of the chemical phenlthiocarbamide.

2. Determine the percentage of the class that belongs to each category and compare this with known percentages for population groups.
3. Determine the percentage of the class who can identify the four basic tastes at the threshold level.

Directions*

1. From your instructor obtain litmus paper impregnated with the standard phenlthiocarbamide solution for testing of tasters. Record the number of tasters and nontasters in your class. Take enough litmus paper to test the members of your immediate family; record the results. What percentage of your class are tasters? Is there a pattern of tasters and nontasters in your family?
2. Prepare solutions in concentrations 5 percent lower than the established taste threshold levels, at the established levels, and 5 percent above the established levels for glucose, sodium chloride, citric acid, and caffeine or quinine. Administer the solutions to ten students, using established sensory procedures, and record their reactions. Compare your data with data collected by others in the class, and discuss taste threshold differences in the class as they relate to the development of individual food behavior.

EXERCISE 4

Objectives

1. To become familiar with the complexities of measuring food preferences.
2. To identify specific food preferences and patterns of preference.

Behavioral Objectives

After finishing this exercise you should be able to:
1. List factors that affect food preferences.
2. Cite difficulties in measuring preferences in the manner used for this exercise.

Directions

This is only one of many ways in which food preferences can be measured. If you could choose your food, how often would you choose this food when it is available? Check the appropriate box.

*The following articles may be useful for this exercise: "Getting Fullest Value from Sensory Testing: Part 1. Use and Misuse of Testing Methods" by N. L. Hirsch (1974) in *Food Product Development* 8 (10):33, and "Taste Sensitivity and Food Aversions of Teenagers" by S. C. Jefferson and A. M. Erdman (1970) in the *Journal of Home Economics* 62:605.

	Every Time	Most of the Time	Some of the Time	Seldom	Never	Have Never Tasted the Food	Do Not Know the Food
Hot dogs							
Apple sauce							
Orange juice							
Macaroni and cheese							
Butter beans							
Milk							
Cottage cheese							
Bananas							
Turkey							
Green beans							
Lettuce salad							
Black-eyed peas							
Poke salat							
Chili							
Rice							
Fresh peaches							
Cornflakes							
French fried potatoes							
Peanut butter cookies							
Pork liver							
Okra							
Fried chicken							
Blackberries							
Chicken and dressing							
Chocolate cake							
Fish sticks							
Collards							
Spaghetti with meatballs							
Oatmeal							

	Every Time	Most of the Time	Some of the Time	Seldom	Never	Have Never Tasted the Food	Do Not Know the Food
Bologna							
Vanilla ice cream							
Fried eggs							
English peas							
Corn							
Baked beans							
Beef liver							
Scuppernongs							
Chocolate pudding							
Nut ice cream							
Sausage							
Buttermilk							
Yellow squash							
Chocolate pie							
Fresh apples							
Broccoli							
Pizza							
Jell-O salad							
Tomatoes							
Hot tea							
Mashed potatoes							
Watermelon							
Strewberry ice cream							
Deer meat							
Cabbage slaw							
Coffee							
Grits							
Hamburger							
Biscuits							

	Every Time	Most of the Time	Some of the Time	Seldom	Never	Have Never Tasted the Food	Do Not Know the Food
Cooked carrots							
Iced tea							
Fresh strawberries							
Sweet potatoes							
Country fried steak							
Corn bread							
Pork chops							
Rolls							
Fresh oranges							
Bacon							
Soda pop							
Turnip greens							
Spinach							
Chicken and dumplings							
Cantaloupe							
Scrambled eggs							
Carrot strips							
Hominy							
Tang							
Banana pudding							
Potato salad							
Chocolate ice cream							
Cheddar cheese							
Vegetable soup							
Blackberry cobbler							

Note the questions you had about each food — How is it prepared? What other choices do I have? etc. Evaluate the effectiveness of this method of measuring food preferences. Are there any patterns in your food preferences?

EXERCISE 5

Objectives

1. To illustrate the complexities of using the 24-hour recall to assess food intake practices.
2. To ascertain the difference in food behavior and food habits relative to your own food intake.

Behavioral Objectives

After finishing this exercise you should be able to:
1. Develop a method for administering the 24-hour recall.
2. Use data provided by 24-hour recall to identify behavior that would be a habit.
3. Recognize that the particular situation influences food behavior at a given time.

Directions

1. Beginning with what you ate this morning, record what you ate and drank during the past 24 hours. Repeat this exercise for 3 days.

   What did you eat and drink this morning? Where? With whom?
   What did you eat and drink before going to bed last night? Where? With whom?
   What did you eat and drink at the evening meal yesterday? Where? With whom?
   What did you eat and drink between the evening meal and the noon meal yesterday? Where? With whom?
   What did you eat and drink at the noon meal yesterday? Where? With whom?
   What did you eat and drink between the noon meal and breakfast yesterday? Where? With whom?

2. Circle behaviors on the 24-hour recall that are habits of yours, and list any other behavior associated with your food behavior that you consider a habit.
3. How and why does your intake this day differ from your usual pattern?
4. Who did you eat with? Why? Did this association make the meal more enjoyable or less enjoyable? Discuss.
5. Discuss techniques for ensuring the accuracy of data collected using the 24-hour recall. What can data from the 24-hour recall be used for? List advantages and disadvantages of using this technique to research food intake and food behavior.

CHAPTER 4   Food Behavior throughout Life — Pregnancy and Infancy

EXERCISE 1

Objectives

1. To become familiar with methods for obtaining statistical information concerning the population.
2. To become familiar with the food and nutrition education material available to pregnant women.

Behavioral Objectives

After finishing this exercise you should be able to:
1. List sources of statistical information concerning the population.
2. List sources of nutrition education information available to pregnant women.
3. Evaluate the adequacy of the nutrition information available to pregnant women.

Directions

1. Find the number of live births, miscarriages, and stillbirths in your county. Compare your figures with national averages and averages for other developed countries and try to account for any differences.
2. Make observations in a prenatal clinic, in a local hospital, and in an obstetrician's office to discover what information is generally available to pregnant women concerning food intake and weight limitations. Evaluate the availability and the adequacy of the information. Can the quality and accessibility of the information be correlated with the infant mortality rate in your county?

EXERCISE 2

Objectives

1. To learn what feeding practices local physicians recommend for infants.
2. To find out what infant foods are available in local groceries.
3. To become familiar with local infant feeding practices.

Behavioral Objectives

After finishing this exercise you should be able to:
1. List infant foods and feeding practices recommended by local physicians.
2. List infant foods available in local grocery stores.
3. List infant feeding practices.
4. Compare and critique recommendations of physicians and actual infant feeding practices.

Directions

1. Interview a local nurse or pediatrician about the pediatrician's views on feeding infants.
2. Check the infant foods available in a local grocery store and observe what mothers buy.

3. Interview five mothers of infants.
   a. What do their doctors suggest they feed their infants?
   b. What do they actually feed the infants?
   c. Complete a 24-hour recall on what the infant ate yesterday.
   d. Tabulate your findings. Evaluate the nutritional adequacy of the infants' diets. Critique feeding practices relative to the development of food behavior in each instance.

CHAPTER 5   Food Behavior throughout Life — The Young Child

EXERCISE 1

Objectives

1. To become familiar with the eating behavior of the preschool child.
2. To use observations and interviews to obtain information about the preschool child's eating behavior.

Behavioral Objectives

After finishing this exercise you should be able to:
1. List the foods eaten by local preschool children.
2. Describe the preschool child's eating pattern.
3. List the permissions and procedures necessary to gain access to the situation you wish to observe.
4. Make a form for recording your observations.
5. Describe the setting of the meal and document the child's responses to the foods served.
6. Develop criteria for evaluating your own participation and be able to critique your own learning performance.
7. Evaluate a 24-hour dietary recall with respect to nutrient adequacy and development of appropriate food behavior and recommend changes to improve nutrient intake or food behavior.
8. Cite some reactions of a preschool child in an eating situation.
9. List the physical and emotional factors relevant in this situation.

Directions

1. Obtain permission to observe a preschool child eating in a nursery school situation. Record your observations. Describe the setting. What foods were served to the child? Who ate with the child? How did the child respond to the food served? Record the foods and amounts eaten by child. Record any conversation about food. Analyze and critique the situation relative to what you learned.
2. Interview three mothers of preschool children. Complete a 24-hour dietary recall for each child to ascertain nutrient intake and food intake pattern. What are the mothers' attitudes toward feeding their children? Do they think that the children eat well? What would they like to change about their children's eating behavior? Evaluate.
3. Repeat 1 and 2 above with kindergartners and with elementary school children.

CHAPTER 6   Food Behavior throughout Life — Preadolescence and Adolescence

EXERCISE 1

Repeat the exercise for chapter 5 with fifth and sixth graders; with junior high students; with high school students.

CHAPTER 7   Food Behavior throughout Life — The Adult Years

EXERCISE 1

Adapt the exercise for chapter 5 for college students in a college residence hall.

EXERCISE 2

Adapt the exercise for chapter 5 for use with middle-aged people in a restaurant situation. Interview three middle-aged persons and have them complete a 24-hour dietary recall.

EXERCISE 3

Adapt the exercise for chapter 5 for use with elderly persons in a group feeding situation and in their homes.

CHAPTER 8   Impairments as Modifiers of Food Behavior

EXERCISE 1

Adapt the exercise for chapter 5 for use with a group of physically handicapped persons; for use with a group of mentally impaired persons.

CHAPTER 9   Food Behavior and Obesity

EXERCISE 1

Objectives

1. To find the meaning of food for a group of obese persons.
2. To find the food preferences of a group of obese persons.
3. To investigate correlations between the meanings obese persons attach to food and their food preferences.

Behavioral Objectives

After finishing this exercise you should be able to:
1. Find a research sample and obtain the necessary cooperation and permission to administer questionnaires on food preferences and the connotative meanings of food.
2. Administer questionnaires to determine food preferences and connotative meanings of food.
3. Tabulate and analyze data on food preferences and connotative meanings of food.
4. Apply the information you have obtained to food and nutrition evaluation.

Directions

Find a TOPS (Take Off Pounds Sensibly), Weight Watchers, or other organized group of people who are trying to lose weight. (You may organize your own group on campus.) Obtain the group's permission and cooperation. Develop and administer an instrument to determine food preferences and connotative meanings of food. (You may pattern the instrument after those in the Student Exercises for chapter 3.) Tabulate and analyze your data. How might the information you have obtained be used in planning an educational project?

CHAPTER 10   Food Behavior Research

EXERCISE 1

Objectives

1. To investigate some sociocultural and demographic characteristics of a community.
2. To become aware of the food and services available in local grocery stores and of sources of special dietary items.
3. To learn what available resources offer nutrition counseling and food and nutrition education.

Behavioral Objectives

After finishing this exercise you should be able to:
1. List some sociocultural and demographic characteristics of the community.
2. List foods and services available in the local grocery stores.
3. List sources of services and information needed for food and nutrition education purposes.

Directions

1. Use the public library, the Cooperative Extension Service office, and the chamber of commerce. Ask for information about the community's population.
   a. What is the population of the community? What is the population of preschool children? Elementary school children? Junior high students? High school students? Young families? Middle-aged persons? Elderly persons?
   b. List the ethnic groups and populations represented in the community. What is the percentage of blacks? Of whites? American Indians? Orientals? Mexican Americans? Others?
   c. List the religious groups and populations represented in the community.
   d. What are the income ranges in the community? How many families are below the national poverty level? At poverty level? One and one-half times above poverty level? Where do the low-income families live? Where do their children go to school? Where do the high-income families live? Where do their children go to school?
2. Use the telephone book to find information. Some books contain a section of information about the community. Turn to that section and answer the following questions.
   a. What is the population of the community?
   b. What is the major agricultural crop, if agriculture is part of the community?
   c. What are the major industries?
   d. Turn in the yellow pages to the section on churches, and see what religions and sects are represented (e.g., Baptist, Roman Catholic, Latter Day Saints, Lutheran, Methodist, Seventh-Day Adventist, Presbyterian, Church of God, Episcopalian, Unitarian, Black Muslim, Muslim, Jewish).
3. Remember that people spend their money differently according to what they value. Observe the homes, schools, and churches. Are there vegetable gardens? If so, are there many or few?

4. Stop at a grocery store and observe. Is this store a large chain store, a small chain store, an independent store, an affiliated store, or a neighborhood grocery? Go into the store. Do not take your pad and pencil; wait until you are outside the store to write down your observations. If you have trouble remembering, go back into the store and check you remembered observations.

a. Note the date and time of your observations, the name of the store, and the type of store. Count the people you see. Does the store seem empty, moderately full, or crowded? Count the people in each of the following categories, and think of other categories you might use.

Women	Children alone
Men	Well-dressed persons
Couples	Casually dressed persons
Women with children	Poorly dressed persons
Men with children	Hurried shoppers
Elderly persons	Leisurely shoppers
Adolescents	

How many checkouts are open? How many checkouts are there?

b. *Fruits and Vegetables.* Which fruits and vegetables occupy the largest displays?

Apples	Lettuce
Oranges	Other salad vegetables
Bananas/Grapes	Celery
Pears	Beans
Peaches/Nectarines	Asparagus
Grapefruit	Broccoli
Strawberries	Potatoes (white and sweet)
Cherries	Tomatoes/Turnips
Tropical fruits	Onions/Mushrooms
Melons	Carrots/Okra
Corn	

Which fruits and vegetables look the freshest and as if they have quick turnover? Which look the least fresh? In a casual manner, ask someone at the checkout or in produce which vegetables and fruits they sell the most.

c. *Canned Goods and Frozen Foods.* Run your hand over the tops of the canned goods. Which are dusty, indicating slow turnover? Check the front window and permanent display areas. What canned and frozen foods are on sale this week?

d. *Cereals and Starches.* Find the area of the store displaying products used in baking. List items that you find there, such as the following.

Unbleached flour	Unenriched cornmeal
Self-rising flour	Self-rising cornmeal
Bleached flour	Rye flour
Enriched flour	Whole wheat flour
Cornmeal	White cornmeal
Royal baking powder	Yellow cornmeal
Enriched cornmeal	Phosphate baking powder

Are there any especially large purchase units of rice, oatmeal, cornmeal, self-rising flour, or similar products?

e. *Meats.* Do meats generally appear fat, lean, or moderate? Do they look bony? Are they brown? Do meat prices seem low, moderate, or high? Check the meats you find displayed.

Liver	Cornish game hen
Tongue	Goose
Sweetbreads	Duck
Brains	Squab (pigeon)
Kidney	Pheasant
Lamb	Rabbit
Veal	Fatmeat (streak of lean)
Fatback	Venison

What kinds of cold cuts (bologna, salami, spiced ham, dutch loaf, etc.) occupy the largest display?

f. *Dairy.* Check the dairy items you find displayed prominently.

Cheddar cheese	Yogurt
Italian cheeses	Buttermilk
Unripened cheeses	High-butterfat milk
Snack cheeses	Homogenized milk
Sour cream	Low-butterfat milk

g. *Beverages.* What brands of coffee, tea, cocoa, and soft drinks occupy the largest displays? Does the store carry beer, wine, or hard liquor?

h. *Other Foods.* Do they have a gourmet section? Are the items dusty? Does the store have a special place for ethnic foods? What nationalities are represented? Italian? Jewish? Chinese? Japanese? Mexican? Others? Does the store have a display of fats and oils? Note whether the display includes shortening, lard, vegetable oils, butter, or margarine. Find the diet section, and notice if the items are dusty. Write down the brand names that the store carries of the following items.

Low-cholesterol eggs	Meat analogs
Salt substitute	Sugarless beverages
High fiber	Decaffeinated coffee
Sugarless ice cream	Sugarless candy
Coffee whiteners	Milk substitutes
Sugarless canned fruit	Salt-free canned goods
Milkless baby formula	Vegetables

i. *Services.* Which of the following services does the store offer? Does it offer any other services?

Delivery service	Package pickup
Check cashing	Telephone available
Special order items	Parking
Butcher on duty	Credit
Easy access to bus service	Rest rooms
Unit pricing	Package carryout
Catering	Accept food stamps
Restaurant or snack bar	Accept WIC coupons
Delicatessen	

5. a. Discuss these questions after completing your observations in the grocery store.

(1) Is the area urban, rural, suburban, or a small town? How does that influence the types of items available in the store? How does this influence the socializing within the store?

(2) Do you find influence of a religious group in the grocery store (vegetarian foods, kosher foods, etc.)?

(3) Do you think a change in the population would result in a change in items in the store? Why?

(4) Were you surprised by any of the items available? Did any items have larger displays than you expected? Why?

(5) After thinking over the food and nutrition education you have had, would you suggest this store as a place to shop? Why or why not? Think about people with low incomes, handicaps, diabetes, sodium-restricted diets, food allergies, cholesterol-restricted diets, and transportation problems; think of vegetarians, small children, the elderly, and those who are homebound.

b. Write eight generalizations about food behavior that you can devise from information gained in this period of observation.

c. Write eight generalizations about the community's sociocultural composition.

d. Write eight specifics about food behavior in the community.

e. Write eight specifics about the community's sociocultural composition.

EXERCISE 2

Objectives

1. To use participant observation to learn about food behavior in the community.

Behavioral Objectives

After finishing this exercise you should be able to:
1. Write up an observation of a community event, using field-note techniques.
2. Describe the functions of food in the community event.
3. Identify the foods served at a community event, the methods of preparing and serving them, and the terminology associated with them.

Directions

From the references at the end of chapter 10 choose one that deals with observation and read it. Participate in a community event and note the functions of food in the event, the foods used, the methods of preparation and service, the terminology used, and so on. Write the information up as field notes.

EXERCISE 3

Objectives

1. To become familiar with the tools of observation.
2. To acquire experience in writing assumptions, objectives, and questions based on observations.

Behavioral Objectives

After finishing this exercise you should be able to:
1. Make an assumption or hypothesis about eating behavior that can be tested.
2. Develop objectives and questions to obtain information in order to test your assumption or hypothesis.
3. Develop questions for interview schedules and for handout questionnaires.

Directions

Read some of the references for research techniques given at the end of chapter 10. Observe for half an hour in a restaurant catering to a specific age group, and make an assumption about the eating behavior of that age group based on what you have observed. Then write objectives and develop five questions to test your assumption. Submit your work to the class for a critique, and then revise your instrument. Using your questions as an interview schedule, interview six people of the same age group as those in the restaurant. Do these questions provide the information necessary to meet your objectives or test your hypothesis? How would you improve the questions? Rewrite the questions for use as a handout questionnaire. Hand the questionnaire out to six people. How do the questions differ from the ones you used in the interview schedule?

EXERCISE 4

Objectives

1. To develop the research skills needed for addressing a food and nutrition problem in the community.

Behavioral Objectives

After finishing this exercise you should be able to:
1. Design a research project to obtain the knowledge necessary for developing a nutrition education program in the community.

Directions

Design a research project, using the Summary of the Research Process (chapter 10, p. 158 as a guide. Use the information you have gained from previous student exercises to develop your hypothesis and objectives.

CHAPTER 11   The Community Food and Nutrition Professional

EXERCISE 1

Objectives

1. To become familiar with the educational background needed by a food and nutrition professional.
2. To relate knowledge obtained in your professional training to the food and nutrition concerns of individuals.

Behavioral Objectives

After finishing this exercise you should be able to:

1. Describe the training required of the food and nutrition professional in each of three positions.
2. Provide information shown by the food and nutrition knowledge and misconception test to be lacking.
3. Recognize the difference between knowledge and misconceptions about food and nutrition.
4. Recognize problems that an individual might have in answering specific questions in the community or that a professional might have in developing questions to ascertain the community's need for food and nutrition education programs.

Directions

1. Read three of the references given at the end of chapter 11. Discuss the type of training that would be needed for the food and nutrition professional in each position.
2. It is important that community food and nutrition workers have a firm knowledge of their subject. Test yourself and then check the accuracy of your answers. A wrong answer with a degree of certainty of 1 or 2 indicates wrong information. A wrong answer with a degree of certainty of 4 or 5 indicates lack of knowledge. The tests that follow are adapted from unpublished dissertations by Doris Phillips (University of Tennessee, 1974) and Lois Ann Wodarski (University of Tennessee, 1976).

Read each of the following statements about food and nutrition. If you believe a statement is true, circle *T;* if you think it is false, circle *F.* Then indicate your degree of certainty by circling one of the numbers that appear on the right of the answer column. If you are very certain about your answer, circle 1; if you are very doubtful, circle 5. If the number 2, 3, or 4 better describes your degree of certainty or uncertainty, circle that number. Be sure to circle both a letter and a number after each statement.

1. Organically grown vegetables are richer in vitamins than those grown by conventional means.   T   F   1   2   3   4   5

2. The Stillman, Atkins, and "Mayo" diets are completely safe ways to lose weight quickly and permanently.   T   F   1   2   3   4   5

3. Grapefruit, cottage cheese, yogurt, lemon juice, and protein bread have positive powers to take off weight.   T   F   1   2   3   4   5

4. Honey is less fattening than sugar.   T   F   1   2   3   4   5

5. A slice of toast is lower in calories than a slice of bread.   T   F   1   2   3   4   5

6. A medium-sized baked potato has fewer calories than a 4-ounce portion of beef.   T   F   1   2   3   4   5

7. A teenager requires more calories than an adult of equal weight and activeness.   T   F   1   2   3   4   5

8. A peanut butter sandwich and a glass of milk is a good substitute for meat.   T   F   1   2   3   4   5

9. Bread and potatoes are fattening foods.   T   F   1   2   3   4   5

10. A serving of the gelatin dessert Jell-O is higher in protein and more nutritious than the same amount of ice milk.   T   F   1   2   3   4   5

11. A food additive cannot be approved for use if it is found to cause cancer when ingested by people or animals.   T   F   1   2   3   4   5

12. Cyanide and arsenic occur naturally in some foods.   T   F   1   2   3   4   5

13. The U.S. RDA (Recommended Daily Allowance) represents the amount of nutrients needed every day by healthy people plus an excess of 30 to 50 percent to allow for individual differences.   T   F   1   2   3   4   5

14. Sweets cause adolescent acne.   T   F   1   2   3   4   5

15. One gelatin capsule a day builds stronger fingernails and healthier hair.   T   F   1   2   3   4   5

16. Organically grown foods are not necessarily free from pesticides.   T   F   1   2   3   4   5

17. Poor diet among teenage mothers seldom affects their babies.   T   F   1   2   3   4   5

18. Some foods a nursing mother eats can cause digestive problems in her infant.   T   F   1   2   3   4   5

19. A teenage mother should "eat enough for two" during pregnancy.   T   F   1   2   3   4   5

20. Tooth decay is often related to poor food habits.	T	F	1	2	3	4	5
21. Pizza has little nutritive value.	T	F	1	2	3	4	5
22. A combination of lecithin, vinegar, and kelp helps burn body fat.	T	F	1	2	3	4	5
23. Unbleached flour is nutritionally superior to bleached flour.	T	F	1	2	3	4	5
24. Mental work significantly increases your body's need for calories.	T	F	1	2	3	4	5
25. You must eat 2,500 kilocalories more than your body uses to put on 1 pound of body weight.	T	F	1	2	3	4	5
26. Vitamins and minerals do not have any calories.	T	F	1	2	3	4	5
27. The greatest danger in following fad diets is that they may cause deficiency or imbalance of one or more nutrients.	T	F	1	2	3	4	5
28. The only disease of humans that is known to be associated with eating foods from poor-quality soil is simple goiter.	T	F	1	2	3	4	5
29. A calorie is a substance found in food which causes weight gain.	T	F	1	2	3	4	5
30. You must eat 3,500 kilocalories more than your body uses to put on 1 pound of body weight.	T	F	1	2	3	4	5
31. Most diseases are related to improper diet.	T	F	1	2	3	4	5
32. Acne in teenagers is related to the condition of the blood.	T	F	1	2	3	4	5
33. It is not harmful to drink milk and eat fish at the same time.	T	F	1	2	3	4	5
34. Fish builds brain cells.	T	F	1	2	3	4	5

Circle the letter of the correct statement. Indicate your degree of certainty by circling one of the numbers at the right — 1 indicates the greatest certainty, 5 the greatest uncertainty.

1. Calories and fats are not assigned a Recommended Daily Allowance because:
                                                                                     1 2 3 4 5
    a. Vitamins and minerals should be of greater importance in food selection.
    b. They are dependent upon the person's weight, age, sex, and height.
    c. They are not considered to be nutrients.
    d. They are not needed by the average person.

2. When a food is labeled "imitation," it: 1   2   3   4   5
   a. Means the food is nutritionally inferior to the food prod-
       uct for which it is a substitute.
   b. Means the food is nutritionally equal to the food product
       for which it is a substitute.
   c. Means the food is nutritionally superior to the food
       product for which it is a substitute.
   d. Is not referring to the nutritional value.

3. When Mrs. Kessler went to the grocery store last week, she   1   2   3   4   5
   found the following label on a can of beef stew.

   > Beef stock, potatoes, carrots, beef cubes, peas,
   > enriched wheat flour, nonfat dry milk, margarine,
   > cornstarch, tomatoes, sugar, monosodium gluta-
   > mate and flavoring.

   From reading the label, Mrs. Kessler learned that in the
   product:
   a. There are twice as many potatoes as beef cubes.
   b. The beef stock is the most abundant ingredient by weight.
   c. Chunks of vegetables will include potatoes, carrots, peas,
       and tomatoes.
   d. The combination of carrots, peas, and tomatoes will be
       greater than the amount of potatoes.

   Questions 4, 5, and 6 are concerned with the following situation. Mrs. Rhorer wants to feed her
family a balanced diet. She planned the following three meals to be served to her husband, 5-year-old
son, and 14-year-old daughter. (Assume that each person would have only one serving of each item.)

Breakfast	Lunch	Dinner
Orange juice	Peanut butter sandwich	Meat loaf
Toast/butter	Canned peaches in gelatin	Cole slaw
Fried egg	Celery sticks	Cooked carrots
	Milk	Hot muffins/butter
		Lemonade
		White cake with lemon sauce

4. Which of the food groups is inadequately represented for her   1   2   3   4   5
   5-year-old son?
   a. Meat.
   b. Bread and cereal.
   c. Milk.
   d. Vegetables and fruits.

5. Which food substitution would make the day's menus more   1   2   3   4   5
   nutritionally adequate?
   a. Vanilla pudding instead of white cake with lemon sauce.
   b. Tossed lettuce salad instead of cole slaw.
   c. Ham sandwich instead of peanut butter sandwich.
   d. Soft-cooked egg instead of fried egg.

6. Now that you have made a substitution (write it in the menu)   1   2   3   4   5
   to improve the nutritive quality of the menu, what addition
   should be made to make the diet more adequate for Mrs.
   Rhorer's 14-year-old daughter?
   a.   More meat.
   b.   More milk.
   c.   More fruits and vegetables.
   d.   More bread and cereals.

   Indicate whether you think the following statements are true or false. Circle *T* for true and *F*
for false. Indicate your degree of certainty by circling the appropriate number at the right (1 for the
greatest certainty, 5 for the greatest uncertainty).

7. Mrs. Hopkins is planning to make beef stew. When   T   F   1   2   3   4   5
   considering cost, it would be better to buy neck
   bones at $.89 per pound than round steak at
   $1.89 per pound.

8. Buttermilk and lemon-soured milk can be used   T   F   1   2   3   4   5
   interchangeably for baking.

9. A german chocolate cake made from scratch is   T   F   1   2   3   4   5
   less expensive than one made from a mix.

10. If fresh carrots (without tops) and frozen carrots   T   F   1   2   3   4   5
    are both $.25 per pound, they will be the same
    price per serving.

11. If instant rice costs $.63 per pound and regular   T   F   1   2   3   4   5
    white rice costs $.82 per pound, the regular white
    rice will cost less per serving.

12. A 10-pound bag of sugar costing $4.23 is less   T   F   1   2   3   4   5
    expensive than two 5-pound bags costing $2.09
    each.

13. Canned orange juice at $.49 for 46 ounces is a   T   F   1   2   3   4   5
    better buy than frozen orange juice at $1.19 for
    six 6-ounce cans (each can reconstituted by
    three cans of water).

14. Mrs. Thompson can plan to get two to three serv-   T   F   1   2   3   4   5
    ings per pound from a chuck roast (bone-in).

15. Synthetic nutrients are not as useful to the   T   F   1   2   3   4   5
    human body as are natural nutrients.

16. Fresh apples are an excellent source of vitamin C.   T   F   1   2   3   4   5

17. The average American diet is frequently deficient   T   F   1   2   3   4   5
    in calcium.

18. Orange juice is a good source of riboflavin.   T   F   1   2   3   4   5

19. A large percentage of the ready-to-eat cereals   T   F   1   2   3   4   5
    are fortified with vitamins and iron.

20. A 4-ounce serving of cooked oatmeal has more vitamins than 4 ounces of uncooked oatmeal.   T   F   1   2   3   4   5

21. Brown-shelled eggs are inferior in quality to white-shelled eggs.   T   F   1   2   3   4   5

22. Citrus fruits and tomatoes make the blood acidic.   T   F   1   2   3   4   5

23. Most people living in the United States do not require vitamin pills.   T   F   1   2   3   4   5

24. Vitamin E and vitamin B complex capsules have little therapeutic value for healthy persons.   T   F   1   2   3   4   5

25. Excess vitamin A and vitamin D can be toxic.   T   F   1   2   3   4   5

26. The only way to lose weight safely is to eat fewer calories than the body uses.   T   F   1   2   3   4   5

27. Supplementing an already adequate diet with vitamin pills can result in supervitality, greater endurance, freedom from illness, and resistance to infection.   T   F   1   2   3   4   5

28. The government requires fortification of cereal products.   T   F   1   2   3   4   5

29. Skim milk contains about the same amounts of body-building protein and minerals as whole milk.   T   F   1   2   3   4   5

30. One ounce of bologna has half as much protein as 1 ounce of lean hamburger.   T   F   1   2   3   4   5

31. Sugar provides necessary energy for children.   T   F   1   2   3   4   5

32. The Cooperative Extension Service provides food and nutrition information to the consumer.   T   F   1   2   3   4   5

33. The nutritional content of packaged food is required to appear on the label.   T   F   1   2   3   4   5

34. The food and nutrition information presented in books by Adelle Davis is totally reliable.   T   F   1   2   ·3   4   5

35. Jean Mayer, a newspaper columnist, is a renowned nutritionist.   T   F   1   2   3   4   5

36. A person's need for calories depends partly on weight and height.   T   F   1   2   3   4   5

37. The nutritive values listed on food product labels are those of the raw product.   T   F   1   2   3   4   5

38. The contents of some foods, such as canned pears, are legally defined.   T   F   1   2   3   4   5

This exercise illustrates the application of knowledge of nutrition and the physical and chemical properties of food, and of resources available to inform and protect the consumer. The community food and nutrition professional must be able to apply such knowledge in everyday contacts with individuals in the community. Some of the questions were repeated. Notice and discuss the way in which the questions are designed.

CHAPTER 12   Food and Nutrition Education in the Community

EXERCISE 1

Objectives

1. To become familiar with the published reports of food and nutritional professionals working in the community.
2. To obtain knowledge of the types of programs food and nutrition professionals in the community are involved in.
3. To critique a situation presented in a journal article.

Behavioral Objectives

After finishing this exercise you should be able to:
1. Find an article in a professional journal and determine the following.
   a. Who the client is.
   b. What problem is being addressed.
   c. How the problem was identified.
   d. The method used to approach the problem.
   e. The evaluation technique used to assess the effectiveness of the approach.

Directions

Choose recent issues of the *U.S. Public Health Journal*, the *Journal of Nutrition Education*, and the *Journal of the American Dietetic Association*. Write an abstract of one article in each journal that concerns nutritional care in the community. In each situation, Who are the clients? What problem is being addressed? How was the problem identified? What methods are used to approach the problem? and What evaluation technique is used to assess the effectiveness of the approach?

CHAPTER 13   Programs and Agencies Providing Nutritional Services and Education in the Community

EXERCISE 1

Objectives

1. To observe community nutrition programs in action.
2. To ascertain the role of the community food and nutrition professional in established programs.
3. To evaluate the effectiveness of established programs.

Behavioral Objectives

After finishing this exercise you should be able to:
1. Describe the role of the community food and nutrition professional within the community.
2. Evaluate the effectiveness of an established program.
3. Make recommendations for improving the effectiveness of the program you have evaluated.

Directions

1. Identify all established programs or agencies in the community that have a food and nutrition component.
2. Choose one agency and identify the professionals working in its food and nutrition component. What are the educational requirements of their jobs?
3. Obtain job descriptions of the personnel in the agency's food and nutrition component. Draw a diagram depicting the interaction of these persons. Diagram the actions of the food and nutrition professional in achieving a set goal.
4. Find information about the agency's organization and its mission. Complete an organizational chart for the agency, including lines of authority.

EXERCISE 2

Objectives

1. To plan a new nutrition education program for a community.

Behavioral Objectives

After finishing this exercise you should be able to:
1. Assess a community's need for nutrition education programs.
2. Plan and develop a program to meet the need.
3. Implement the program.
4. Evaluate the effectiveness of the program.

Directions

1. Chart the existing food and nutrition programs that have an impact on the community. What is the training of the food and nutrition professionals involved?

2. Develop an educational program to meet the needs of a segment of the community. Base it on your previous experiences in the community and apply the criteria outlined in chapter 12.
3. Observe food and nutrition professionals on-the-job for the agency for a period of 2 weeks. Keep a detailed log of activities that they engage in. Whom do they interact with? What is the nature of the interactions?
4. Read journal reports of the agency's past performance. Interview five clients of the agency's food and nutrition service. What are the problems of the service? What are its successes? How might the successes be increased?
5. How could the agency enhance the work of its food and nutrition professionals? What might the professionals do to be more effective in their role? Identify other professionals that contribute to the success of the food and nutrition professional.
6. Generally speaking, is the agency accomplishing its mission? What are its limitations? Is the agency's food and nutrition component accomplishing its goals? List specific goals of the food and nutrition component. List means of accomplishing the goals and analyze their effectiveness.

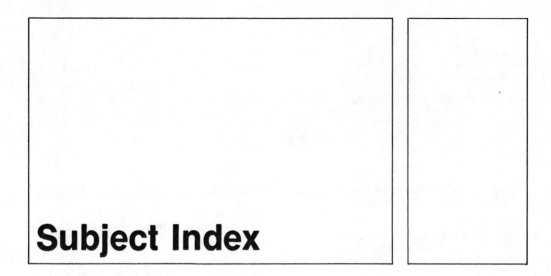

Subject Index

Italic page numbers indicate tables or illustrations.

Author Index